COSTUMES & TEXTILES OF AWADH

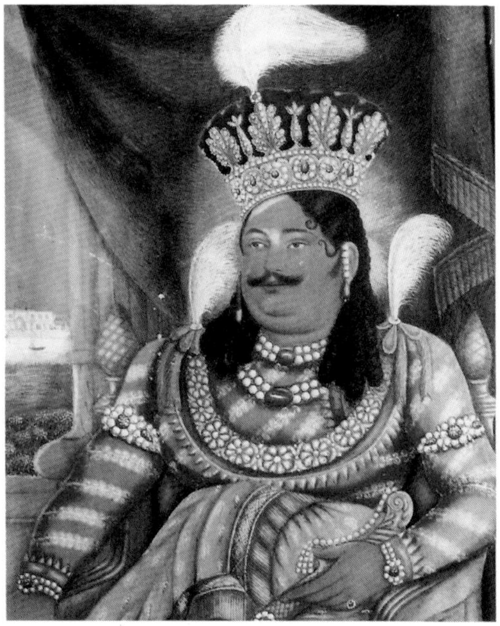

From the Era of Nawabs
to Modern Times

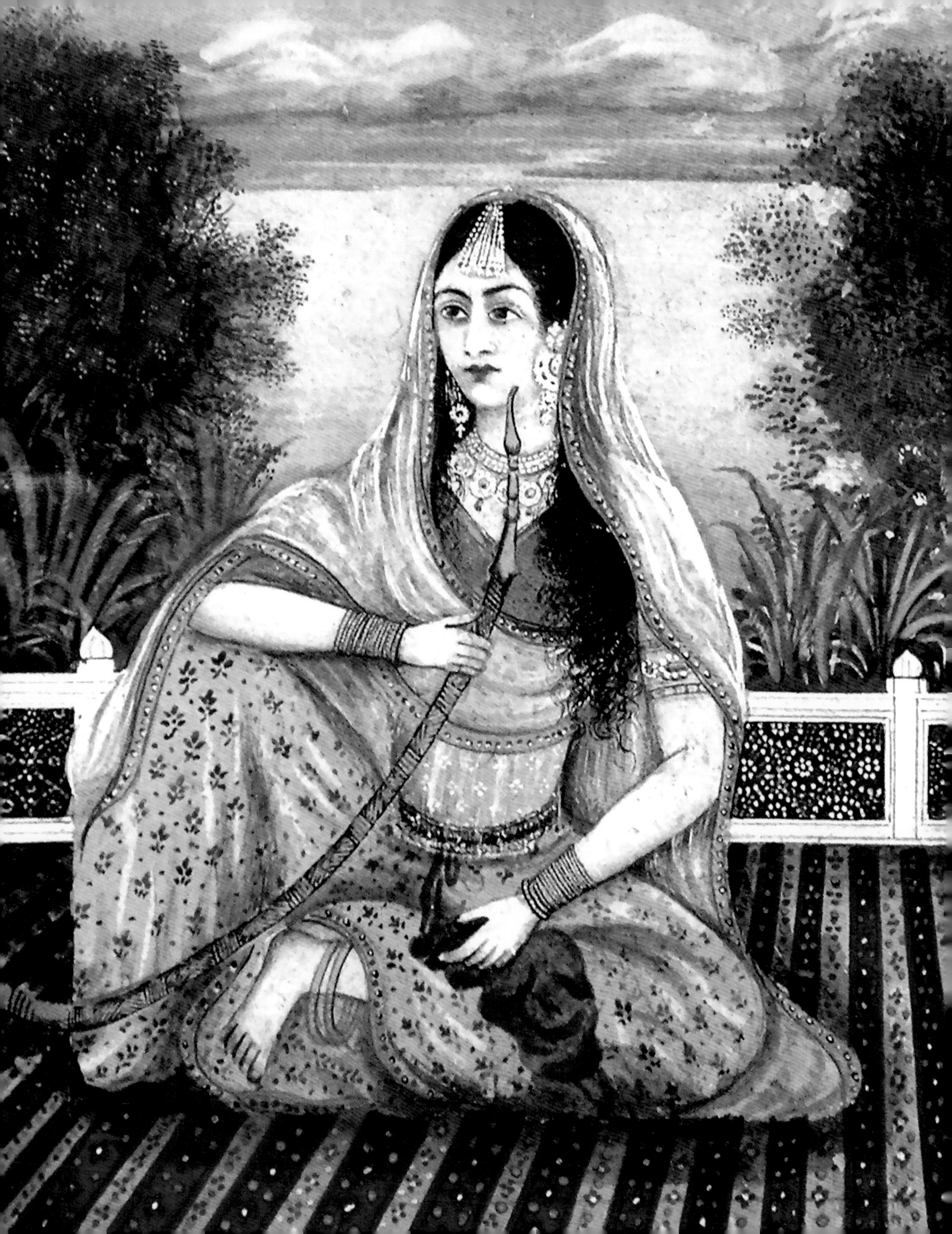

COSTUMES & TEXTILES OF

AWADH

From the Era of Nawabs to Modern Times

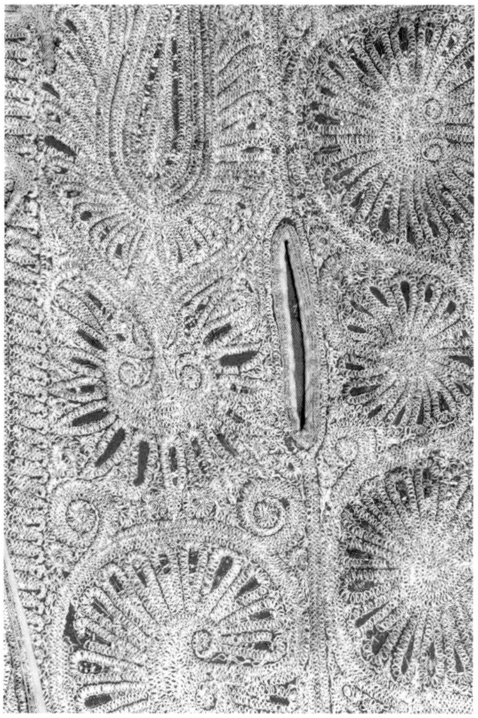

SUSHAMA SWARUP

Lustre Press
Roli Books

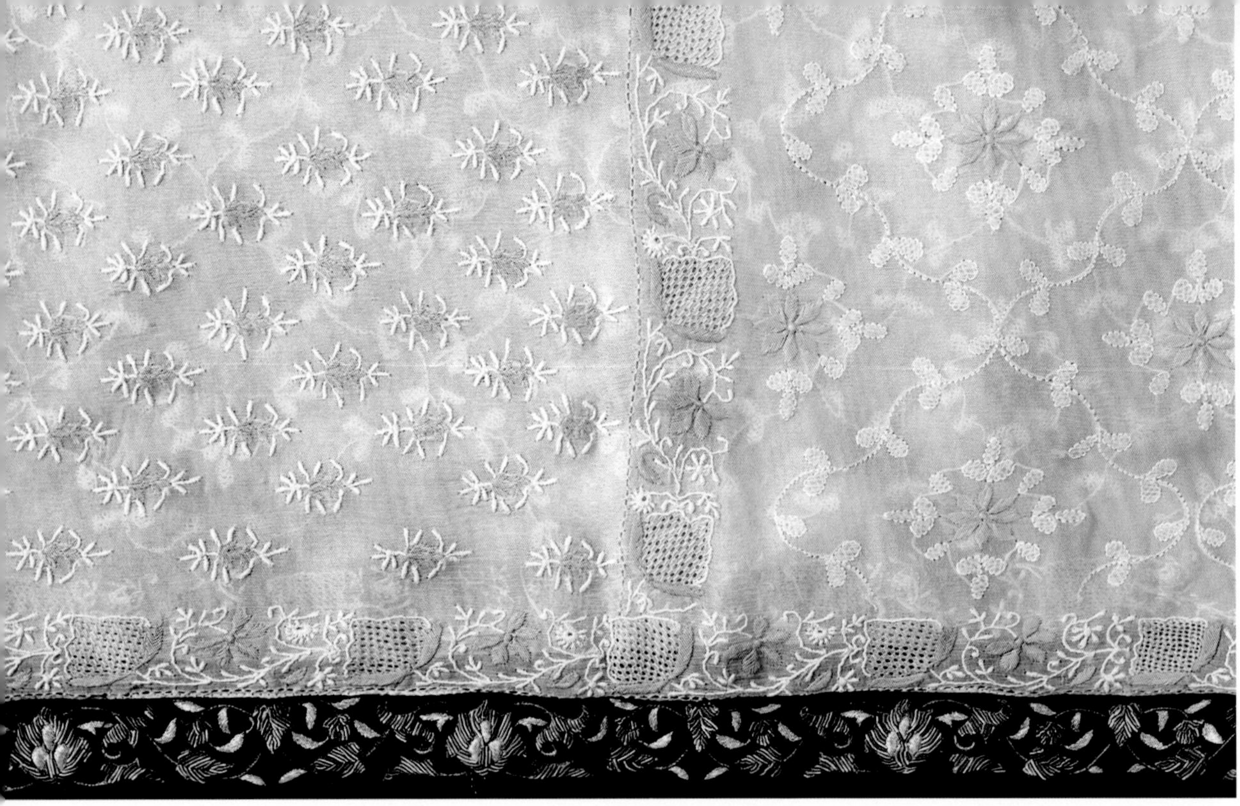

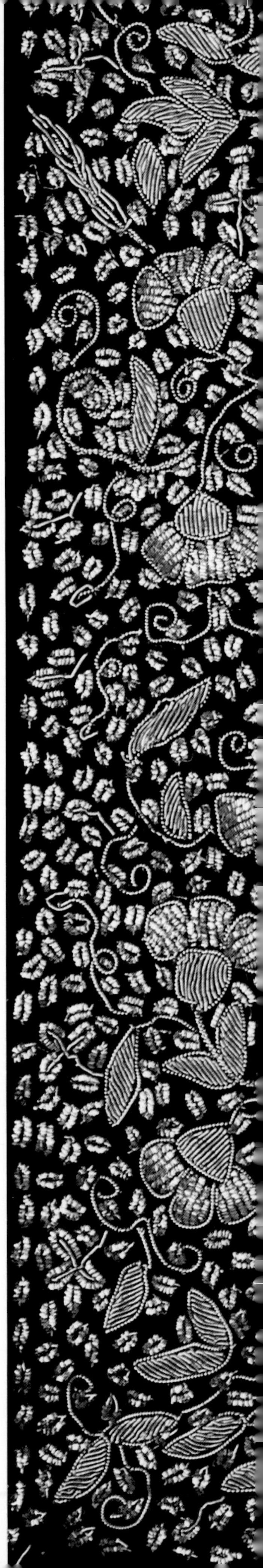

Published in India by
Roli Books
M-75, Greater Kailash II Market
New Delhi-110 048, India
Ph: ++91-11-40682000, 29212782
Fax: ++91-11-29217185
E-mail: info@rolibooks.com
Website: www.rolibooks.com

ISBN: 978-81-7436-891-1

Editors: Priya Kapoor and Jyotsna Mehta
Design: Bonita Vaz-Shimray
Pre-press: Jyoti Dey
Production: Naresh Nigam, Shaji Sahadevan

Printed and bound at Thomson Press, India

Above: *Chikankari* with zardozi on border.
Facing page: Zardozi work studded with semi-precious stones.
Previous pages: Page 1: Nawab Wajid Ali Shah wearing a traditional,woven *jamdani angarkha* with *adi-bel* motif.
Page 2: Courtesan wearing lehenga, choli and a *jamdani odhni* with floral *butis*. The *odhni* borders are decorated with *minakari* work.
Page 3: This red silk and cotton-lined *choga* is densely embroidered with stylized flowers in gold *kalabattun*. The rich gold embroidery (done on deep red fabric) was popular at the Delhi Court as well as in Awadh.

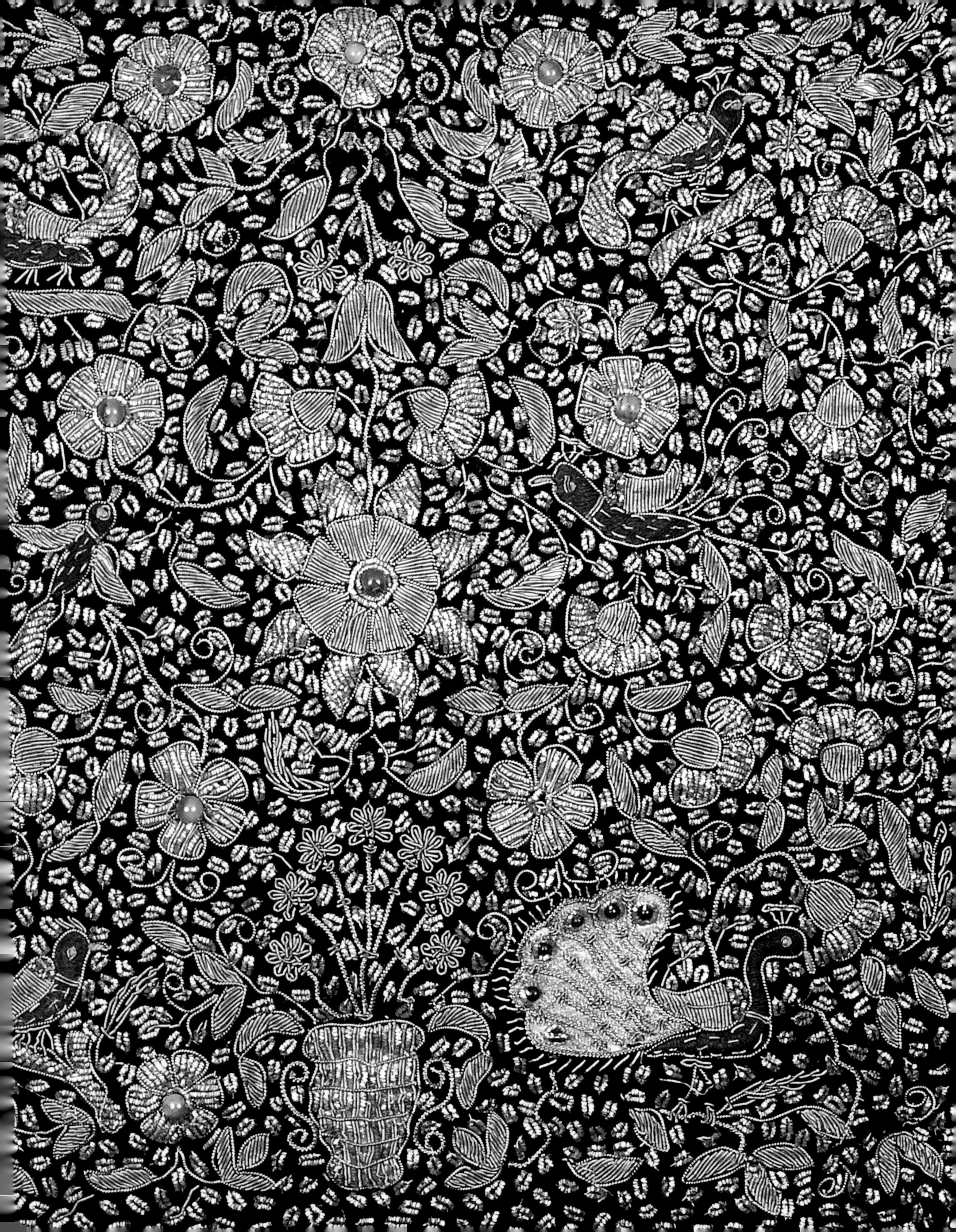

CONTENTS

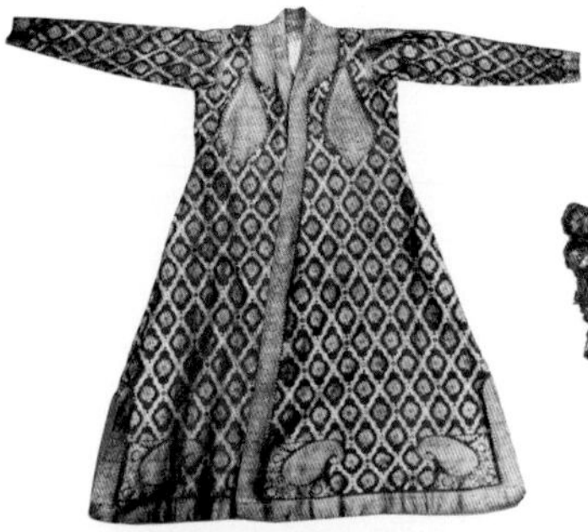

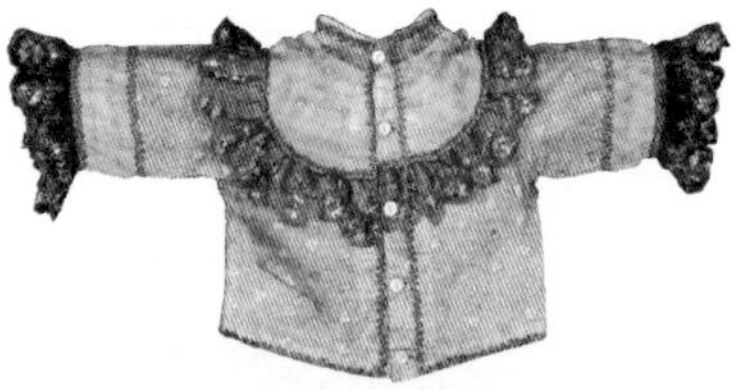

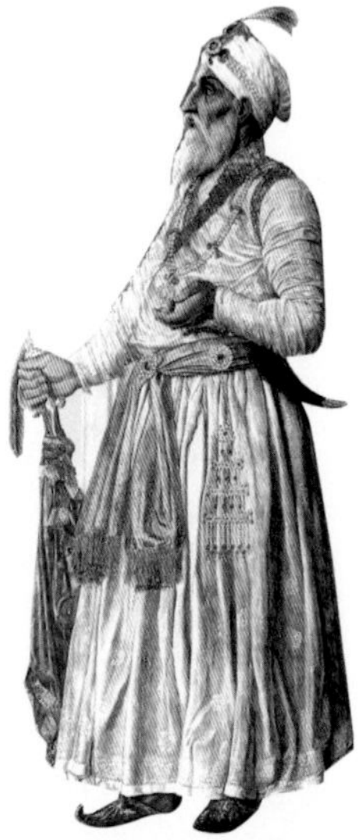

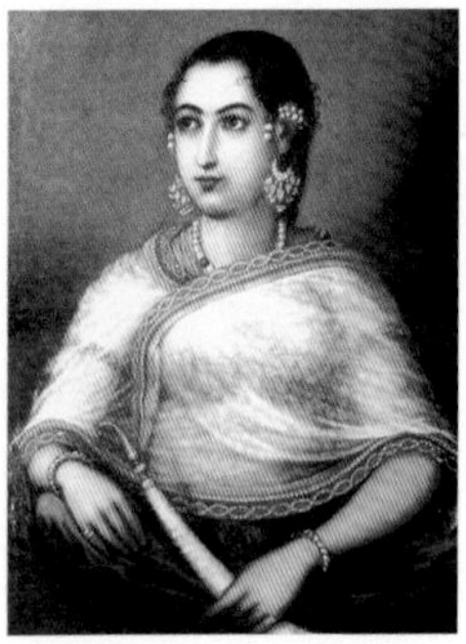

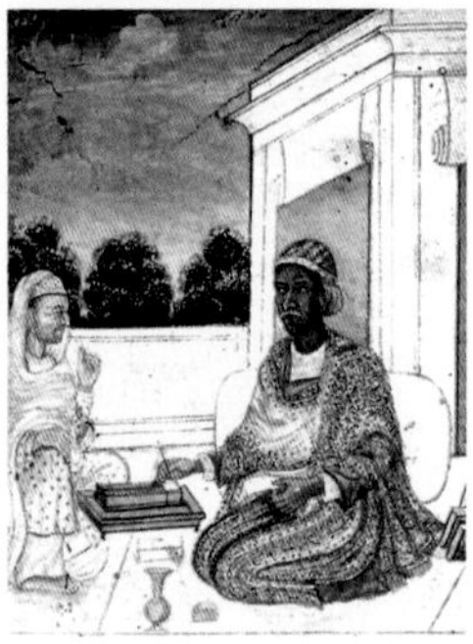

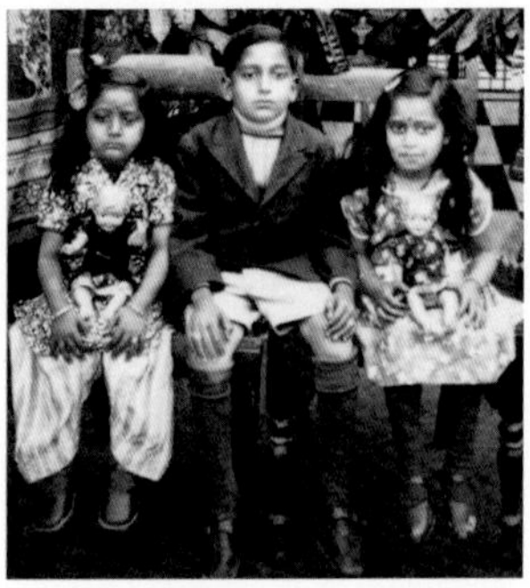

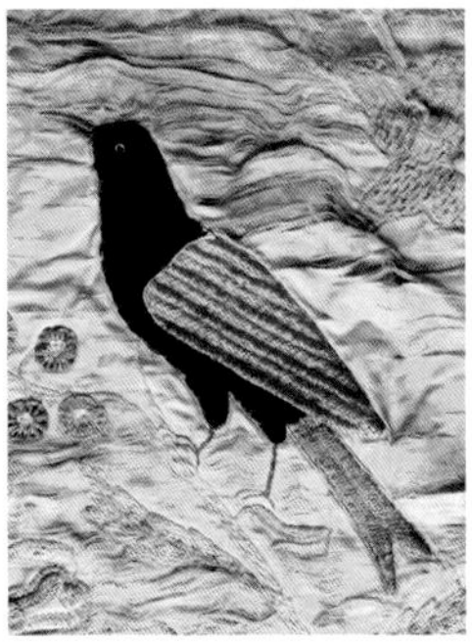

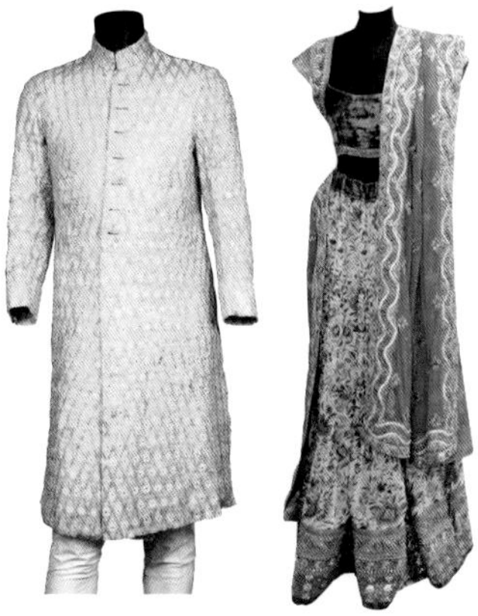

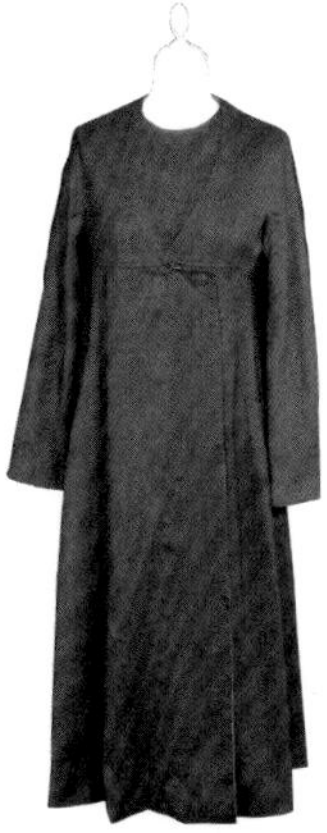

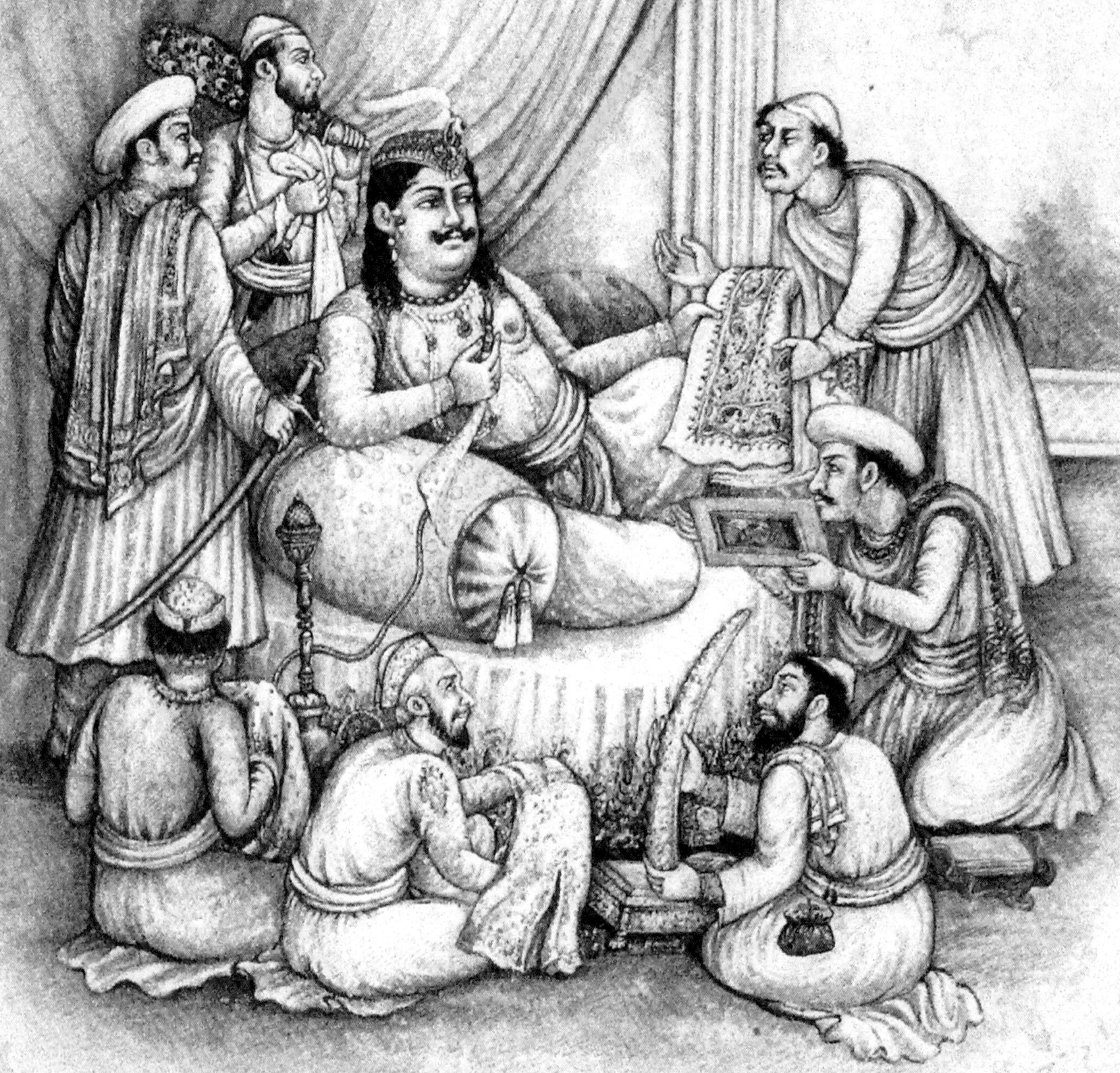

یہ لکھنؤ کی چکن، یہ زری کے شام و سحر ہر ایک تار پہ سو بار الجھے تارِ نظر
یہ جام دانی ہے یا کھکشاں کی راہ گزر یا کوئی تختۂ گُل رات بھر کی اوس میں تر
سیاہ رات بھی آئے تو صبح گلشن ہے طلسمِ شامِ اَوَدھ کا چراغ روشن ہے

— ڈاکٹر راہی معصوم رضا

ये लखनऊ की चिकन, ये ज़री के शामों सहर, हर एक तार पे सौ बार उलझे तारे नज़र
ये जामदानी है या कहकशां की राहे गुज़र, या कोई तख़्तए-गुल रात भर की ओस में तर
सियाह रात भी आए तो सुबह गुलशन है, तिलिस्में शामें अवध का चिराग़ रौशन है
- डा० राही मासूम रज़ा

PREFACE

Beyond the view of India as the land of spiritual enlightenment lies another unexplored India that unfolds with a charm. Between its exotic heritage and its modern-day image, lies an India that is vast and rich, textured and intricately woven with cultural history. This book is a mere glimpse—through textiles, fabrics and costumes—into the splendour and romance of one such culture- the culture of Awadh.

Since childhood, I held a fascination for the costumes worn by my mother, grandmother, and aunts, but it was only about fifteen years ago that I grew really attentive to the exquisiteness of their clothes. They evoked lush images in my mind. The many names of the cotton cloth muslin, such as *ab-e-rawan* (running water), *shabnam* (dew) and *baft hawa* (woven air), sounded like the whisper of a cool breeze; the sensuality of *jamdani*, the passion of *kinkhwab*, seemed like woven enamel; the grace of *chikankari*, splendour of zardozi, playfulness of *gota-kiran*, and grandeur of *kalabattun* elevated the embroideries to exquisite forms of art.

I have always been aware of Lucknow's magnificence and have lived in the city that was the capital of the nawabs of Awadh. To have experienced its culture, characterized by *nazakat* (elegance), *nafasat* (refinement) and *tehzeeb* (etiquette), is a privilege I hold dear to my heart. I have felt the city's *taraanah* (symphony), created jointly by Hindus and Muslims, living happily alongside each other, sharing common interests and habits, and speaking a common language. Lucknow has been the 'melting pot' of various cultures – Hindu, Persian and British. Through centuries, these communities have created a rhapsody of colours, patterns and textiles; each telling a unique story, yet all blending together in a sweet melody.

This book is my homage to the creativity, artistry, finesse, finery, music and poetry of that bygone era; and to the legacy of the exquisite workmanship that still lives on in the narrow alleys of Lucknow. It is a humble contribution to the city of dreams.

Facing Page: [Translation] This is chikan and zari artwork of Lucknow has its days and nights resplendently weaved into them. Each yarn has the human sight struggling a hundred times, fathoming its beauty. This *jamdani* is the trail of the milky or a bed of roses refreshingly bathed in the night long dew. Here even the dark night is fragrant, bright like a garden of morning. The magic of Awadh evenings remain candle-lit.

INTRODUCTION

Fashion is but the reflection of the contemporary tastes of society, preferences, trends and styles. Understanding fashion and its evolution becomes even more interesting when viewed through the lens of history and its significant events and moments. As such, fashion and history are not mutually distinct, but rather intricately intertwined, and the richness of the textiles and the costumes of Awadh (it is a region of the modern state of Uttar Pradesh around Ayodhya, west of Varanasi) has its roots in its history.

This book portrays a special journey through Awadh, connecting dates and events to the evolution of gorgeous and delicate costumes, textiles, colours, motifs and ornamentations from the eighteenth century up to present-day India. It attempts to recapture the ambience of the Nawabi Era (1722-1856) and of the British Raj (1856-1947) in Awadh, through the luxurious lives of wealthy nawabs, their begums, courtiers and courtesans. A glimpse of its reflection in modern times will also be portrayed.

The Nawabi Era is known for its court culture, especially in the capital city of Lucknow, which became the centre of political, cultural and leisurely activities of the nawabs. This period was one of growing wealth and opulence. The refined court sophistication and the glorious era of Lucknow gave birth to a specific costume style. Great importance was given to the art of dressing, apparels and jewellery. The effect was attained by combining *nazakat* with *nafasat*, or elegance with refinement, such that it permeated every aspect of nawabi life, and was particularly reflected in the costumes of the time.

The fashion of Awadh, under British Raj, reflected Western influences brought by the annexation of Awadh to the British Empire in 1856. In order to integrate with the ruling class, Indians adopted British costumes, and Western-style clothes gained importance. Elements of European style, such as structured tailoring, collars, cuffs and buttons, were introduced. Hand-woven fabrics were replaced by machine-made, imported fabrics, and machine-stitching took over hand-stitching. Today, in twenty-first century India, there is fusion of Indian and Western fashion.

Most of the vernacular terms used in this book, including some Awadhi names of textiles, remain without a corresponding English term.

Facing Page: A taluqdar wearing silk brocade floral-patterned sherwani with churidar paijama and formal Oxford shoes or balmorals. The sherwani has a band collar fastened with buttons and button-holes. A pocket-watch with chain is seen in a vertical pocket, specially designed for the accessory of the time. An umbrella completes the formal outfit.

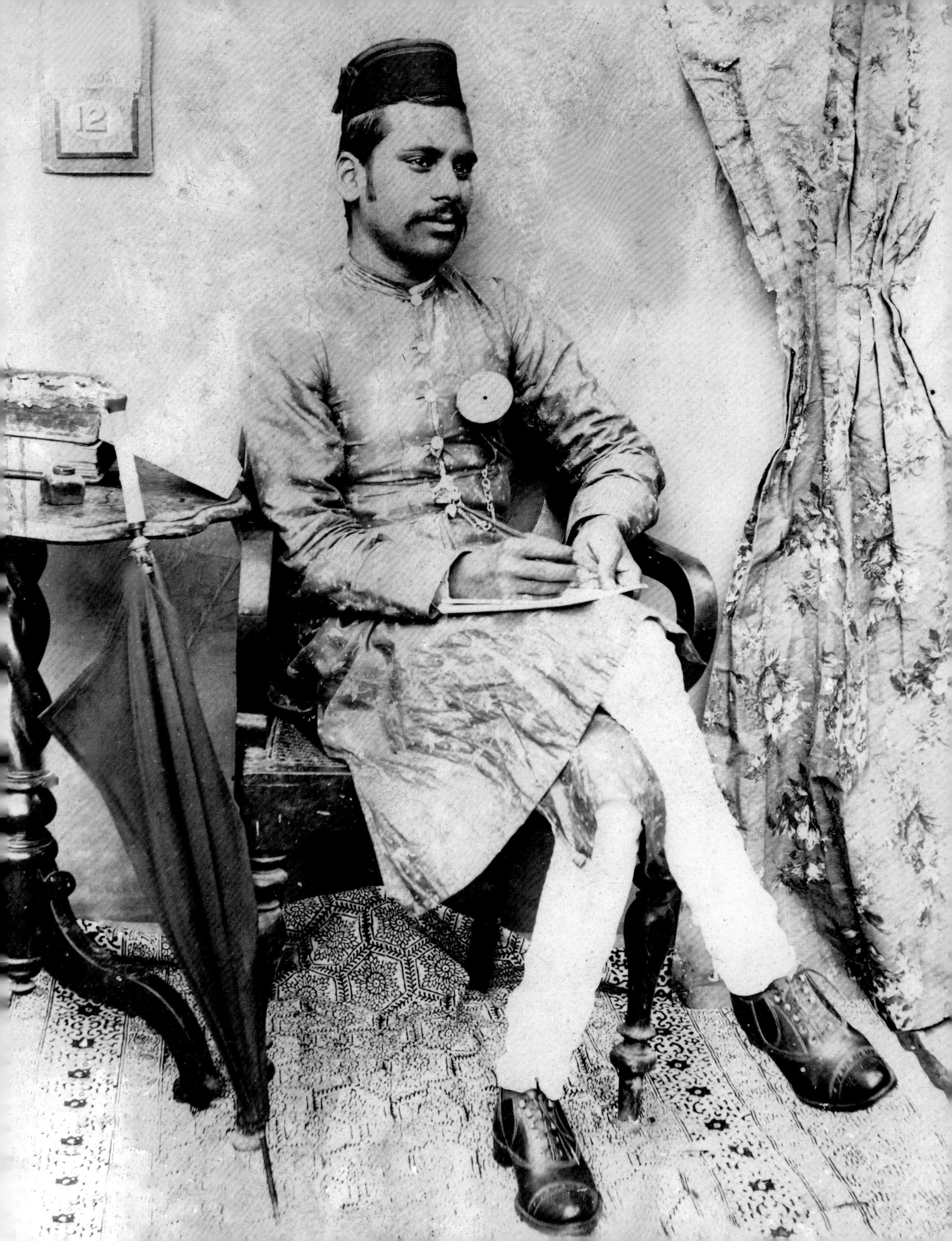

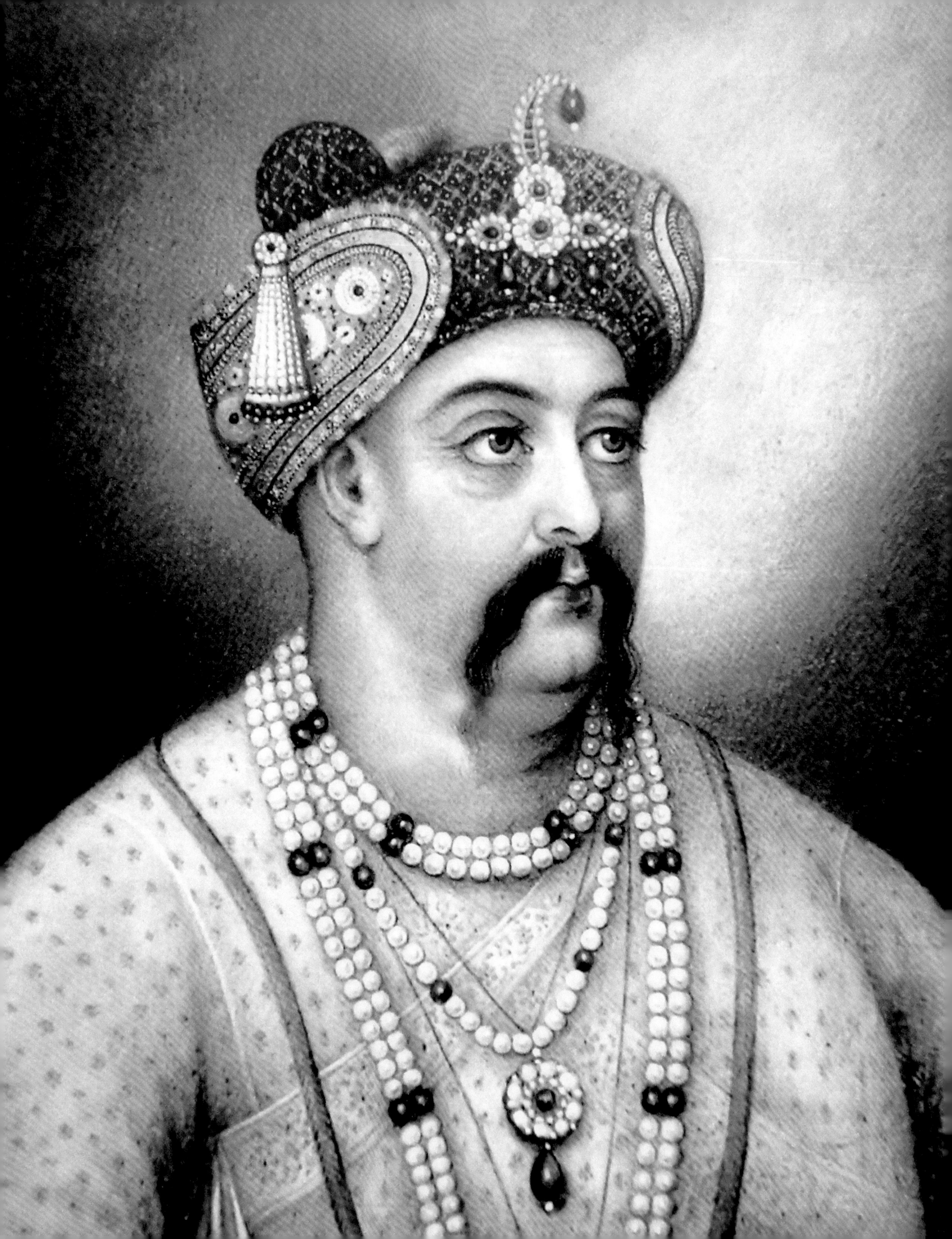

AWADH-NAMA

1722-1947

AWADH NAMA
The Chronicle of Awadh

'[Awadh] ... is situated at the root in the heart of the Indian peninsula. Interposed between the Ganges and the Himalayas, its fertility is so remarkable amongst the principalities of this prolific land that it is commonly referred to as the "Garden of India".' R.W. Bird (the Assistant Resident at the court of Awadh during the reign of Wajid Ali Shah) in Lucas et al. (1923).

Since time immemorial, Awadh has been one of the richest regions of India, both in terms of wealth and culture. It was the cradle of Indian civilization, the object of many invasions, and the melting pot of different religions and people.

Around 800 BC, the Aryans moved towards the Ganga and Jamuna doab (Gangetic plains) to avail of the vast fertile land suitable for settlement. By the late Vedic period, *mahajanpadas* (kingdoms) had started to form. Ayodhya was the capital of one such *mahajanpada*, the kingdom of Kosala, and is regarded as one of the seven holy places of the Hindus. In fact, the Mahabharata and the Ramayana, the two great Indian epics, both originated in this region. The Ramayana was written by Tulsidas in Awadhi, the language of the region.

In 1580, during Mughal Emperor Akbar's reign, Ayodhya and its neighbouring cities became one of the twelve *subas* (provinces) of the Mughal Empire, and became known as Awadh. The *suba* was governed by a subedar. In 1720, Emperor Muhammad Shah of Delhi appointed Sadat Khan of Nishapur (Persia) as the Subedar of Awadh (Lucknow State Museum). After he successfully brought together–under one administration– the inhabitants of the region, which included mainly Hindus, Muslims and Afghans, Sadat Khan was conferred the title of Burhan-ul-Mulk (Credit to the Country) by the Mughal emperor (Sharar, 2001). In addition, although the title of 'Nawab' was usually bestowed upon a high ranking official or governor of a province under Mughal rule, it was added to his name as an honorific title. After him, the title of Nawab came to be transferred in a hereditary manner rather than being conferred by the Mughal rulers (Sharar, 2001).

In 1722, Sadat Khan Burhan-ul-Mulk (r. 1722-1739), the first nawab, made settlements called mohallas for his

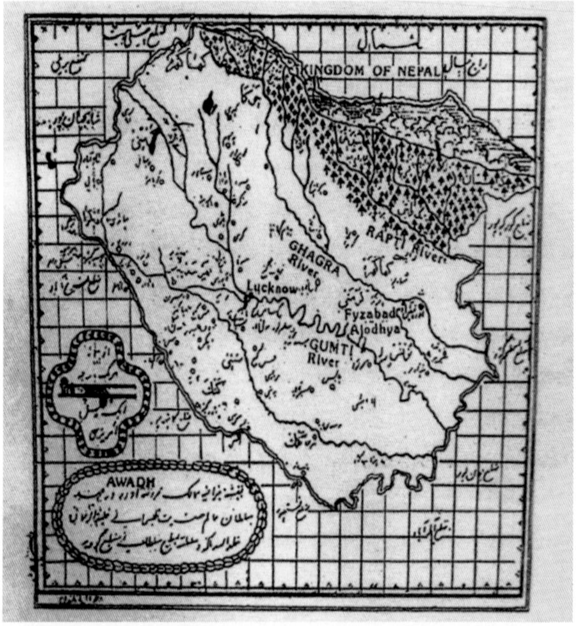

Above: The geographical map of Awadh issued by the Awadh imperial court in 1849.
Page 13: Nawab Asaf-ud-Daula wearing cross-over *jamdani jama* and a turban with *kalgi* and *turra*.
Facing page, Left: Official emblem of the founder of the Court of Awadh, Sadat Burhan-ul-Mulk. It consists of two winged mermaids, a shield with four knobs, a crown and a royal umbrella, topped by a bird and two swords. The umbrella is a symbol of spiritual leadership.
Facing page, Right: A bow representing King Ram of Ayodhya, a pair of fish and the confluence of the rivers Ganga and Yamuna, symbol of Uttar Pradesh.

army and administration, laying the foundation for the elegant court for the nawabs of Awadh in Faizabad. It is said that when he was crossing the River Gomti, a fish fell into his lap. He took it as an auspicious omen and made the fish (*jalpariya*) his royal emblem. This symbol appeared on textiles of the period and can be seen on the gates of several residential and official buildings even today.

Asaf-ud-Daula (r. 1775-1797), the fourth nawab, shifted the capital from Faizabad to Lucknow, which was to become one of the most magnificent cities ever. It was during this period that the court of Awadh saw an era of cultural renaissance. The nawabs were living

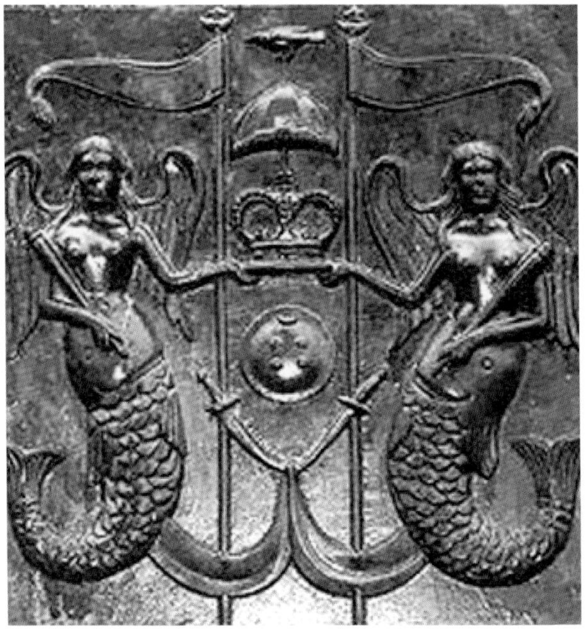

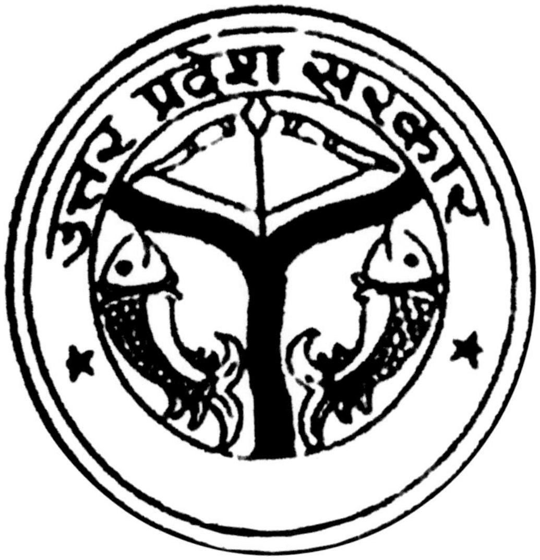

in opulence, endorsing cultural endeavours, especially in the performing arts, and built architectural masterpieces.

During this period, however, the British steadily gained increasing administrative and military powers. Nawab Ghazi-ud-Din Haider (r. 1819-27) was the last ruler of Awadh to bear the title of nawab, as he was conferred the title of 'King' by Lord Hastings in 1819. From then onwards, the rulers of Awadh lost their sovereignty to the Delhi Court and became puppet kings in the hands of the British. They had almost no authority over the administration of Awadh and became dependent on the Delhi Court. The lifestyle of these kings was strongly influenced by the Western ways of living. Patronage was given to many of the Western artists who in turn adopted traditional costumes of the court.

King Wajid Ali Shah (r. 1847-56), the tenth and the last king of the Court of Awadh spent large amounts of money on the welfare of his subjects and on beautifying the city. He built a palace complex called Qaisar Bagh, which was the centre of administrative and cultural activities. He was a great patron of music, art and dance, and was trained in singing and dancing himself. It was during this period that Lucknow reached its zenith of culture.

'Not Rome, not Athens, not Constantinople, not any city I have ever seen appears to me so striking and beautiful as this, and the more I gaze the more its beauty grows upon me.'

–Sir William Howard Russell reporting, on Lucknow, in the *London Times*, 1857

In 1856, with the British firmly established in India, General James Outram dethroned Wajid Ali Shah and annexed the province of Awadh to the growing British empire. This marked the formal end of the rule of the nawabs of Awadh and the beginning of British Raj, which then extended until the independence of India in 1947.

On 15 August 1947, the province of Awadh became one of the states of independent India, and on 26 January 1950, when India became a republic, it was given the name of Uttar Pradesh with its capital in Lucknow. Monarchy and the feudal structure were replaced by a democratic political system, and all titles, including 'nawab', were abolished. The interesting fact is that the state emblem of Uttar Pradesh keeps alive its legacy by incorporating a bow representing King Ram of Ayodhya (original name for Awadh), a pair of fish – the insignia of the nawabs of Awadh – and the *sangam*, or confluence of the rivers Ganga and Yamuna, in the doab region.

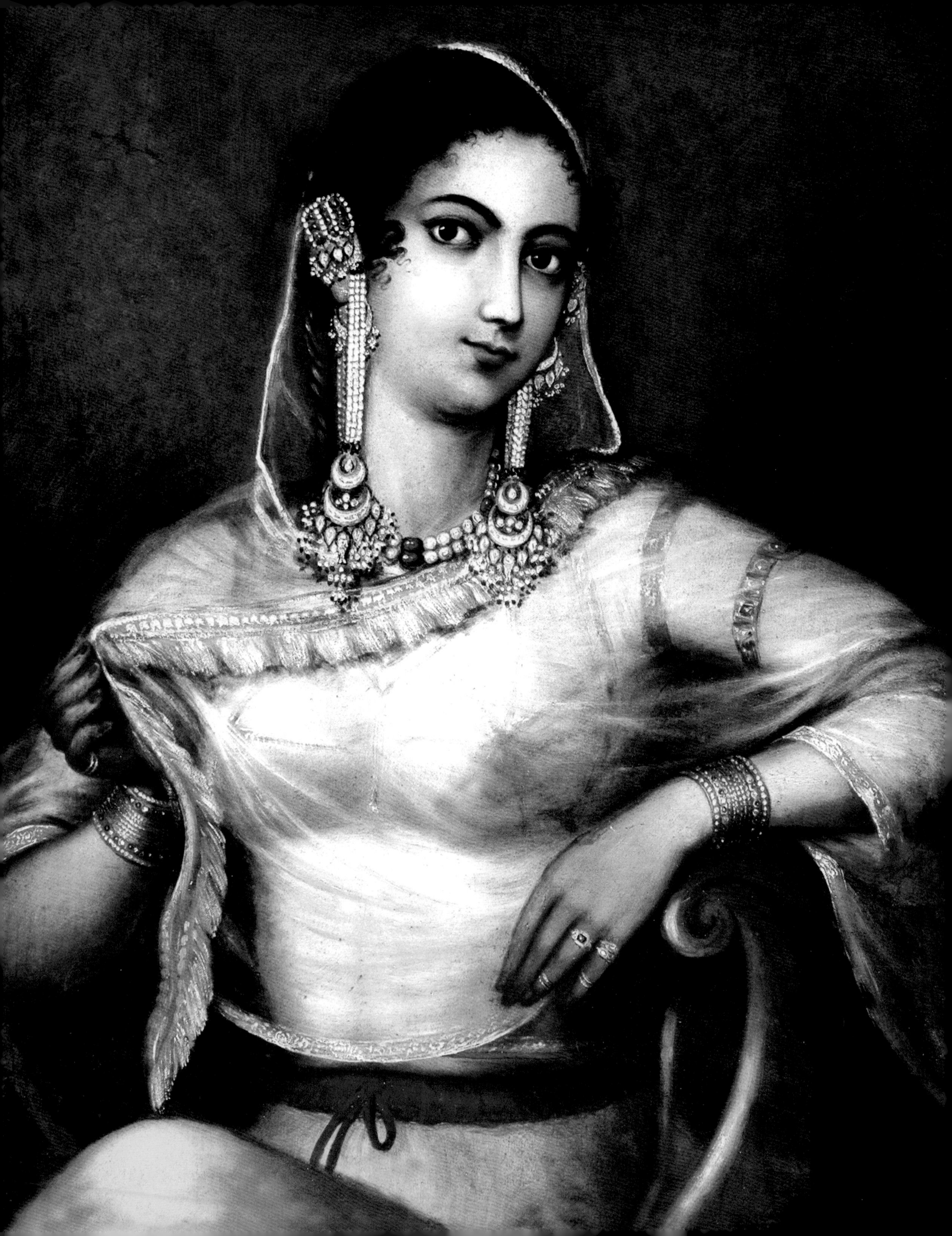

SHAN-E-AWADH

1722-1856

SHAN-E-AWADH
Splendour of the Court of Awadh

History made the nawabs and the nawabs defined the culture of Awadh. It was a peculiar period in history, when the rulers' wealth increased through continued tax collections but at the same time, their power decreased with the arrival of the British. The nawabs continued to pay large amount of revenues to the British through various treaties, in exchange for their security. In this peaceful atmosphere, palace life was filled with imperial extravagance.

'The nawabs were proud and surrounded themselves with paraphernalia such as titles, elephants, horses, sarpesh decorated with jewels, insignias, jewel-studded swords, daggers and other weapons, fringed palanquins, howdahs, trappings, garlands of pearls, beautifully embroidered shawls, handkerchiefs and other clothes of costly works' (Aseh-ul-Matabai, 1927).

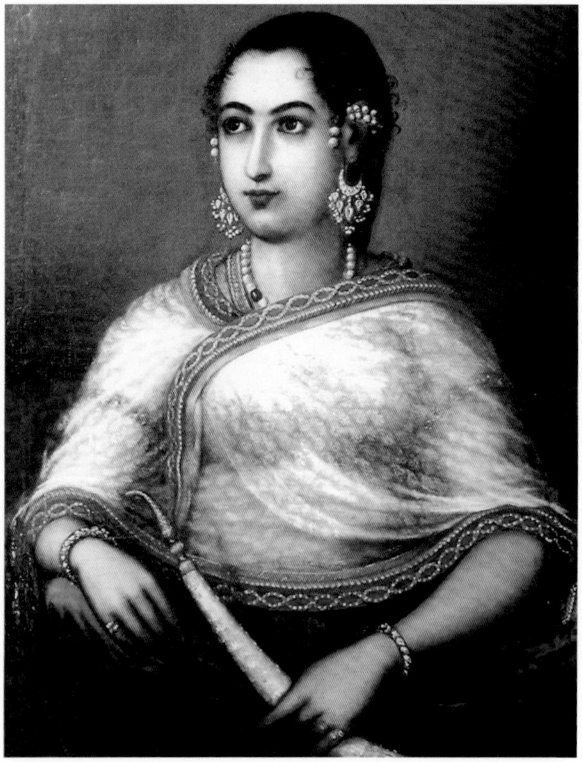

Above: The begum is seen wearing a paijama where *izarband* is visible below the zamdani *odhni* edged with green border and embroidered in heavy zardozi work.
Previous page 16: Begum wearing *lehenga*, *choli* and *mulmul odhni*. The edges are decorated with gold and silver *gota-kiran*.
Facing page: Nawab Asaf-ud-Daula is seen mounted on a gold hauda in a royal procession. Men are seen wearing colourful *jamas*, *sidha* paijamas, *patkas* and turbans. The elephant is decorated with caparison, necklaces and *turra* (formal decoration for head). Interestingly the ears of elephants are decorated with fish pattern, insignia of nawabs of Awadh. The horses are also richly decorated with jewels.

BAHAR-E-AWADH: COURT OF AWADH IN FULL BLOOM

The palaces were at the centre of all political, professional, cultural, religious and personal activity. Elegance, graceful manners, extreme politeness, lyrical speech and legendary hospitality distinguished the nawabi distinct court culture. The romantic and courtly culture often spread beyond the court and became a part of the people of Awadh. During the nawabi period (1722-1856), smaller towns including Unnao, Rai Bareilly, Farrukhabad, Bahraich, Sultanpur, Sitapur, Hardoi, Lakhimpurkhiri and Barabanki, also came under the influence of the nawabi-Awadhi culture.

Patronage was given to artists, poets, jewellers and master textile artisans from all over India, as well as those from places like Tashkent, Samarkand, Isfahan and Bukhara. Western artists were also attracted to the magnificent court of Awadh. This brought a wave of innovation as Indian artists, experts in miniature paintings were now exposed to realism on large oil canvases. Thus European influence became more marked in Indian art during the later period of nawabs.

GULISTAN-E-AWADH: AMALGAMATION OF CULTURES IN THE COURT OF AWADH

Awadh became the most important region of India to witness the fusion of cultural diversity and harmonious coexistence of Persian and Indian cultures, as well as the two main religions of the time: Islam and Hinduism. The nawabs also showed a positive tolerance towards Hinduism by participating in Hindu festivals like Basant, Holi, Diwali and Dussehra. Hindus and Muslims adopted each other's religions through various practices: a Muslim crescent adorns the top of a Hanuman temple in Aliganj; orthodox Muslim women observed the Hindu festival Navratri and

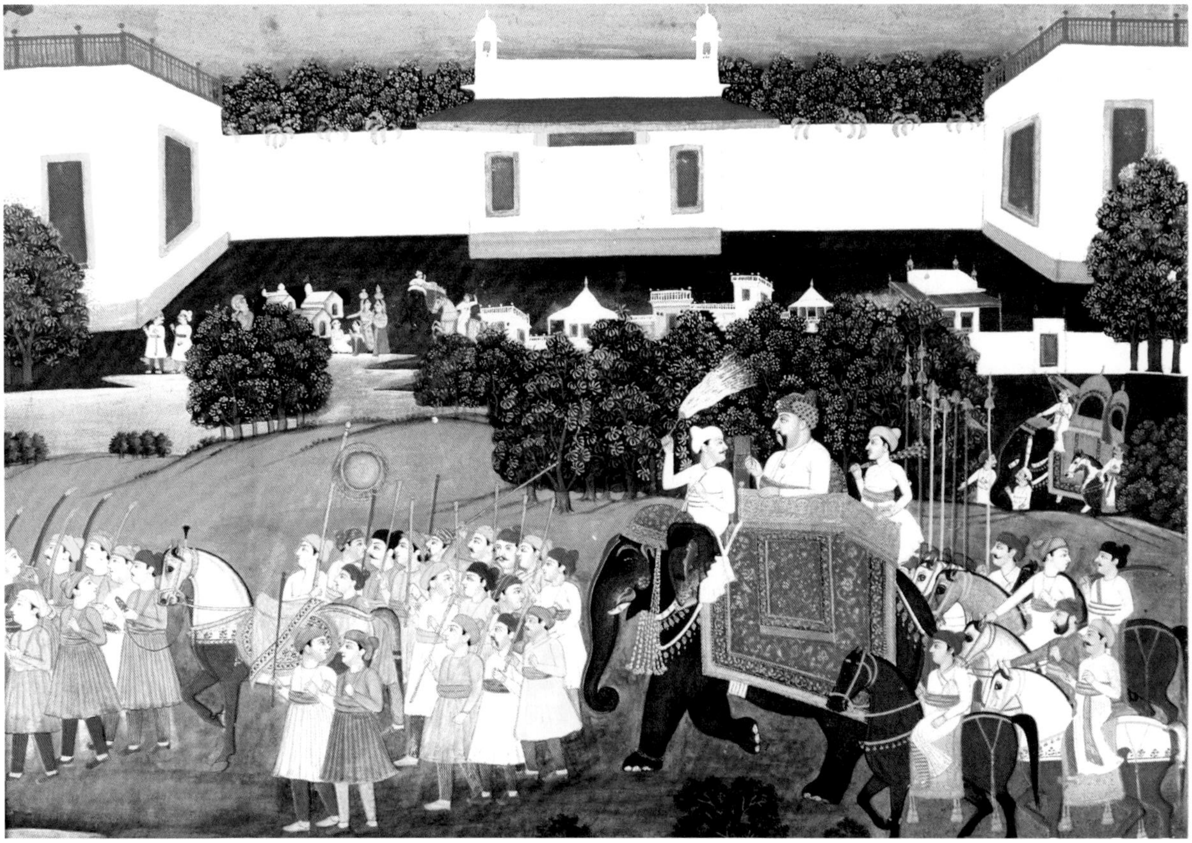

conservative Awadhi Kanyakubj Brahmins (belonging to Kannauj) ate meat (Mishra, 1999).

Hum ishq ke bande hain mazhab se nahi vaqif
Gar kabaa hua to kya butkhana hua to kya
(I am a devotee of love and unacquainted with religion;
To us it does not matter, whether it is the Kaba or a temple.)
—Wajid Ali Shah in Sitaram (1932).

The coexistence and intermingling gave rise to a culture of mutual respect and tolerance called Ganga-Jamuni *tehzeeb*. The expression is borrowed from the names of the two important rivers (Ganga and Yamuna) in this region, which converge at Prayag (present-day Allahabad). The essence of the expression is that when the rivers, each having its own colour (the Ganga being turbid and light yellow and the Yamuna being green), amalgamate and flow into each other, the integration is so seamless such that no difference can be noticed. This cultural synthesis had a particular influence on the costumes. The brocades woven with gold and silver threads were described as Ganga-Jamuni. In parts of India this term is also borrowed to refer to a sari having upper and lower borders in two different colours.

ANDAZ-E-AWADH: STYLE IN THE COURT OF AWADH

Every passageway of the palace was perfumed with rose and *kewra* water during the *saawan* (monsoon) festival. *Jhulas* (swings) were suspended from the branches of trees with strings made of silk and *kalabattun* (metallic thread made by wrapping gold or silver gilt thread around silk or cotton yarns). The seats of the swings were decorated with *gota-kiran*.

In Lucknow, *itr* or attar (natural perfume extracted from flowers) had a special place in everyday life, and it was considered fashionable and sophisticated to use it. Nawab Ghaziuddin Haider was a great connoisseur of *itr* and even had fountains of perfumed water in his bedroom. The use of *itr* also became popular in the zenana and in the court as courtesans had their kothas perfumed with it. Sweet smelling flower petals were used to make *itrs* and oils, that were applied to skin and hair. Best *itrs* were made of *gulab* (rose), *kamal* (lotus), *chameli* or *juhi* (jasmine), *champa* (magnolia), *kewra* (pandanus flower) and *chandan* (sandalwood).

It was during the nawabi period that the popularity of paan reached its peak. In Lucknavi culture, even offering the paan to guests was an expression of *nazakat*. The risen veins on the back of the betel leaf were in fact levelled to

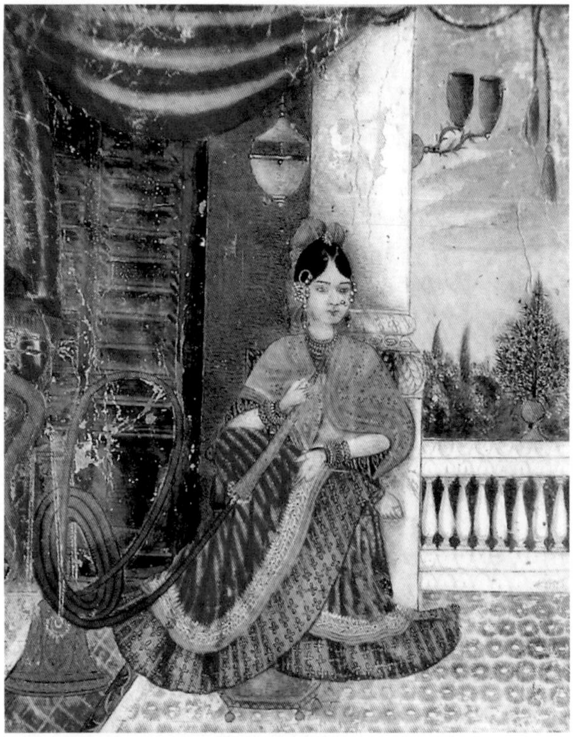

Above: The begum, is dressed in gorgeous *kalidar* brocade paijama embroidered in zardozi work and yellow *odhni*, is seen enjoying the hukkah. The length of the pipe and the silver chain hanging from the top determined the status of the person smoking it.

Facing page: The courtesan Umrao Jaan in the famous film by Muzaffar Ali, is wearing tight-fitting *anarkali* dress with churidar paijama and long-flowing *odhni*. The typical ornaments like *jhumar, tika, hathphool, payal* and five-stringed *haar* (necklace) complete the outfit and enhance her beauty. The *alta* (red paint) applied to her hands and feet makes her attractive and desirable. Nawabs and courtiers are wearing *jamawar* woollen shawls worn in various ways on their *jamas* and their flared paijamas of silk and precious brocade. The headdresses show great variety in material and ornamentation.

prevent the harm they could do to the delicate palates of nawabs and begums. In addition to the usual ingredients such as *chuna* (lime), *kattha* (catechu), cardamom and *supari* (areca nut) special silver, gold and pearl powders were also used. The *chuna* used for paan was dipped in milk and *kattha* was diluted in rose water. The paan was finally wrapped in silver foil and served on silver plates.

The court of Awadh cannot be imagined without the hukkah – a sign of prestige and richness. The hukkah was very popular in the Mughal court of Delhi but when it came to Awadh, it reflected fineness. Extra attention was paid to the details. The cords were made of silk and *kalabattun* and the base was made of bidri work in pure silver. Generally, the cords were three metres long, but for the nawabs they measured up to thirty metres. Nawab Sadat Ali Khan and King Nasir-ud-din's love for the hukkah bordered on addiction. The favourite hukkah of Wajid Ali Shah was made of pink hand-blown glass. Hindu hukkahs were made with one pipe while Muslim hukkahs had two pipes, with the height varying from two inches to two feet. In the late eighteenth and early nineteenth centuries, hukkahs also became popular in the zenanas of noblemen, the rich and also with the British.

Even the tobacco used for hukkahs was prepared with great sophistication. Sugar syrup with apple, pineapple and clove was added to lessen the bitter taste of tobacco. For the nobles, it was then delicately flavoured with rose and *kewra*-water, cardamom, saffron, *jaiphal* (nutmeg) and *javitri* (mace). The base was filled with milk rather than water.

Another example of subtle elegance was that the nawabs were always given water to wash their hands after the meals in *besandani*, besan being a coarse grain helped to take off all the grease from hands. The gold or silver *silabchis* (portable wash-basins) had a metal sieve so that the dirty water was out of sight; these covers were layered with grass, so that when the nawabs or begums washed their hands, the water did not splash out of it.

The indulgent nature of the nawabs was also expressed through pastimes such as chess, cockfights, *bater-bazi, titar-bazi*, *kabutar-bazi* and kite-flying. For a cockfight, roosters were meticulously trained and the Nawabs would pride themselves on possessing the finest specimens in the world. Even the fighter cocks were fed by hand, in the true Lucknavi-style, to protect damage to their beaks. The ideal 'nawabi diet' for them consisted of saffron, almonds, pearl-dust and gold foil to make them strong.

SHAM-E-AWADH: EVENINGS OF AWADH

Under the rule of nawabs, an era of peaceful coexistence and interaction created a cultural synthesis known as *dhoop-chhaiyan* (sunlight-shade), in the fields of literature, music, dance and poetry. Musicians and dancers came to Lucknow, giving rise to new musical forms and instruments under the patronage of royalty. Persian and Indian musical instruments informed each other, giving birth to dance and music forms like kathak, thumri, khayal, dadra, qawwalis, ghazals and sher-o-shairi, which were later perfected.

The language also underwent a gradual change. Awadhi, the original dialect since the time of Tulsidas, was first influenced by Farsi or Persian (brought by the Mughals) and then came to be substituted by Urdu (mix of Persian and Khadi Boli), which was again the result of the intermingling of two cultures and each other's linguistic expressions.

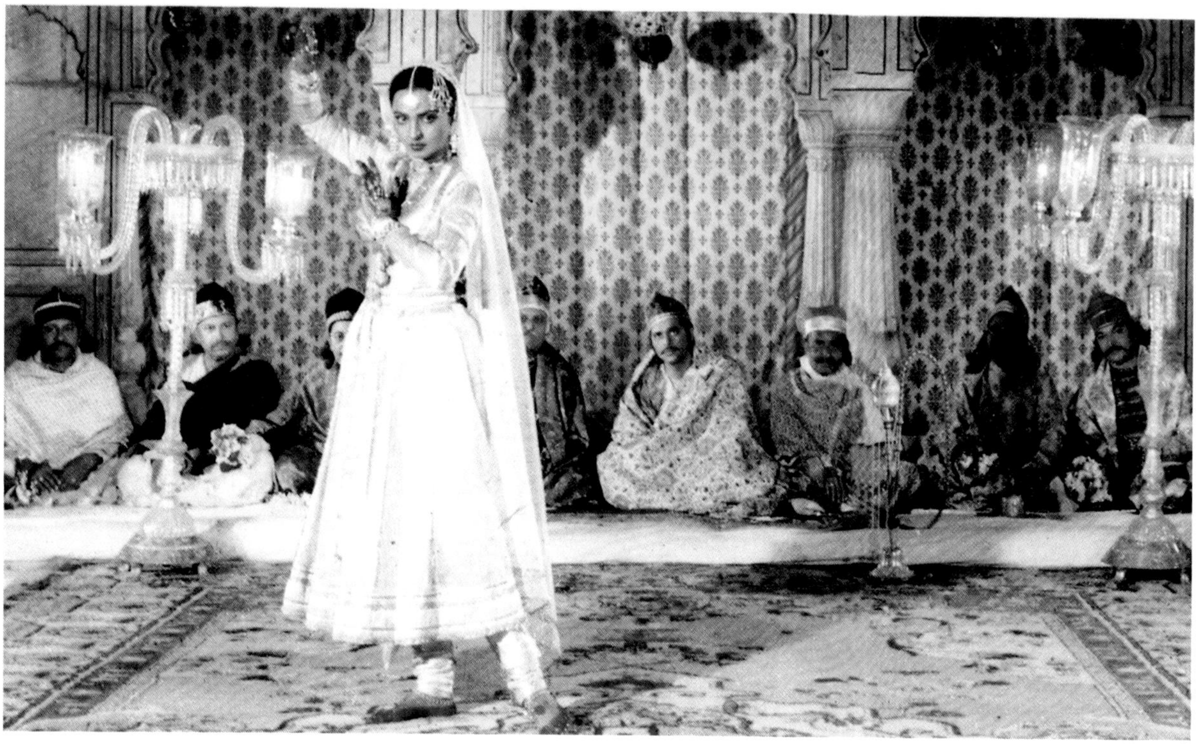

ROLE OF COURTESANS

Imagine taking a walk in the lanes of eighteenth century Lucknow. Your eyes would fall upon the young nawab stepping down from his horse-carriage, dressed in elegant fine muslin clothes and wearing a cap just as delicate. You would find the air full of enchanting perfumes and people greeting you with a *farshi salaam* (traditional, long bowed greeting). You would experience *nazakat* and *nafasat* in every movement of theirs. The whole ambience would give you the feel of the famous *tehzeeb*, for which Lucknow is reputed. You might be served a paan, wrapped in silver foil with ultimate delicacy; the manner of offering being no less exquisite itself.

Accomplished courtesans played an important role in the socio-cultural life of the court of the nawabs. Many of them had emigrated from the Delhi Court of Mohammad Shah Rangeley, after his downfall. They served as a link between town and country, and were able to build bridges between Hindus and Muslims, between the Awadhi and Urdu languages, and between the bhakti cults (particularly that of Krishna) and Shi'ism (Graff, 1999). The courtesans were considered the protectors, preservers and guardians of Awadhi culture and of refined manners. They maintained well-furnished and decorated halls where they gave exquisite dance and music performances. There was no better seminary than a courtesan's *nishatkhana* or kothi for Urdu poetry. Young men of noble families were sent to the kothas to learn composing and reciting poems, for social etiquette and sophisticated manners.

Around the mid-nineteenth century, the courtesans of Awadh began to assert their influence on the nawabs of Lucknow. 'They would accompany the Nawabs on their tours and in turn, received wealth in the form of property and ornaments such as embroidered cashmere wool and brocade shawls, bejewelled caps and shoes, silver-, gold-, jade- and amber-handled fly whisks, silver cutlery, jade goblets, plates, spittoons, hookahs and silver utensils for serving and storing food and drink, and valuable furnishings Graff (1999).' The courtesans strongly influenced the dressing mode in the zenana too with their seductive styles.

During the time of Asaf-ud-Daula and Sadat Ali Khan, Ujagar and Dilruba were two famous courtesans whose performances during the Holi festival were considered unparalleled. The courtesans were famous for their *ada* (style), beauty and sophistication. Inspired by the enchanting shyness of these beauties of Lucknow, a poet has rightly said:

Izhar-e-mohabat kar na sake,
Kuchh keh na sake kuchh sun na sake
Yahan humne zuban kholee hee thee,
Wahan ankh jhukee sharma bhee gaye.

I was not able to express my love,
I could not say anything or hear anything
I had barely opened my lips to speak,
That she cast down her eyes and blushed.

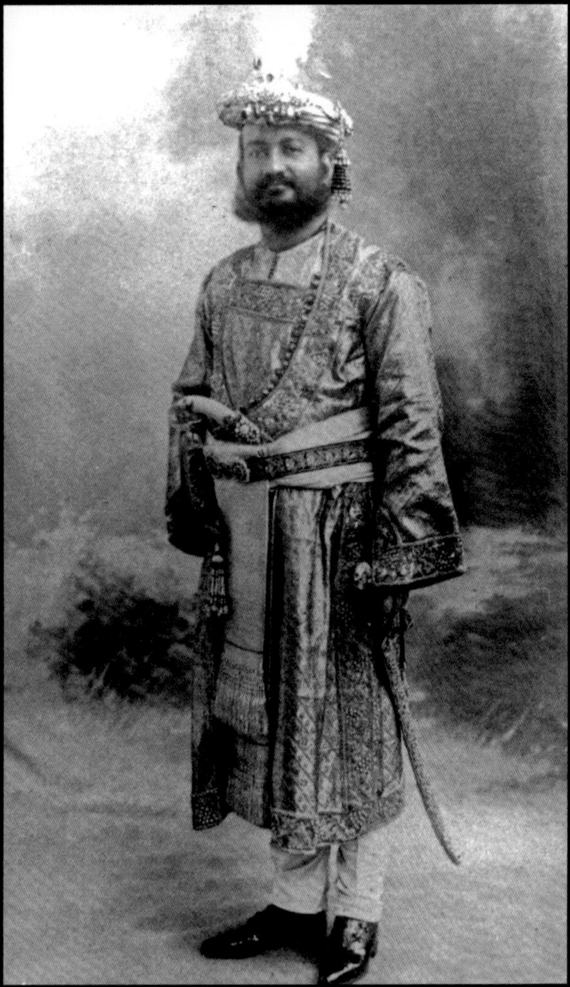

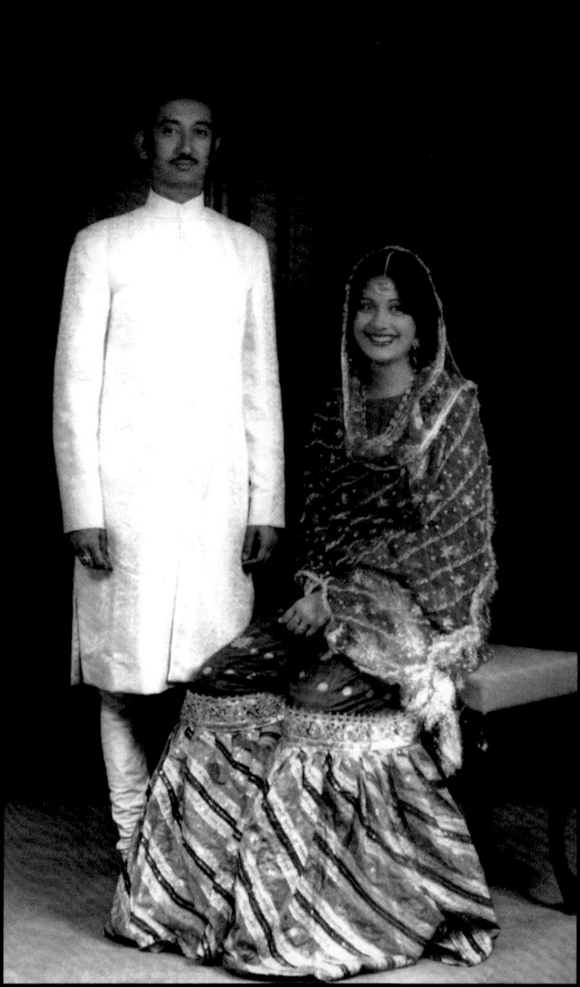

Left: Late Maharaja Sir Mohd. Ali Mohd. Khan (1876-1931) is wearing his ceremonial dress, '*khillat*, *patka,* churidar paijama, heeled shoes and holding the customary sword as a sign of nobility. **Right:** Rajkumar Mohd. Amir Naqi Khan and Kunwar Rani Kulsum in their wedding attire. He is wearing *sherwani* with churidar paijama and begum is wearing *arri khariyon ki gote ka* paijama kurti and *odhni* enriched with zari border. The brocade *paat* of the paijama and the *gote* made of diagonal silk stripes is embroidered with *salma sitara*. A composite *gota* band joins the upper part with the lower part of the garment called *chasak*.

LEGACY OF A NAWAB

Interview with Rajkumar Mohd Amir Naqi Khan of Basha State, Lucknow

My interview with Rajkumar Mohd Amir Naqi Khan of Basha State was an experience in itself. From the moment I entered his palace (Iqbal Manzil, Wazirganj, Lucknow) till the end of the interview, I had a strange sensation of travelling back into the enchanting era of nawabs. His house was full of photographs of bygone days, which showed that the palace was the centre of political and cultural activities at the time of the British Raj and the Independence movement of India.

Rajkumar Mohd Amir Naqi Khan belongs to the royal family of Mahmudabad. He can be considered the preserver of Awadhi culture, as can be seen from his multifarious activities. The most important of these are his contributions to the preservation of historical monuments of Lucknow and the revival of the old arts and restoration of rare paintings. In his own words, 'my life has been dedicated to continuing the legacy of the culture of Awadh and the Ganga-Jamuni tahzeeb.'

My interview started with reminiscences of his childhood memories. He recalled the clothes worn by his grandparents and parents. His grandfather used to wear an *angarkha*, churidar paijama and *patka*; and he wore *khillat* with *patka* and a sword with high-heeled shoes for ceremonial use. The influences

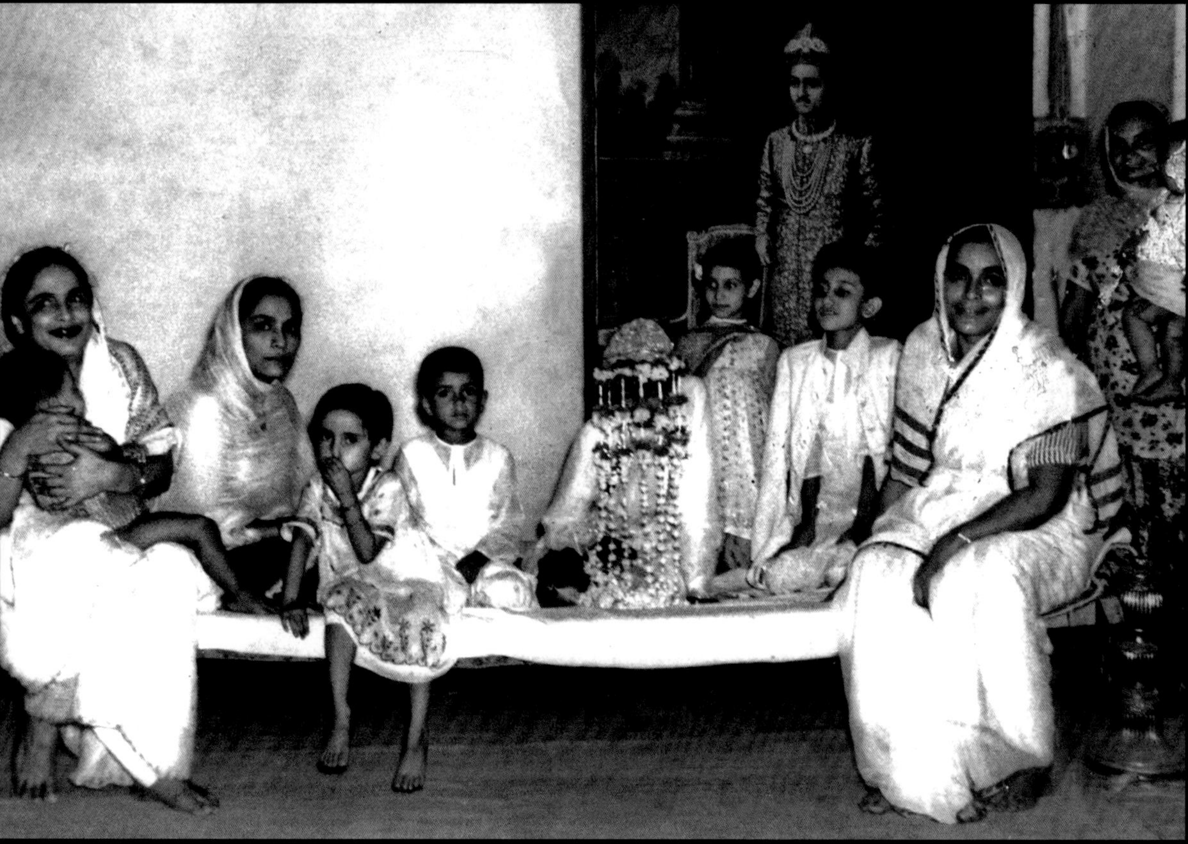

of Hyderabad can be seen in the style of draping the dupatta, and the Awadhi touch in *ghatele* (type of shoes in fashion in Awadh) worn by his respected great grandmother.

The married women of his family wore *bar ka paijama* (also called *bade paichon ka paijama*). *Kali*s determined the volume of the paijama; more *kali*s gave importance to paijamas. Unmarried girls wore *ghuttanas* (knee-length paijama) with kurta and chunni. These were made of muslin for everyday wear in summers and brocades and silks for the winter season. These garments were decorated with zari and *kamdani* for special occasions.

Rajkumar remembers that his mother, aunts and sisters wore many kinds of ornaments like *tika* (ornament for the forehead), *chapka* or *jhumar* (to be worn on the right side of the head), *karnphool* and *bunde* (earrings) in the form of fishes called *machalia*, *guluband* (necklace), *tauk* (a pendant), *haar* (necklace), *satlara* (seven-stringed necklace), *bajuband* (armband), and *dastband* (bracelet), *payal or pajeb* (literally meaning anklet that bestows beauty on the foot). The married women wore *kare* (heavy bangles made of

Birthday celebration of Rajkumar Amir Naqi Khan who is seen wearing *sherwani,* churidar *paijama* and *sehra*. The dress for birthday celebration was as important as a wedding costume. To celebrate the birthday or *saal-girah* of a son, a knot is tied in a string every year, as the term *saal* meaning a year and *girah,* tying a knot. Instead, a silver ring is added to the necklace of a daughter each year.

An interesting revelation he made was that there was an area allocated in the palace for *mughlanias* (artisans) to stitch, dye and embroider cloth. Fabrics were dyed in natural colours and real flowers were added for a pleasing aroma. The flowers were chosen according to the season of the year. For summer, rose, *khas*, *harsingar* were preferred; for monsoons, *bela*, *juhi*, *chameli*, *champa* were favoured; and in winter, *mushk*, *hina* and amber were chosen.

My rendezvous with Rajkumar recreated the era of nawabs, not only through the description of costumes but also through the nawabi *tehzeeb* of Raj Kumar Mohd Amir Naqi Khan. His courteous and gentle disposition and his refinement reaffirmed the continuity of the legacy of Awadh's culture

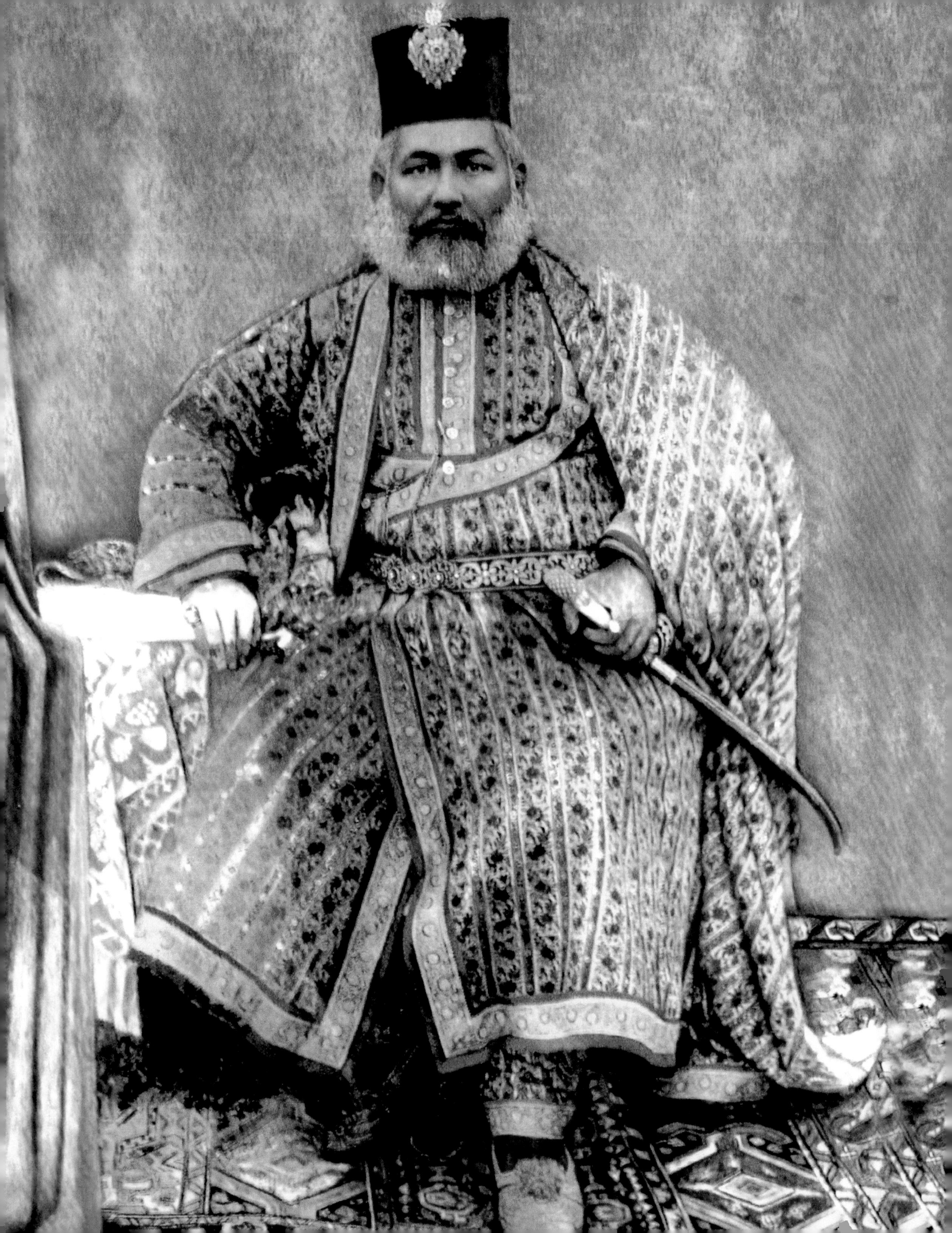

NAWABI ERA

1722-1856

NAWABI ERA

The era of the nawabs was particularly influential in the evolution of fashion. Royalty set traditions, customs and trends in Awadh. The aristocracy of Lucknow gained immense wealth with the feudal system and spent extravagantly on their dresses. This had an impact on the dresses of the courtiers, taluqdars and Awadhi people in general. The emphasis was not only on costumes and textiles but also on how they were worn. In Awadh, stitched clothes were preferred by Hindus on certain occasions. For example, for purposes of cooking and the requirement to be hygienic, the concept of 'ek vastra' (single clothing) was predominant. If the person responsible for cooking was male, he would wear a dhoti (cloth-length); if the person was a married woman from the family, she would cook in 'ek vastra' and then change her clothes after cooking, and wear her lehenga/*angiya*/ chunni at the time of the meal. If the woman was a widow, she would have her meal in the same dhoti.

MEN'S COSTUMES

In 1827, during the reign of Nasir-ud-din Haider, Lord Combermere visited Lucknow and was hosted by the king in a true regal manner. The splendour of his court was described by an officer in attendance of the Commander-in-chief as (Hilton 1911):

On arrival at the palace, we sat down to breakfast with the King and his courtiers. The king was splendidly attired in a tunic of green velvet, and girded with a costly shawl. He wore a turban enriched with diamonds and his person was profusely ornamented with necklaces, earrings, and armlets of diamonds, emeralds and pearls.... The throne is, however, beautifully decorated with embroidery in seed-pearl. Here His Majesty presented the Commander-in Chief with his portrait set in diamonds, suspended by a string of pearls and emeralds.'

The main upper body costumes of the period were *jamas*, *choga*, *angarkha*, *patka* and pagri or topi as important accessories. A *patka* or *kamarband* is 6 to 10 yards long and 20 inches wide, with a border which shows weaving and highly ornamented ends that are left hanging in the front. An expression of the *nafasat* of the period was the sophisticated construction of garments. For example, in the *chogas* of the period, instead of washing the entire garment, only the lining was removed, washed and then reinserted into the *choga*, in order to protect the delicate textiles of the costume.

Other costumes included the *shaluka* (short-sleeved upper garment fastened at the chest with loops), which was worn under the *angarkha*, *farji* or *fatohi*. In winters people wore a full-sleeved quilted garment known as *dagla* and the half-sleeved one was called *mirzai*. The quilting was done artistically in a *barfi* (diamond-shaped) pattern.

The kurta was a popular dress of the Delhi Court and became the *kali*-kurta when it reached Awadh. It was generally

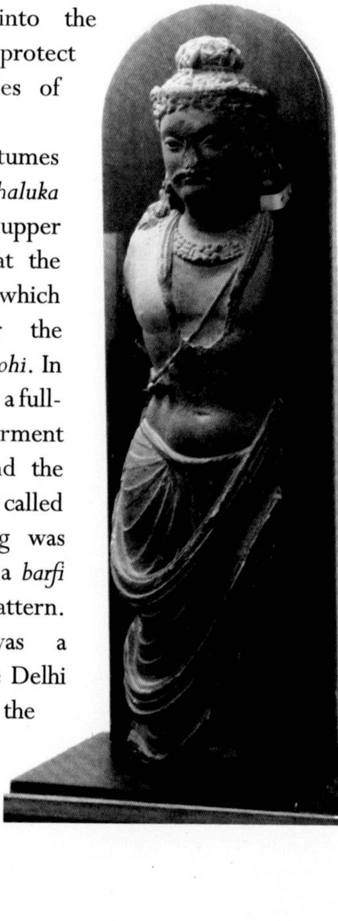

Previous page 24: Late Sir Raja Amir-ud-daula Amir Hasan Khan of Mahmoodabad wearing *choga* over a matching *angarkha*, and a *jamawar* shawl thrown over left shoulder. A plumed *Kalgi* adorns the Turkish cap. An elaborately ornated gold belt completes the attire.

Right: The only piece of costume elegantly draped for rituals, *ek vastra* with the *janeu*, a sacred initiation ritual thread made of three or six cotton strands that hangs from left shoulder. It is celebrated between seven and fourteen years of age, also makes a person eligible to participate in all the family traditions and rituals after this ceremony.

Facing page: Nawab Asaf-ud-daula is wearing cross-over jama of *jamdani* muslin woven with small woven *butis* with wide-legged *paijama*. The border of the *jama* is embellished with a gold border. Pagdi with *sarpesh*, *patka* and *talwar* complete the royal attire.

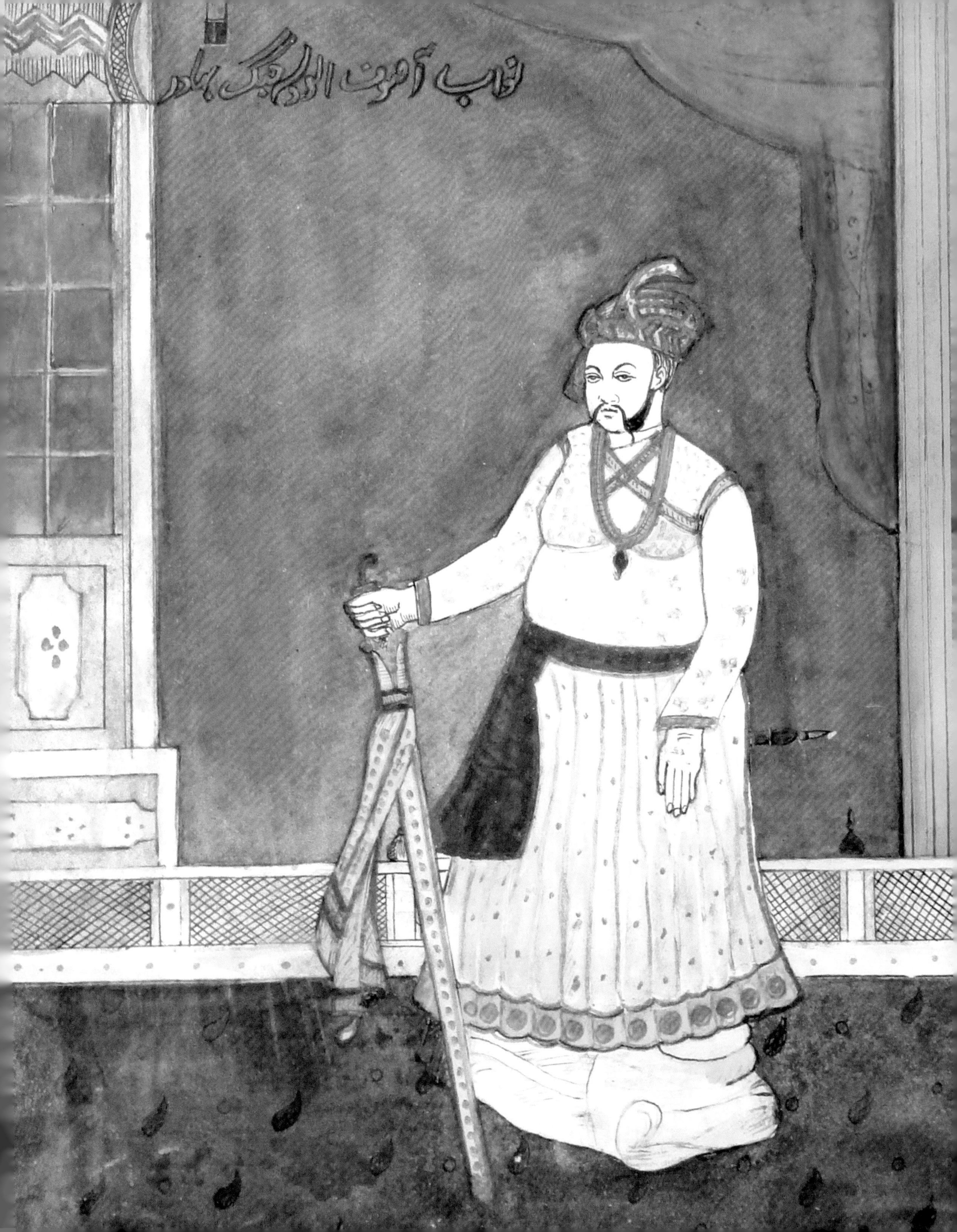
نواب آصف الدوله جنگ بهادر

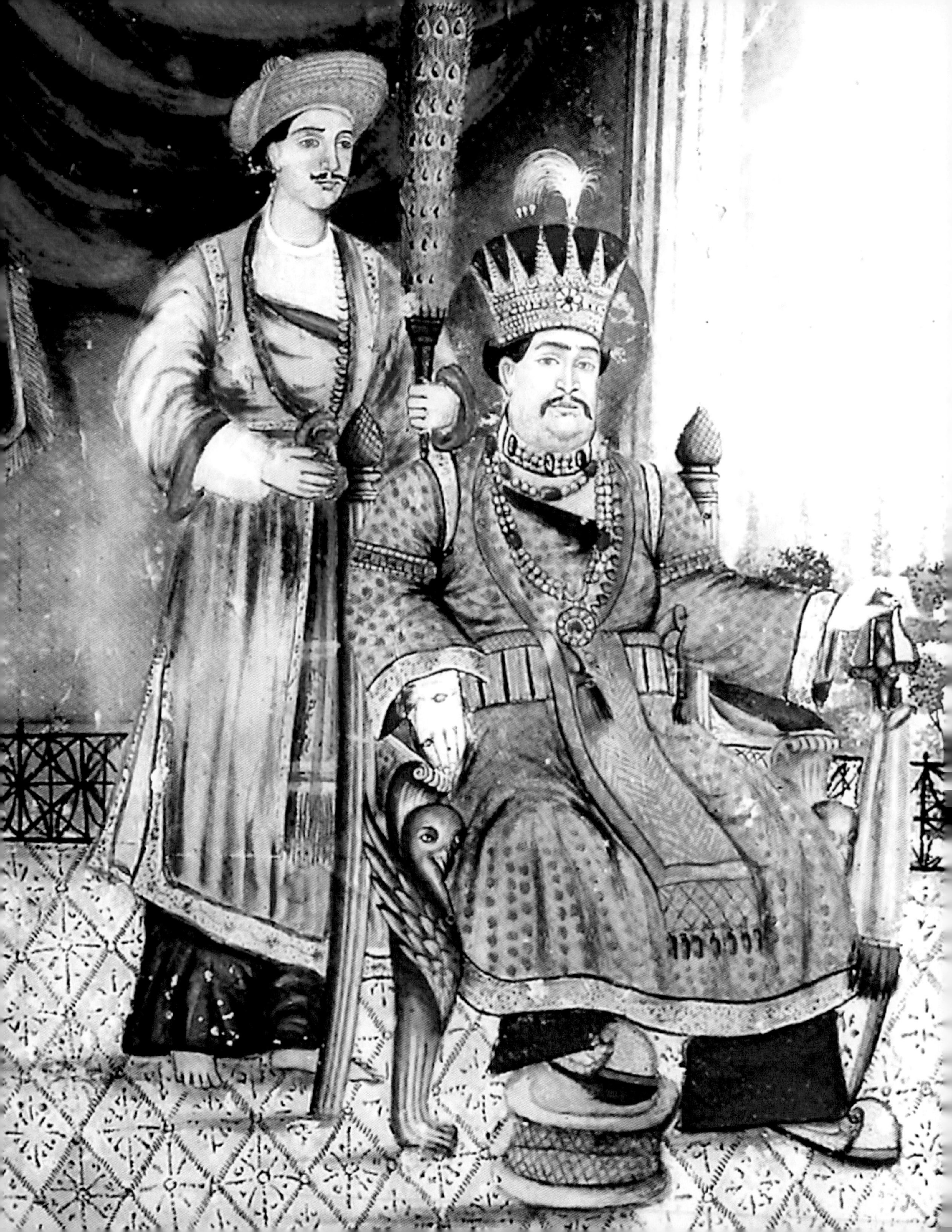

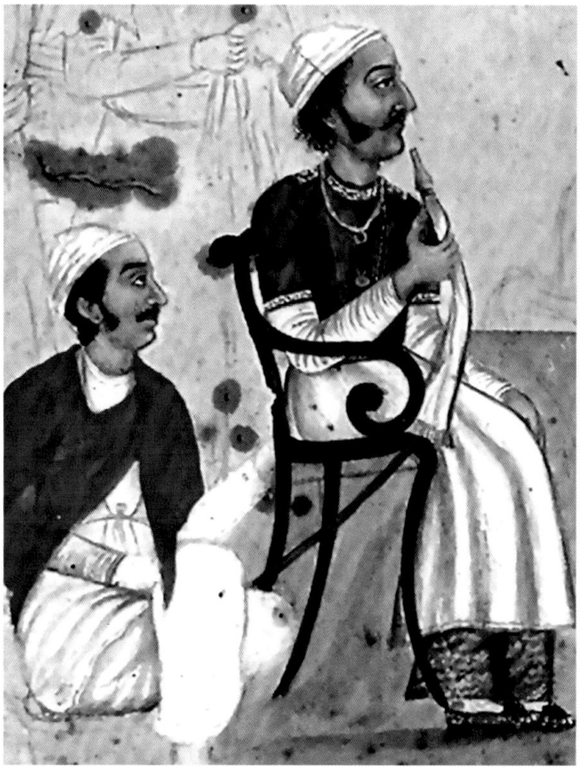

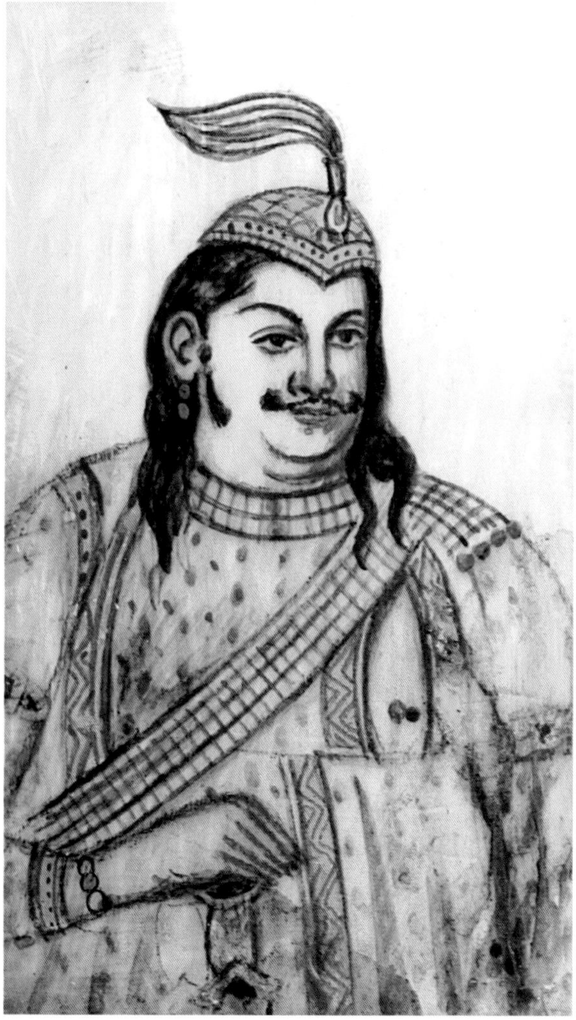

Above: Noble Ali Naqi Khan wearing an *angarkha*, a wide-legged paijama and a *dopalli* cap. The velvet *farzi* is embroidered in zardozi work with *salma sitara*.
Right: Wajid Ali Shah wearing *alampasand topi* introduced by him.
Facing page: The nawab (seen seating) is wearing an elaborate brocaded *angarkha*. A rich zardozi embroidery outlines the border while his *patka* is embellished with tassels. His attendant is also dressed in an *angarkha* and *paijama*, but of simpler material.

made of fine muslin and embroidered with *chikankari*. The *jamas*, *angarkhas* and kurtas were made from the *jamdani* of Tanda, which enhanced the elegance of the costume. Nawabs gave their patronage to these artisans by creating a centre of excellence for *jamdani* weaving in Awadh.

Garments for the upper body were accompanied by paijamas, a trouser-like garment. The paijamas worn in the nawabi period were of three types. The *sharai* paijamas were of ankle-length, tight at the calves but comfortable at the hips. The *arz ke paichon ka paijama* or *sidha* paijama was wide-legged of straight cut. By the mid 1800s, the *ghuttana* type of paijama (*aureb* or bias-cut) came into being which was long tightly-fitted at the calves and with many folds at the ankles, later known as churidar paijama. Nawab Ghazi-ud-Din Haider and Nawab Nasir-ud-Din Haider wore the wide-legged paijamas, which were neither very wide at the hips nor tight at the bottom. They were made of rich brocade and other expensive materials. In continuance of the peaceful coexistence seen earlier in the nawabi era, Hindus adopted paijamas for formal wear, and Muslims adopted the dhoti, usually worn by Hindus, when they were at home. The men's dhotis were 396 cm by 108 cm, with fine borders called *jalchuriya*.

Headgear was exceptionally important and it was considered improper to step outside the house without one. Topis and pagris have always been an important costume for men. Nawab Burhan-ul-Mulk, Nawab Shuja-ud-Daula and Nawab Asaf-ud-Daula used to wear a white dastar, a turban of fine muslin, similar to those worn by the Delhi noblemen and used *kalgi/sarpesh* (gold and jewelled ornaments) in their turbans.

Nawab Sadat Ali Khan wore a new type of pagri, called *shamla*, made of silk or brocade. A length of white cotton cloth was tied underneath, with an opening at the crown, so that the pagri may not slip down. There was also the four-cornered cap, *chaugoshia*, which in Awadh was less elongated and more rounded than the ones worn at the Delhi Court. To give the cap its round shape, special wooden and copper moulds were used. During Ghazi-ud-Din Haider's rule (1814-1827), the *mandel* or *mandeel* type of pagri became popular—it was shaped like a tambourine. It later became more rounded in the front, as well as at the back of the head and was usually embroidered with gold or silver thread. One of the favourite caps among the princes and nobles was the 'General's topi', developed on *mandel*, that became part of the British military uniform. It was round in shape and generally made of black velvet with gold and silver embroidery. At the time of King Nasir-ud-Din Haider (1827-1837) the Shias were in ascendancy in Lucknow. He opposed the idea of the four Caliphs and to show his respect for the Panjtan (the five members of the Prophet's family), adopted a cap with five corners and *chaugoshia* became *panchgoshia*. This became popular after his death as it was meant to be worn only by the king. The *dopalri* cap, introduced at the time of Muhammad Ali Shah (1837-1842), was made of two pieces of cloth to fit the head, with a seam across the top. It was made of fine muslin or *jamdani*, embroidered delicately with *chikankari* and *kamdani*. It was appreciated by the majority because of its elegance and remained popular till the time of the mutiny. *Nukkadar* (pointed), a very small and narrow cap, also called *kishtinuma* (boat-like), embroidered with gold and silver thread was the favourite of King Amjad Ali (1842-47). King Wajid Ali Shah (1847-1856) invented a cap and called it *alampasand*; it had a cardboard base and was worn by people who were honoured with titles in the court, but this did not become too popular.

A large number of people from the lower social classes, such as weavers, dyers, embroiderers, artisans and other craftspeople were employed by the royalty and nobility. There were acrobats, *qawwals* (musicians),

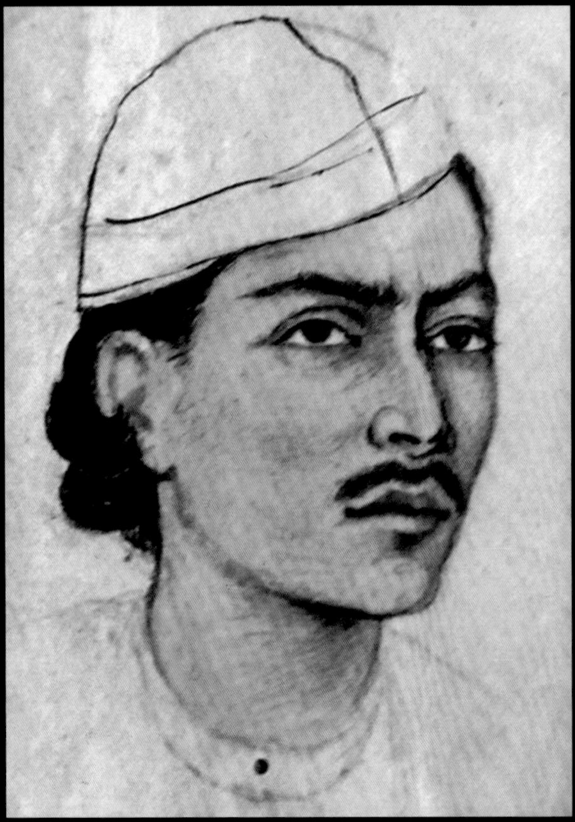

Dandy Style

While referring to Lucknavi fashion, we must not forget the 'banke' (plural of *banka*). The term *banka* (dandy) was given to a man who was fashionable, trendy and honoured his word. These men could be recognized from a distance because by their stylish apparel and fine appearance—they were always dressed in their best clothes and flaunted muslin kurtas in winter to show their indifference to cold. They wore coloured and embroidered net *shaluka*s under their muslin kurtas; *ghatela* shoes, kept their hair long, had trimmed moustaches and used kajal to enhance their eyes. Their lips would be red owing to the constant chewing of paan. These people used to dye the first phalanx of the small finger of their right hand with henna as a fashion statement.

One such famous banka was Ghulam Hussain, after whom a bridge was named. It is said that once he borrowed some money from a moneylender and left a box in his custody as guarantee. The moneylender kept the box without seeing the contents. When the loan was duly paid and the box was opened; it contained only a hair from Ghulam Hussain's moustache, signifying how significant the value of his word was.

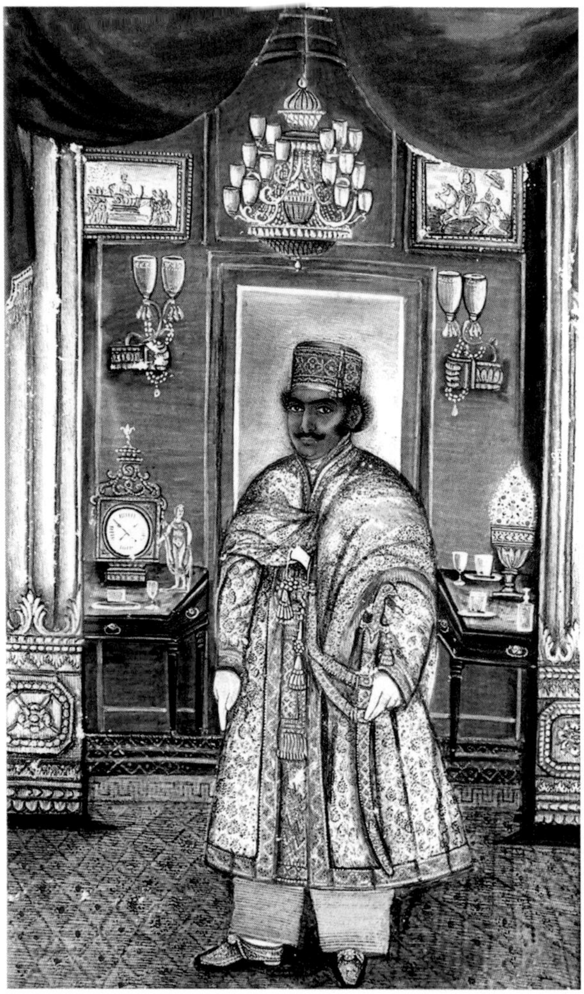

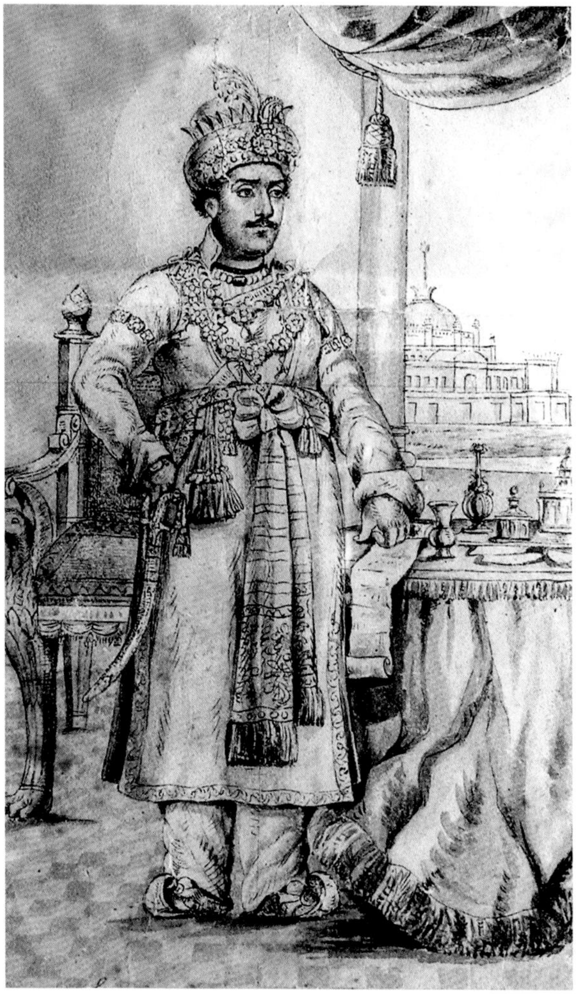

Above: A noble of the court of Awadh, dressed traditionally in brocade *choga*, *arz ka paijama*, round cap, heeled shoes and the *jamawar rumal*.
Right: Nawab wearing *angarkha* with an elaborate *patka* tied in a bow style. His lavish lifestyle reflects in the two-stringed pearl necklace and *bajuband*.

naqqals (imitators), *bhands* (comedians), tailors, bird trainers, *bhishti* (water-carriers) and betel sellers who lived in the villages. These people generally wore dhoti-kurta or paijama-kurta and a *ganji* (vest) and *gamchha/angochhas* (a traditional Indian towel made of loosely woven cotton fabric). *Angochha* is derived from the words *ang* (body) and *gochha* (a root meaning to bind) and it is almost exclusively used by Hindus as a head-wrap in villages.

Lucknavis were particularly fond of shoes and were always inventing new styles of footwear. The Nawabs wore *kafsh* (high-heeled shoes) popular at the Delhi Court; *ghatela*, which was 'long and was shaped like an elephant's trunk, curving over the feet in a large spiral' (Sharar, 2001) and *jootis* (slip-on shoes) with upturned toes, usually elaborately embroidered. In Lucknow, a nobleman or a courtier would step out of the house appropriately dressed in *chaugoshia*, immaculate *angarkha* of fine muslin, wide-legged paijamas, a *rumal* over the shoulders, with a cane in hand, and Lucknow-made *khurdnau* (short-toed velvet shoes) on the feet.

In Lucknow Hindu nobles continued to wear their traditional dhotis and *angavastras* with *khadau*, footwear made of wood as opposed to leather shoes that were brought to India by Muslims. For horse riding they would wear high boots.

An important typical garment of the nawabi period was a scarf called *rumal*. Paradoxically, it was called *rumal* but was bigger than the normal scarf (90 by 90 cm) measuring 110 x 110 cm. It was made of muslin, often embroidered in chikan work for summer use and of *jamavar* for winter use. It was worn over the shoulders. The nawabs of Awadh bestowed doshala as a mark of honour to dignitaries instead of the *khillat* given by Mughals.

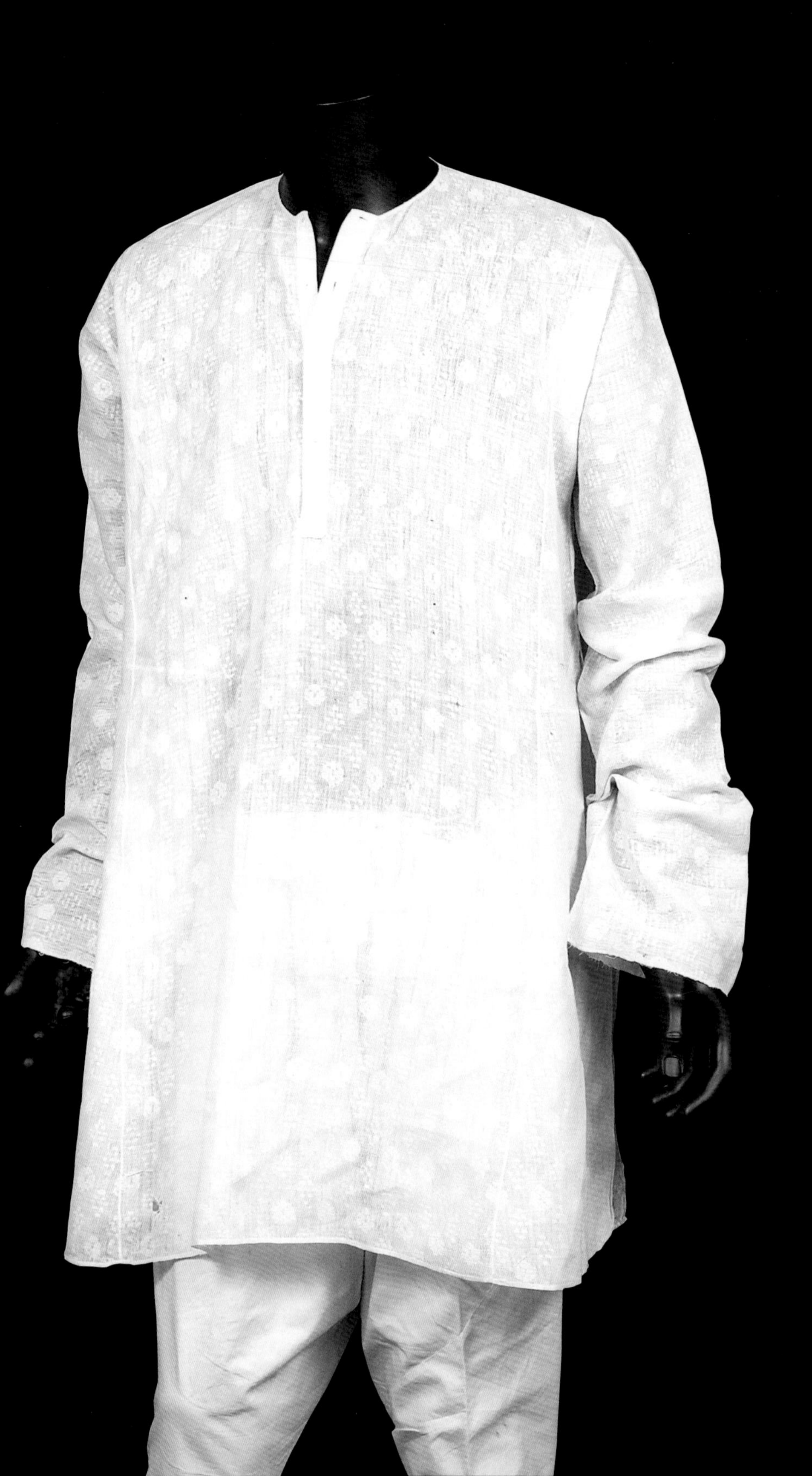

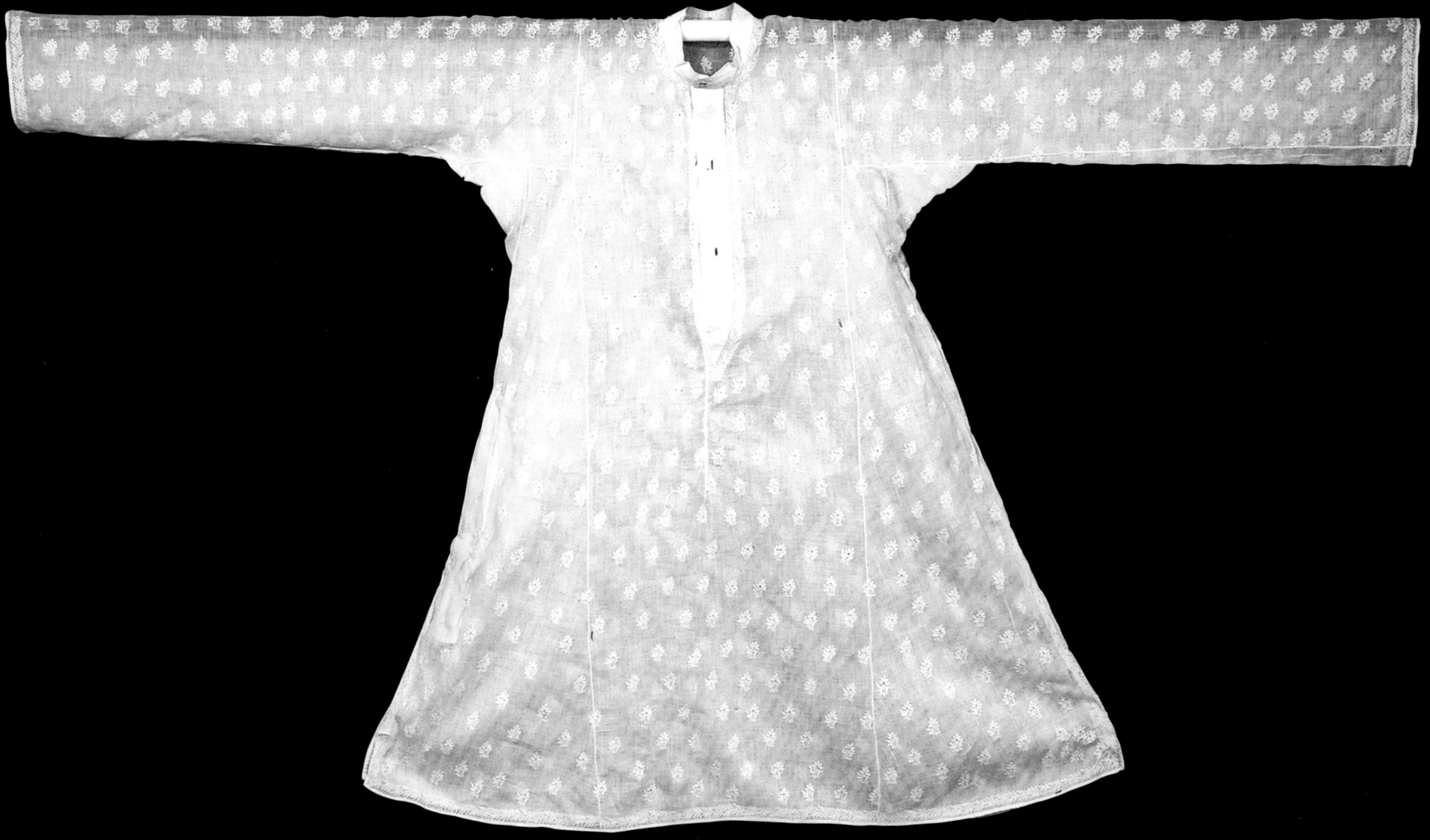

The *kali* kurta is open from the front and has a round neck. The *kalis* or gored panels give a fuller look to the garment. A triangular gusset is sewn under the arm and two suspended pockets are inserted in the side-seams.
Facing page: *Jamdani* kurta with small *butis* was woven at Jais in Rai Bareilly district.

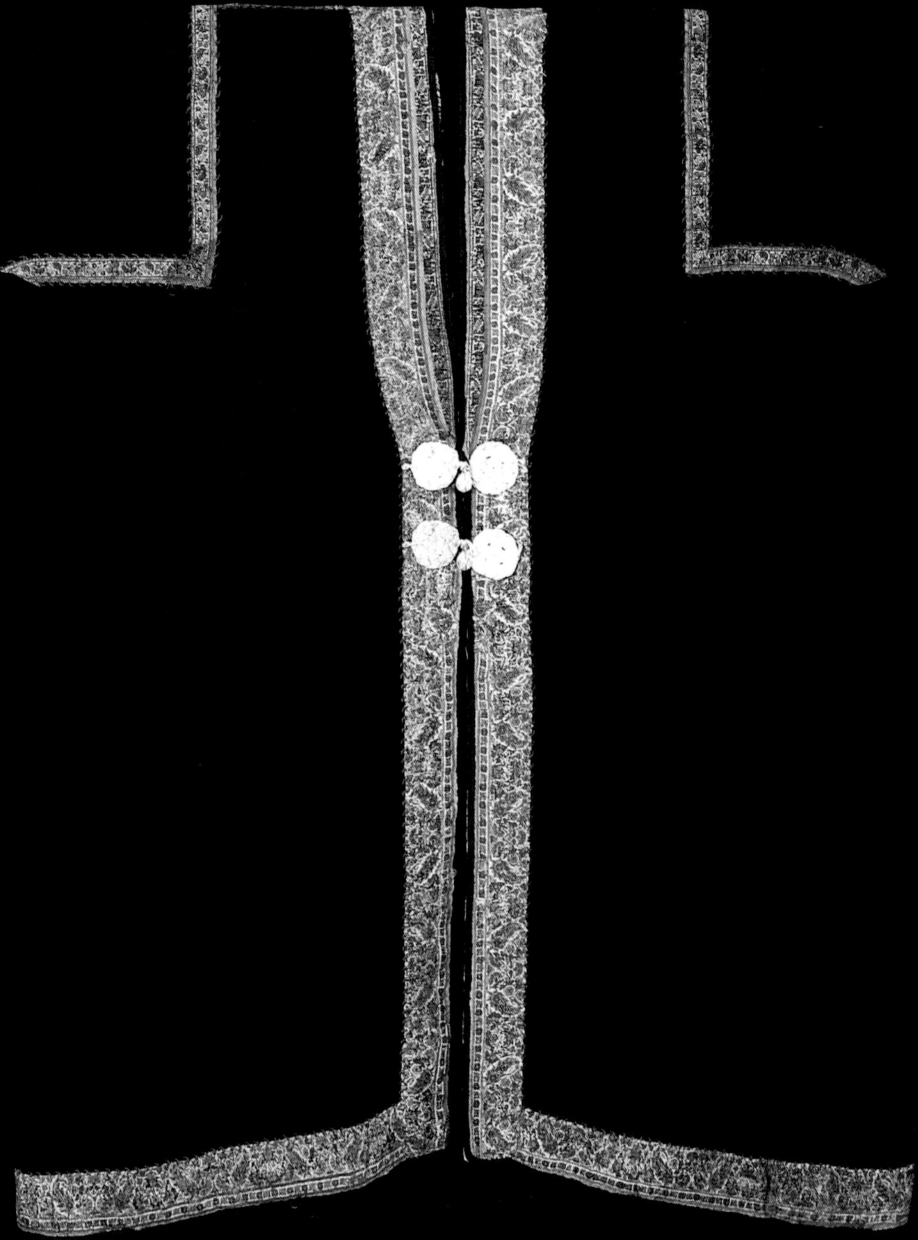

Above: This long-sleeved *choga*, used as an outer garment, is made of soft black *pashmina*, obtained from the fleece of the underbelly of the rare Tibetan wild mountain goat. It is open from the front but fastened at the waist level. Borders are woven in *jamawar*.
Facing page, Above: Detail - A floral motif in eighteenth century appliqué work decorates the *pusht* (back side of the garment).
Facing page, Below: The fastening, with cloth-cased buttons and loops, indicated the rank of the person wearing the garment.

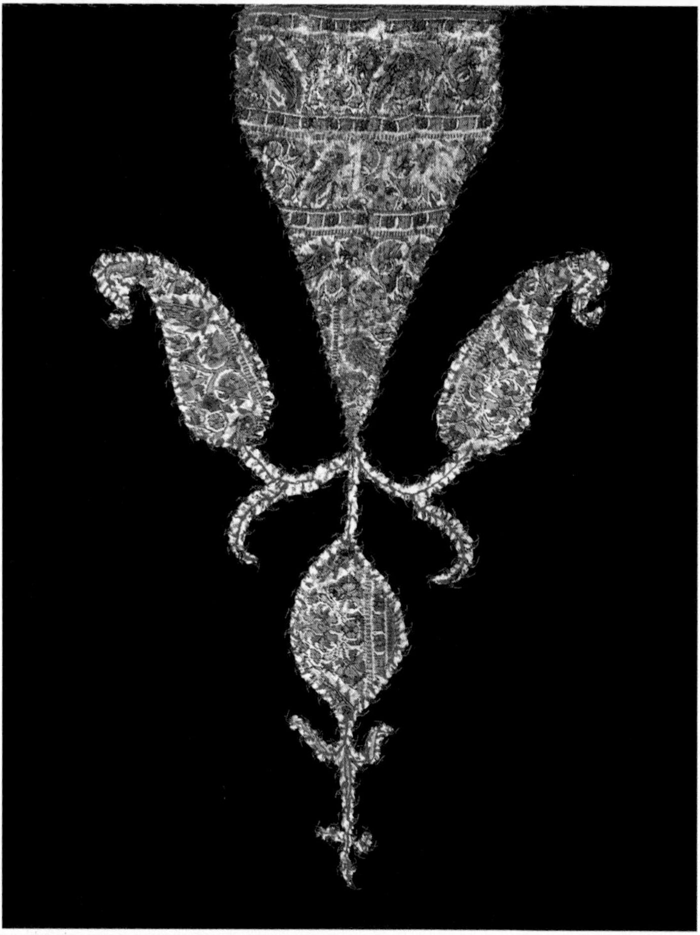

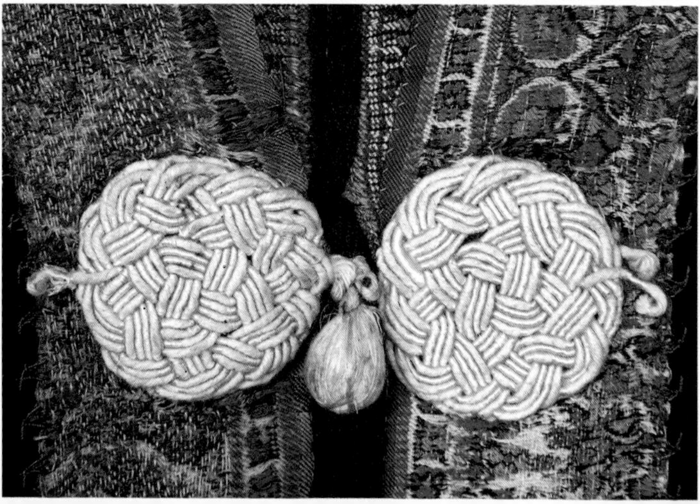

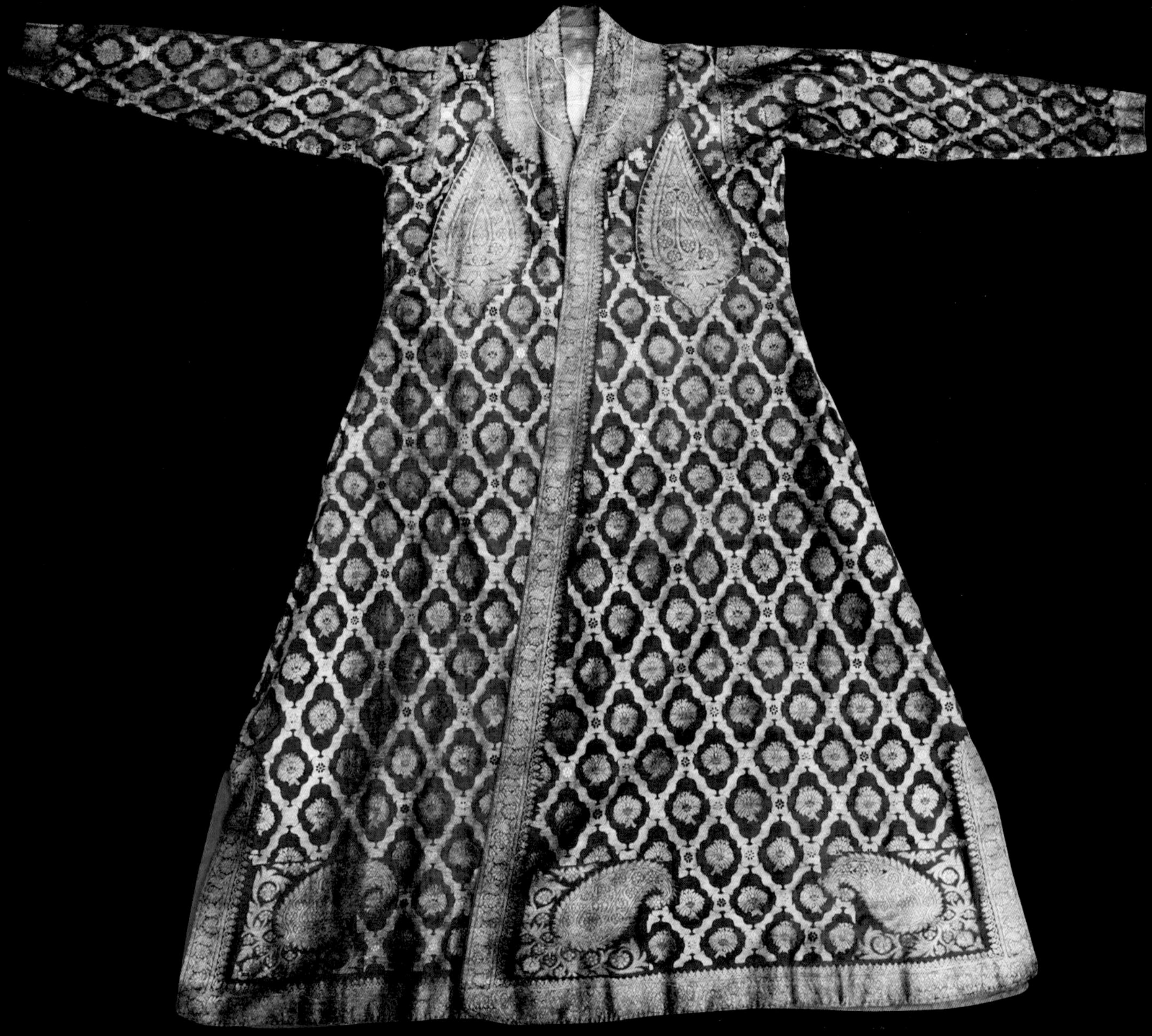

The main ground of the purple *choga* is formed in a trellis pattern of the *burfi* (lozenge) decorative motif, woven in silver zari. The fabric seems to be specially woven with *amiya butis* in the front and corners. The band collar gives it a look that is different to the *choga* without a collar.

Facing page: Brocade *choga* woven at Banaras with intricate decorative motifs of *kairi* and paan at the *pusht*.

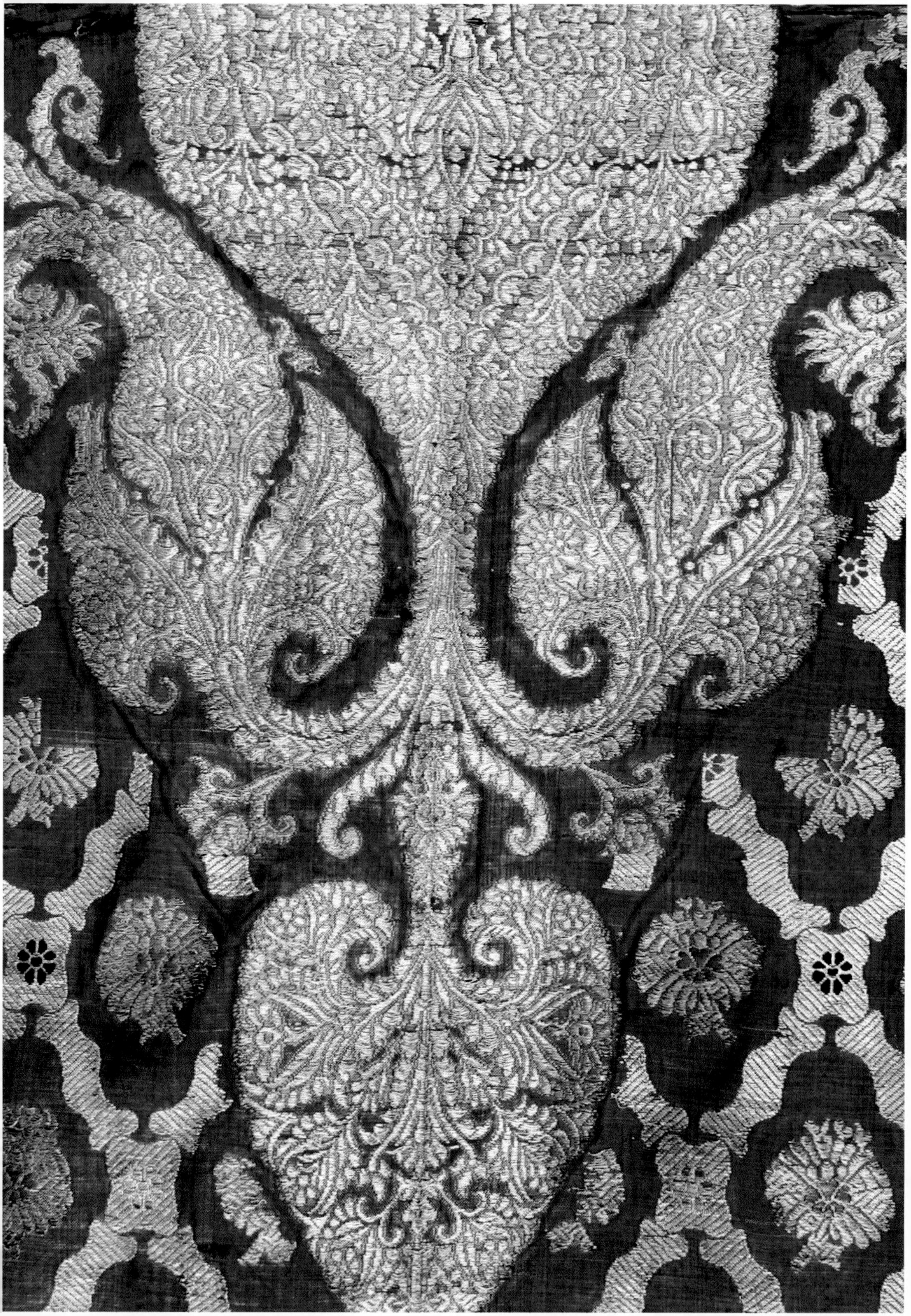

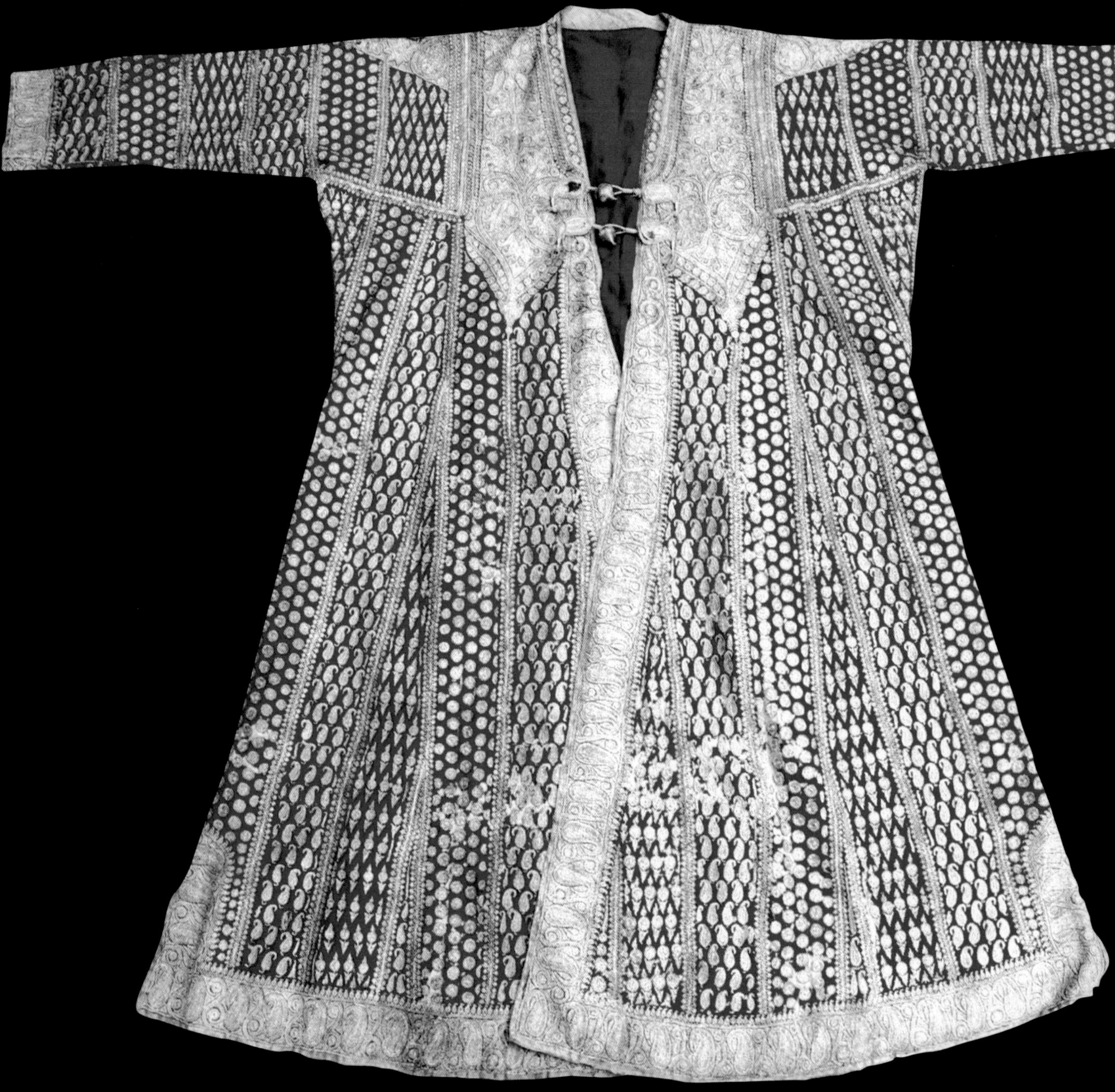

Above: This red and gold *choga* is made of highly prized *pashmina* wool. The ground is embroidered with the typical *amiya* motif of Awadh with *champa-kali* (jasmine buds) and *asharfi* (coin) motifs. The flare has been increased by the insertion of *kalis* with matching lining in red silk. It is said that the clothes of royalty were never washed; only the lining was detached, washed and sewn back again.
Facing page, Above: The fastening with loops and the buttons is in the shape of *amiya*, typical motif of Awadh.
Facing page, Below: Detail of the intricately embroidered *pusht* of the *choga.*

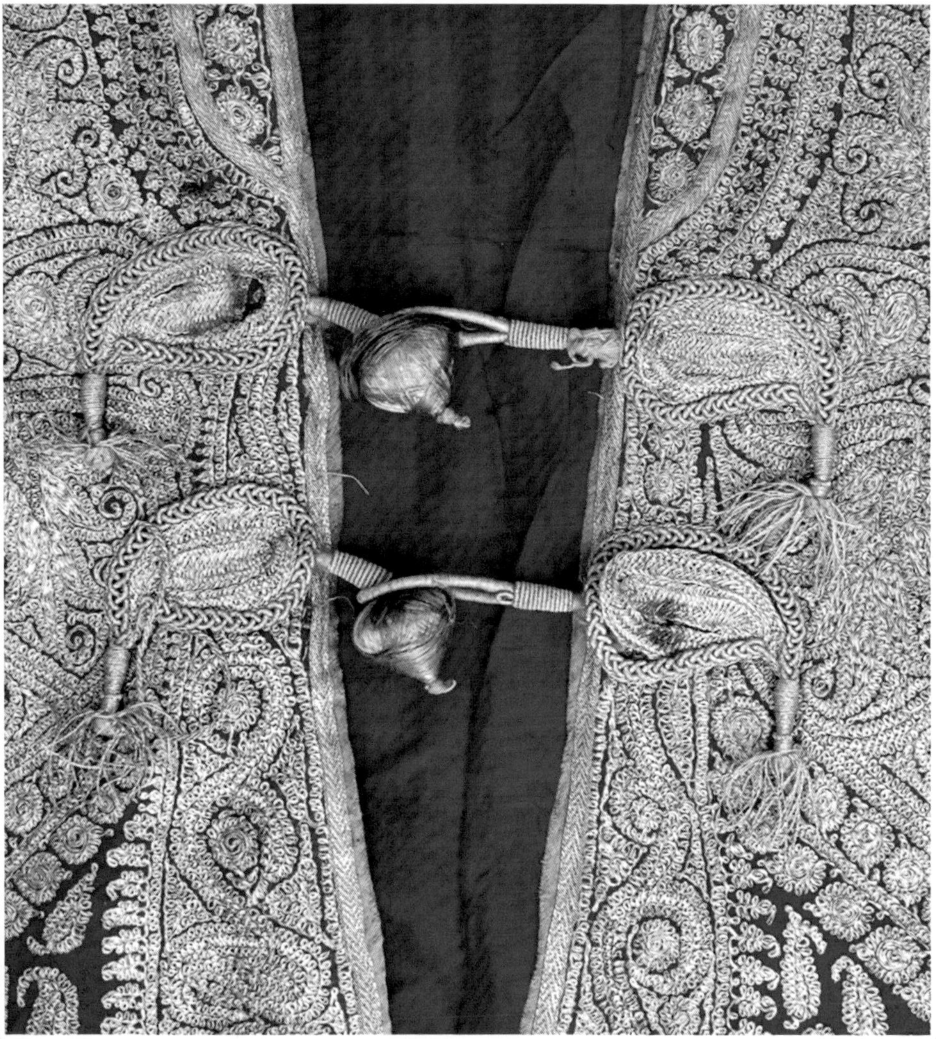
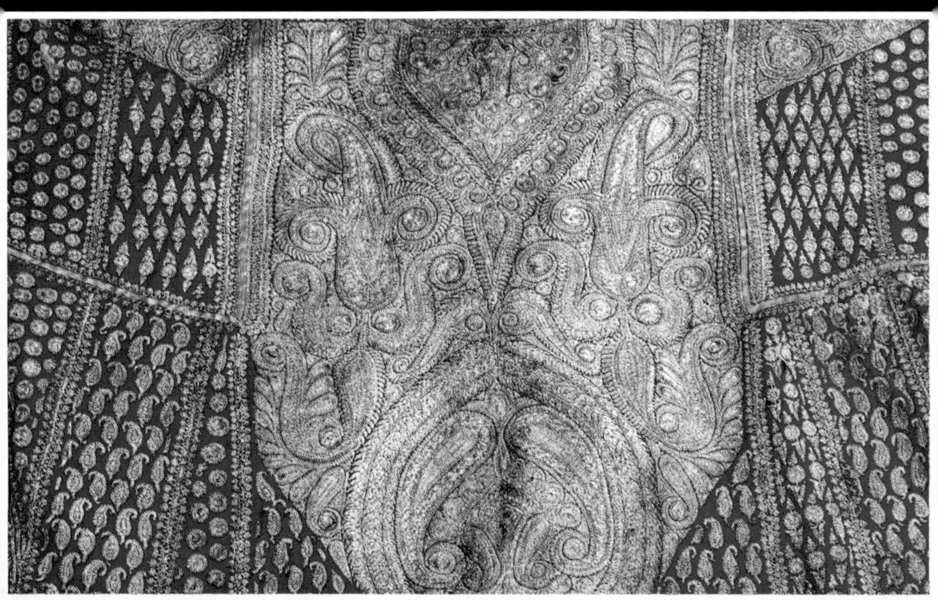

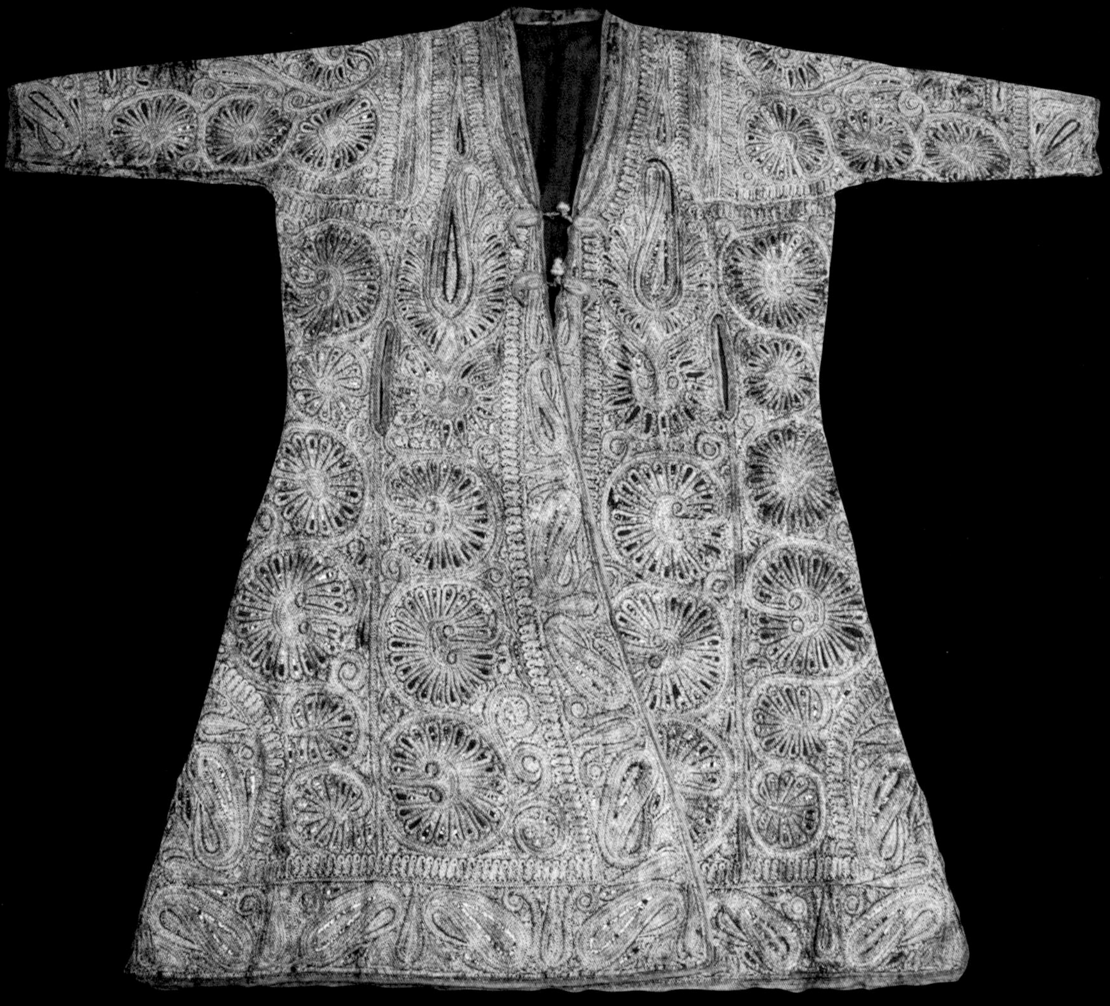

This red silk and cotton-lined *choga* is densely embroidered with stylised flowers in gold *kalabattun*. The rich gold embroidery done on deep red fabric was popular in the Delhi Court as well as in Awadh. Vegetable dyes were used and madder root was used to obtain the red colour.
Two pockets are inserted by making a vertical slit at the waist.

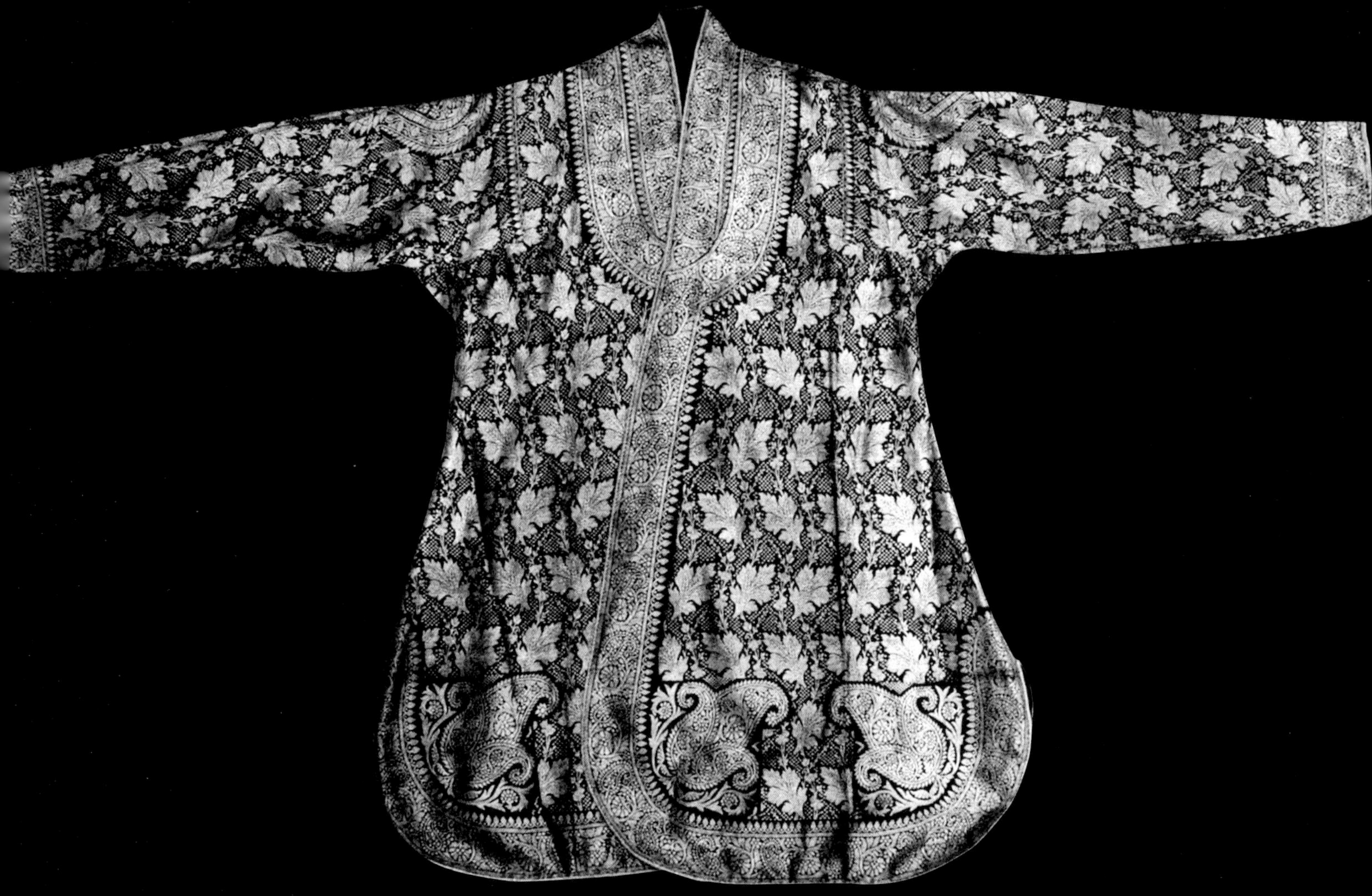

This black *choga* is shorter than the traditional *choga*. The rich silk *brocade* for this *choga* was probably designed and woven in Banaras on a *naksh* loom. Decorated *konias* (corner motifs) adorn the front and back (right). A broad woven border runs along the front edge, hemline and sleeve edges.

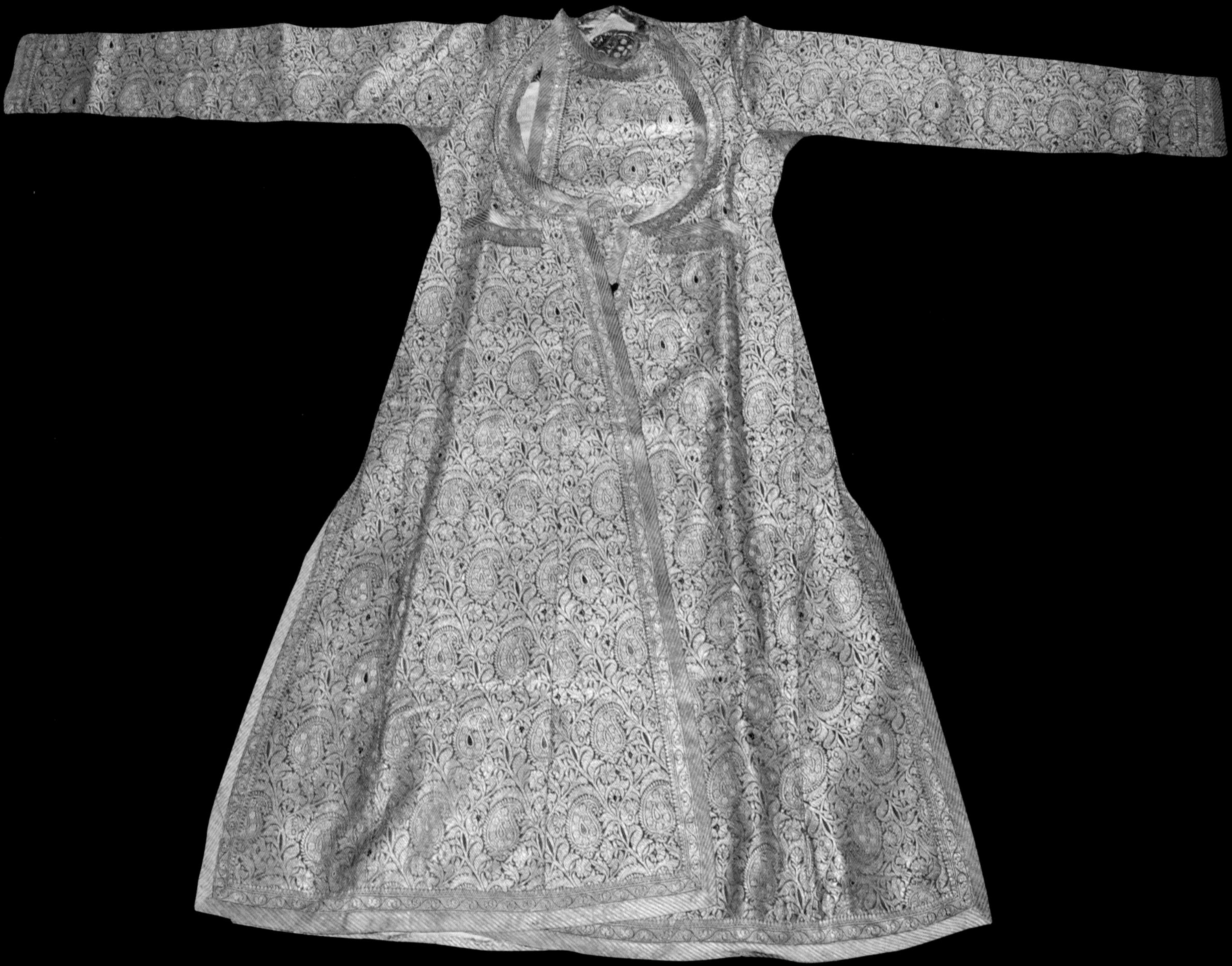

This *angarkha* is made of *kinkhwab* brocade. *Amiya butis* have been woven with flowers and creepers. The use of pink and purple silk threads within gives the effect of *minakari* jewellery, which was popular at the time. An *aureb* (diagonal-cut) edged border in contrasting green beautifies the neck, the *purdah* or the inner flap covering the chest, sleeves and hem.

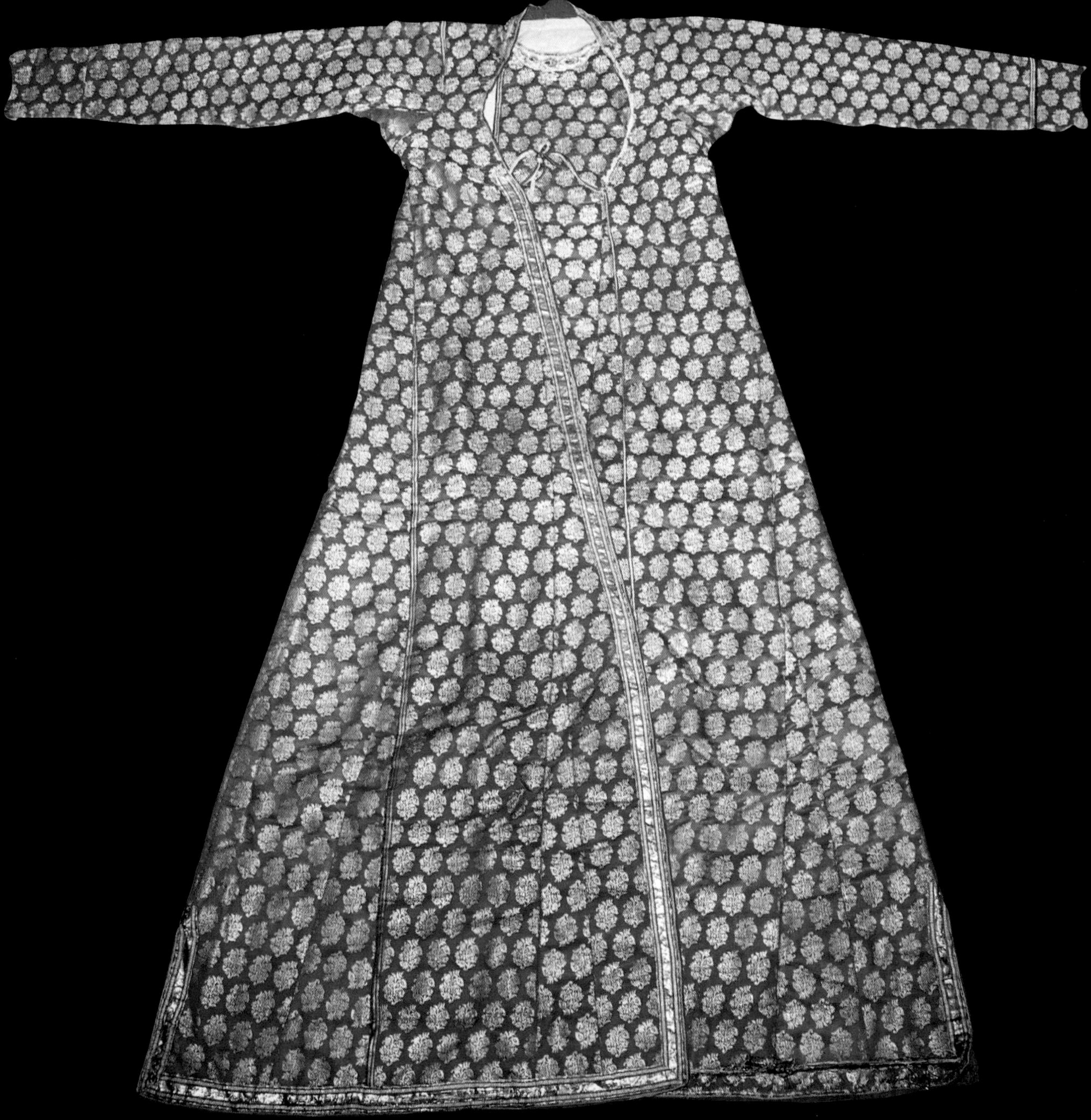

This red *bafta* silk brocade *angarkha* was probably woven in Banaras. The chest opening is higher than in normal *chogas*. The sleeves are tapered at the edges. Gussets have been added at the armpits for easier movement of the arms and it is quilted, making it suitable for winter.

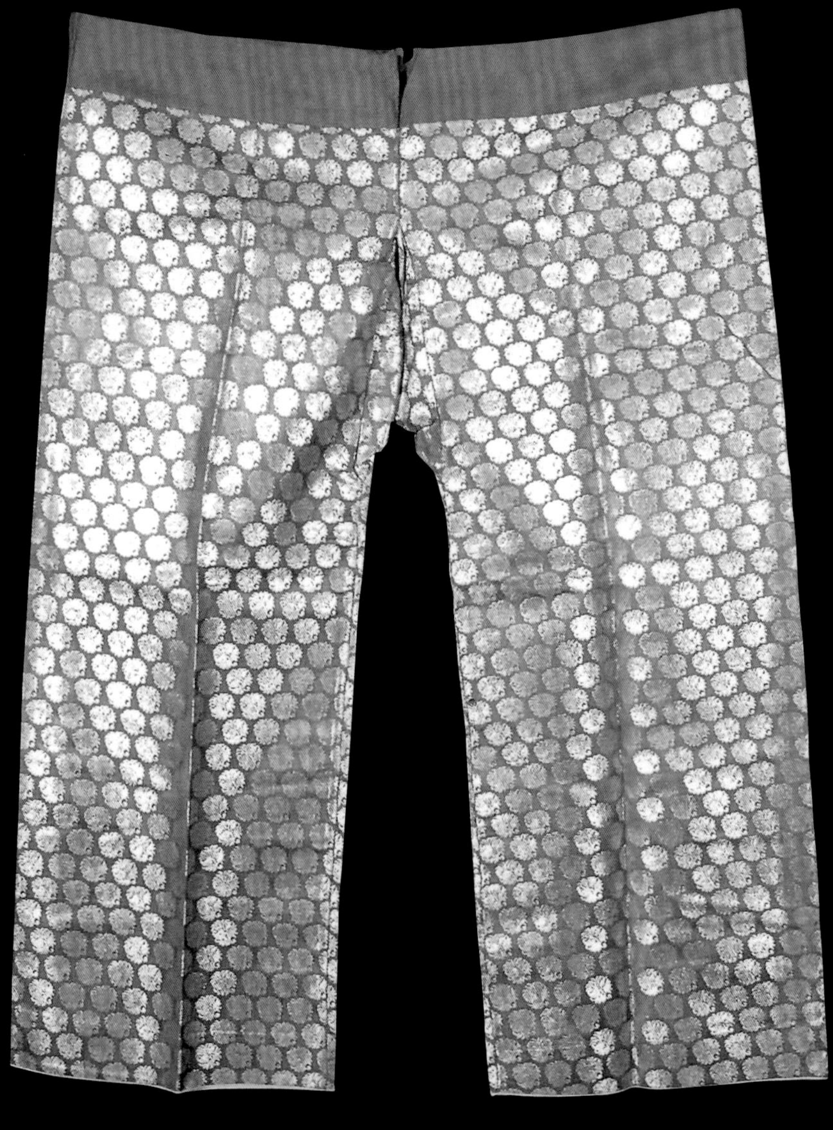

The banaras brocade wide-legged paijama.

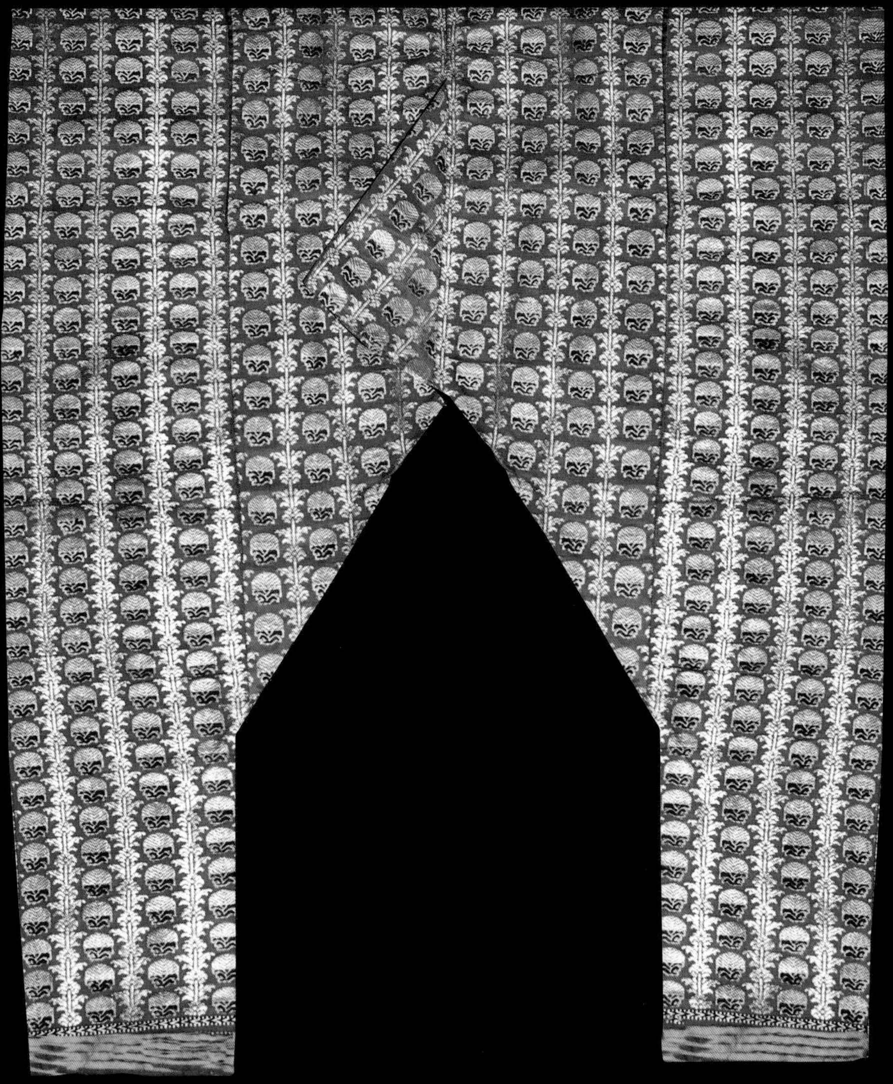

This *sidha-paijama* is woven in *amru* brocade. The repeated floral patterns are enclosed in stripes. The leg pieces are cut straight, just below the knee, a flared panel is attached. The *mohri* is decorated with a geometric pattern in black and white in accordance with the colours of the paijama.

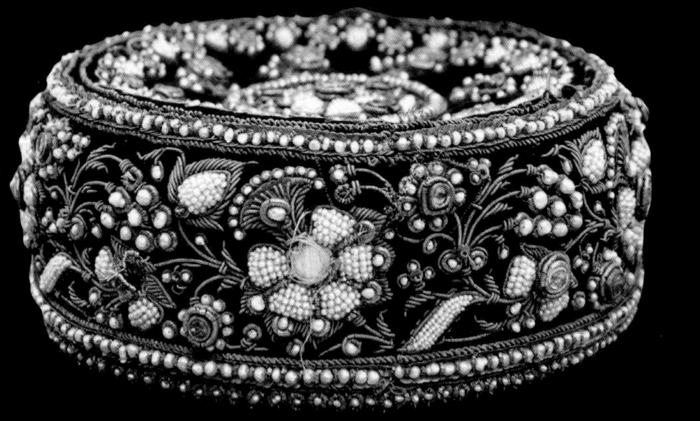

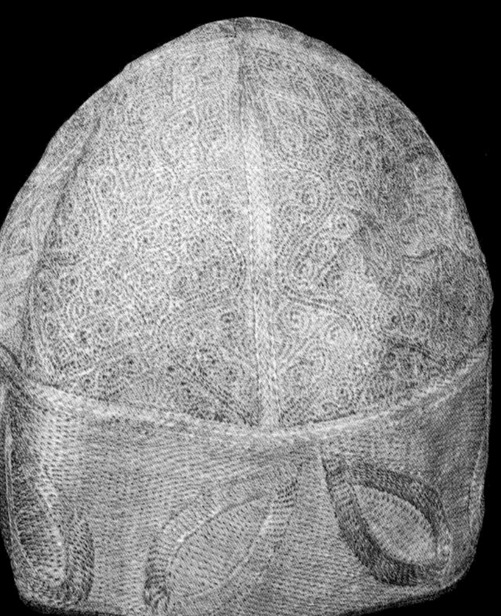

Clockwise from top:

1. This round velvet cap is gorgeously embroidered in zardozi, with silver *tikkis, katoris, badla* and precious stones. The tri-folio pattern is decorated in *kundan*-work. (*Facing page, detail*).

2. The four-cornered cap, *Chaugoshia*, looks like an elongated dome on the head. The four long conical sections joined together and crescent-shaped patterns sewn on at the rim was the modification to the cap when it arrived in Awadh from Delhi Court. It is richly embroidered with gold and silver *kalabattun* giving the effect of Ganga-Jamuni, Ganga stands for gold and Jamuni for silver. It is also described as a combination of sunlight (gold) and moonlight (silver). It was worn by nobles and persons of distinction.

3. This cap is made of silk-brocade, padded with cotton and wool, suitable for winter wear. It was worn by nobles and courtiers at the courts of Delhi, Agra and Lucknow.

4. This elegant *Dopalli topi* is made of *jamdani* fabric and is simply cut into two symmetrical pieces, slightly curving towards the crown. A fine zari piping embellishes the curved edges. The *kamdani butis* in *badla* across the body and a simple border of couched zari thread deep at the hemline gives it a sophisticated look, making it ideal to be worn with a kurta and *angarkha* during the summer season.

5. The *Nukkadar* cap takes its name from the pointed form of the cap at two ends. This richly embroidered cap in pure gold zardozi work was mainly worn by the princes, nobles and wealthy men.

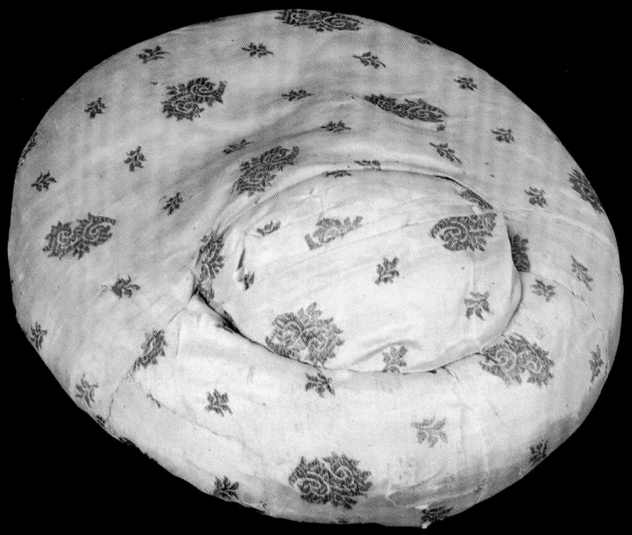

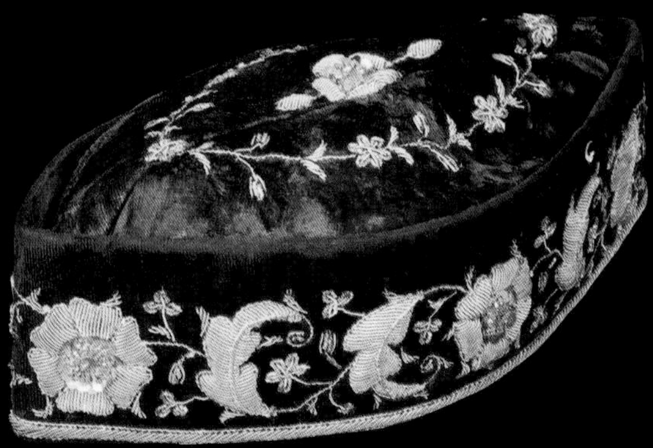

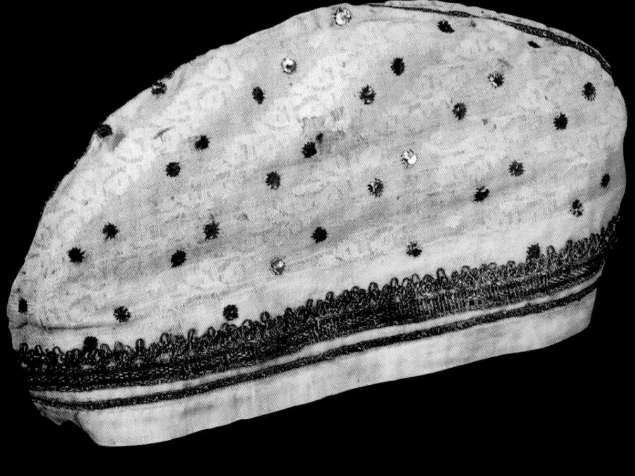

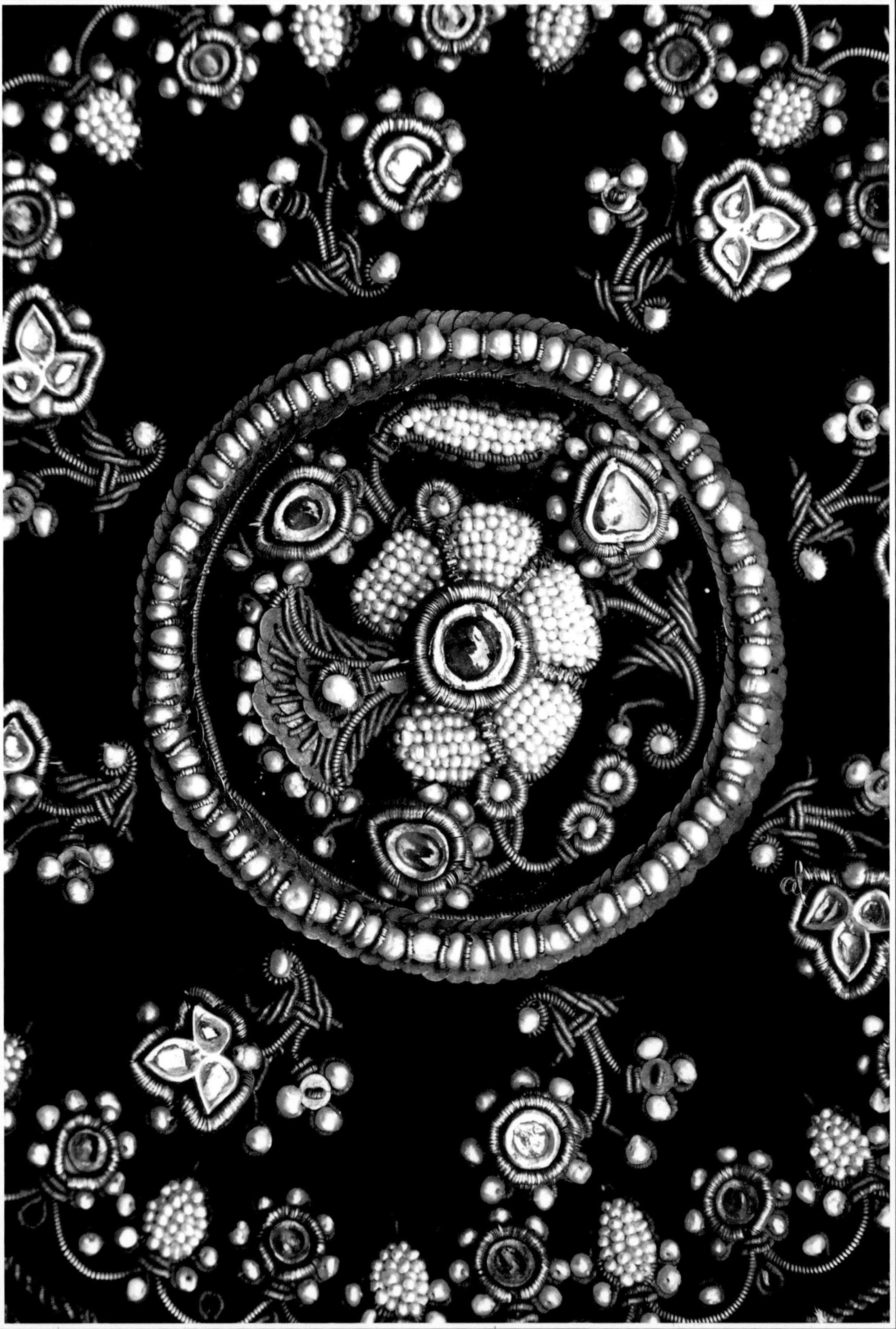

WOMEN'S COSTUMES

A British officer in the court of King Nasir-ud-din Haider referred to Begum Taj Mahal (one of the king's wife) as follows (Hilton 1911):

'Her dress was of gold and scarlet brocade, and her hair was literally strewed with pearls, which hung down upon her neck.....She wore long sleeves open at the elbow, and her dress was a full petticoat with a tight body attached, and open only at the throat. She had several persons to bear her train when she walked; and her women stood behind her couch to arrange her head dress when, in moving, her pearls got entangled in the immense robe of scarlet and gold she had thrown around her.'

With increasing prosperity, greater role of the courts and increasing attention paid by the nawabs to develop their own style, the costumes for women also began to evolve independently. Initially, two distinct fashions coexisted during the nawabi period in women's costumes, reflecting the Hindu and Muslim cultures prevalent at the time. Gradually, the initial differences between the two kinds of costumes were reduced, as there was increased interaction among the two cultures. The most significant change in women's costumes during the nawabi period was that they became distinct from those of men's.

Hindu women generally wore a lehenga with the *angiya*/choli and chunni/*odhni*/fari/*chunri*/dupatta. *Angiya* was also called *chota kapda*, or small cloth. The chunni is not only a veil but also a beautiful expression of the *nazakat* and *nafasat* of Lucknow, owing to the delicate style in which it was worn. In fact, depending on how the woman chose to carry it, the chunni would become a protective or a seductive garment. Worn by gently covering the face, it became the purdah; draped loosely but gracefully around the upper part of the body, it became seductive; and worn traditionally over the head, it became a mark of respect.

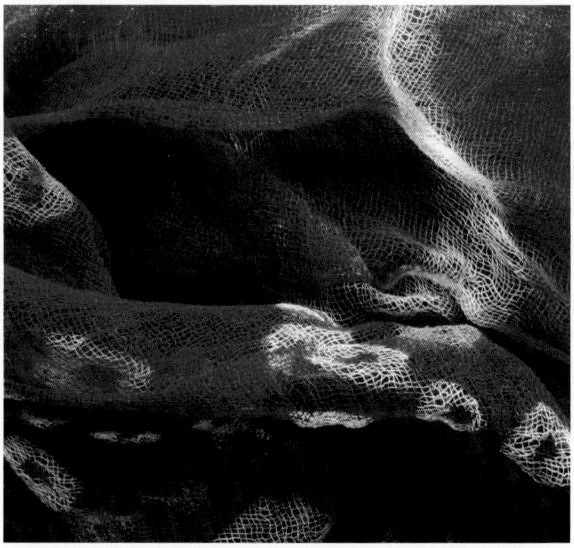

The chunnis of varied dimensions (generally 220 cm in length and 117cm in width) were made of silks as well as various types of muslins, such as *tanzeb*, *nayansukh*, *mainafal* (multicoloured cotton weaving), *doria* (striped) and *laheriya* (wavy). These garments, made of muslin, were so fragile that they had to be discarded after few washes. They were decorated with various types of *gota* (ribbon with flattened gilt wire in warp, and silk in weft, woven out of gold and silver threads), such as *lachka* (crumpled wide *gota*), *dhanush* (crumpled narrow *gota*), *uttu* (a thin strip of plain *gota*), *pattha* (plain *gota*), *chutki-wala* (of pinched form), *champa* (jasmine-shaped) and *gokhru* (hoof-shaped).

Among Hindu brides, there was one special type of chunni, specifically used on the first night of the wedding. It was called a desi *chunri* (locally-made chunni) and was made of roughly woven cotton fabric and then dyed in red and yellow vegetable colour with tie-and-dye technique. This was given as a gift to the bride by the elder brother of the groom, denoting that she was, thereafter, a part of the groom's family and with her rested the honour of the family. The desi *chunri* was sewn inside the pillow after the first night. The child could never see it. It was not considered proper for a child to know about the first night of his/her parents.

Muslim women belonging to the aristocracy in the earlier nawabi period were dressed in clothes similar to those of men. The *peshwaz* (long-sleeved, front-open, loose robe with a bodice and a skirt) was the only outfit which was exclusive to the women and was worn with an inner-vest and *sidha* paijamas similar to that of men. With time, *peshwaz* and the inner vest was discarded. The upper garments began to include the *kurti* (shirt) and the *shaluka* (half-sleeved garment worn over the *angia*).

The women wore the chador and burqa to go outside the zenana. Layered clothing was given preference. With the influence of Hindu women in the harem, their style also changed. The *chador/chadariya* – a long, unstitched sheet of varying materials and measurements – was used to drape the upper body by Muslim and Hindu women alike. It was wrapped over the shoulders or the head. The length of chunnis and chadors varied from 200 to 300 cm and their width from 115 to 165 cm. They were made of muslin for summers, silk, velvet and woollen in shawl material for winters, embellished in many different

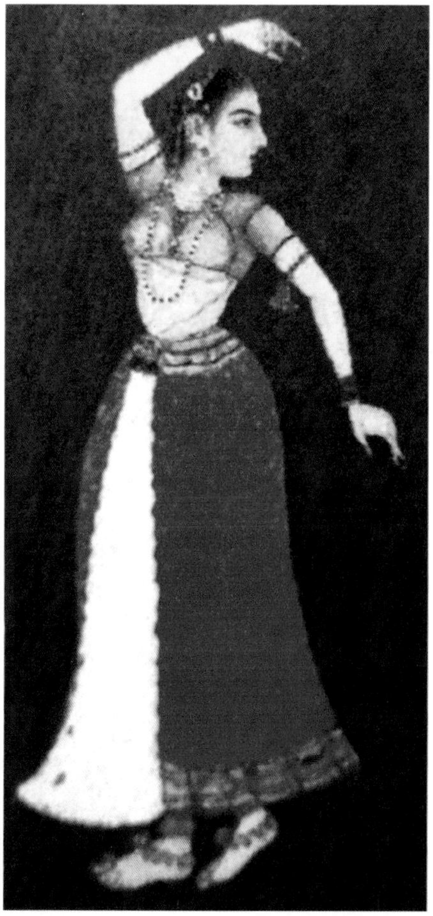

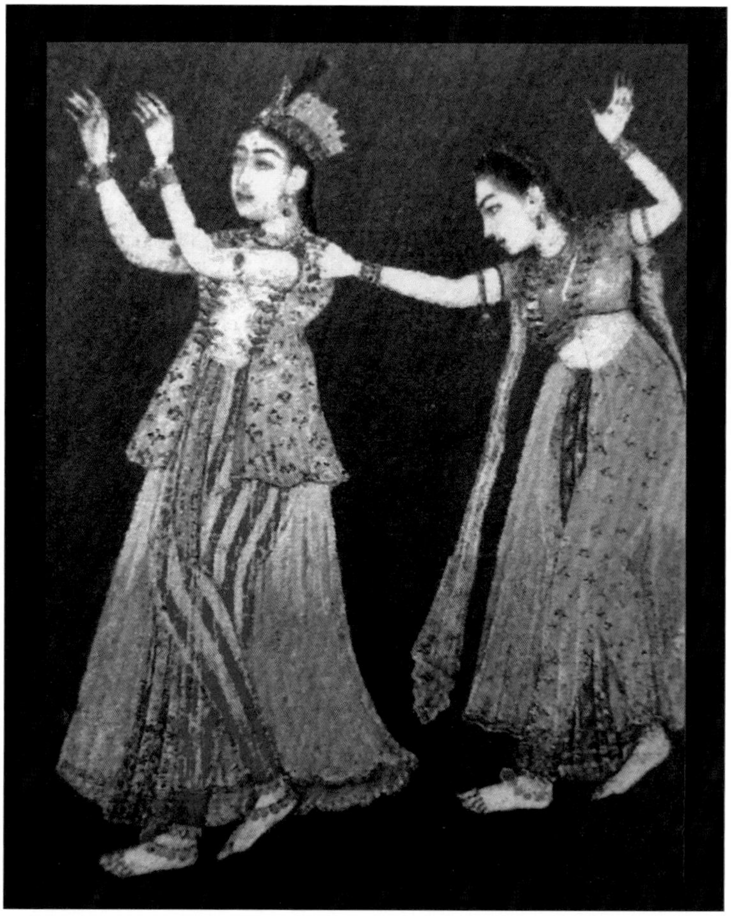

ways of ornamentations. They were embroidered with *kalabattun*, making it suitable for important occasions.

Hindu women wore lehengas as lower garment, made of hand-woven materials; cotton, silk, *gulbadan*, *galta* (*mashru*), in designs of *zozi* (stripes), *choupar* (chequered-squares) and *nimjari* with borders of different colours and cuts. The lehenga is made of three parts: a waistband, a skirt and a border at the hem. There were various patterns of lehengas popular in Awadh, such as *gotdar* (with broad border), *kalidar* (with panels), *aurebdar* (with bias-cut cloth), *jhalerdar* (with frills) and *patdar* (with elaborated skirt). The joints of the skirt and the border were decorated with *gota*. These decorations were referred to as *chasak* and gave the costumes the name of *chasakdar* lehenga. The lehenga had an important role as it was worn for multiple occasions. In a wedding ceremony, a lehenga was sent to the bride as an auspicious gift by the bridegroom's family and the bride was to wear that very garment at the time of *bidai*, when she left her parents' house to become part of her husband's family. The wedding lehenga was called *latbor ka lehenga* and was highly decorated with *gota* and embroidered with *salma*, *sitara* and zardozi in floral designs. Widows did not wear lehengas, but wore a simple cotton dhoti.

Left: Hindu women wearing traditional lehenga-choli-*odhni* combination.
Right: Muslim women wearing muslin *peshwaz*, *angiya* or half-sleeved *shaluka*, striped brocade *paijama* can be seen underneath. The cap is decorated with a plume.
Facing page: *Desi chunni* dyed with natural colours.

Muslim women wore mainly *sidha* paijamas. The lehengas worn by Hindu women and the paijamas worn by Muslim women as lower garments are different. The Muslim lower garment cannot be made without the *miyani* (gusset). According to anecdotal evidence, some Muslims were prohibited from prayers unless wearing a garment that had a *miyani*. It is said that Mughal Empress Noorjahan invented a variation to the lehenga of Hindus by adding a *miyani* (gusset) to it. The upper part was like the paijama, also called *izar*, and the lower part resembled a lehenga.

Paijamas were of various types: *sidha* (straight), *suttana*, churidar (with bangle-like creases on the ankle), *kalidar* (with panels) and *farshi* (trailing). *Sidha* and churidar paijamas reached down to the ankles; *suttana*

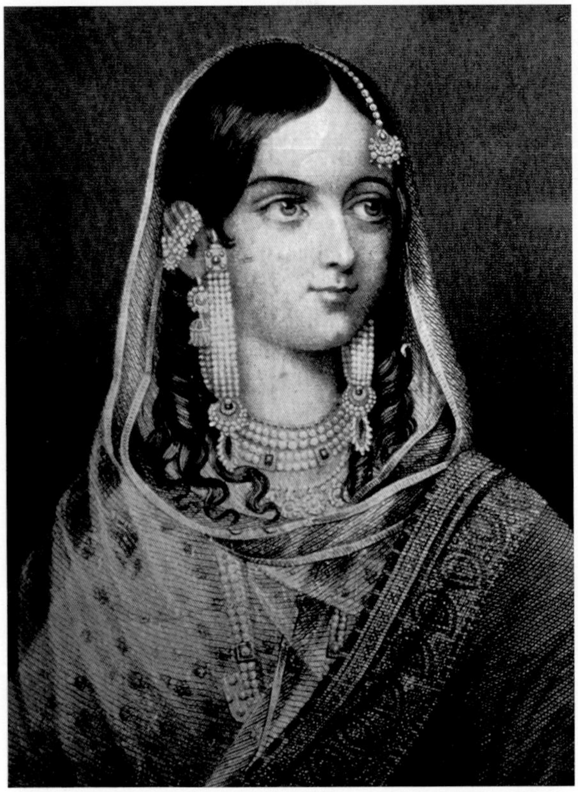

Above: The begum is elegantly and lavishly dressed in *jamdani odhni* and wearing variety of ornaments with pearls and precious stones.
Facing page: The begum is dressed in Awadhi *farshi paijama* and an elaborated *odhni*. The *paat* (upper half) is in red silk and the *gote* (lower half) is in green silk embroidered in a *burfi* (lozenge) pattern. The two separate sections are joined and decorated with crinkled *gota* and a strip of zardozi work. A matching and elaborately decorated *odhni* accompanies the upper garment. The *gote* is gathered up and held at the waist.

was worn wide at the top and comfortably roomy around the legs and ankles; *kalidar* went down to the heels, while the *farshi* paijama was so long that it used to trail on the *farsh* (floor). The *farshi* paijama was an innovation of this period and was designed especially for royal women. They were made of 18 yards of precious material (as opposed to *kalidar* paijamas that were 9 yards). The *gote* (bottom half) was applied either above the knees or just below the knees. *Bandiyas* (servants) helped the begums hold this voluminous, wide-legged farshi paijama, often worn with a kurti. The women employed to help dress royal women were called *mashshata*. Begum of Rampur remembers how gracefully the farshi paijamas were worn (Kumar 1999): 'There was a certain style of wearing the farshi ... the gote was carefully folded by a maid and held by the wearer in her left hand, leaving the right hand free. The pallav of the *odhni*/chunni was draped so long that it almost touched the floor ... the ensemble had such royal grace and elegance that you did not just walk into a room, you made an entrance.'

The gharara (a variation of the paijama) became popular in Lucknow during the reign of the eighth ruler of Awadh, Nasir-ud-Din Haider (1827-1837). He liked the gowns of British women and introduced gharara in the zenana. Mrs. Meer Hassan Ali spent twelve years in Lucknow (presumably from 1816 to 1828), visited the zenana during this period, was fascinated by the costumes of the begums. She says, 'The most fashionable females of Lucknow, wear trousers which are so full below the knee that they almost cover the feet...a very broad silver riband binds the top of the pyjammah; this being double has a *izarband* (a silk-net cord) run through, by which this part of the dress is confined at the waist. The ends of the *izarband* are finished with rich tassels of gold and silver curiously and expressly made for this purpose, which extend below the knees; for full dress these tassels are rendered magnificient with pearls and jewels (Ali 1917) .'

The women of Awadh, like the men, were fond of shoes – they wore *kafsh*, *ghatela* and jootis made of velvet and embroidered with zardozi. In Lucknow, new kinds of shoes were invented for begums, called *aughi*. They were embroidered in gold, silver and coloured threads. Later, *ghatela*s were replaced by *tat-bani*, which were made in Banaras brocades suitable for formal occasions.

To adorn themselves, women loved to wear elaborate rings, nose-rings, earrings, necklaces, armlets, bangles, *jhumar* (hair ornament), *mathapatti* (ornament for the forehead), *paijeb* (anklets), *bichiya* (toe-rings), *kardhani* (waist-band) and *hathphool* (ornament for the hands) and *hansli* (necklace). As gold was used for worship and considered pure, it was not worn on the feet– ornaments for feet were thus usually made of silver. At times, as a sign of respect, brides were gifted gold anklets by the groom's family, depending on the affluence of the family.

The *batua*, or pouch, was an important accessory of this period. These *batua*s had many compartments to carry jewellery, money, *itr*, tobacco and paan and had strings for opening. *Batua*s were made of different materials, varying from expensive makhmal (velvet), silks, brocades, *jamavar*s and *chheents* (printed cotton, literally, 'sprinkles'). They were also decorated with *gota* and *kiran*. For special occasions the name of the person would be embroidered on these *batua*s. Smaller pouches were called *batuiya*.

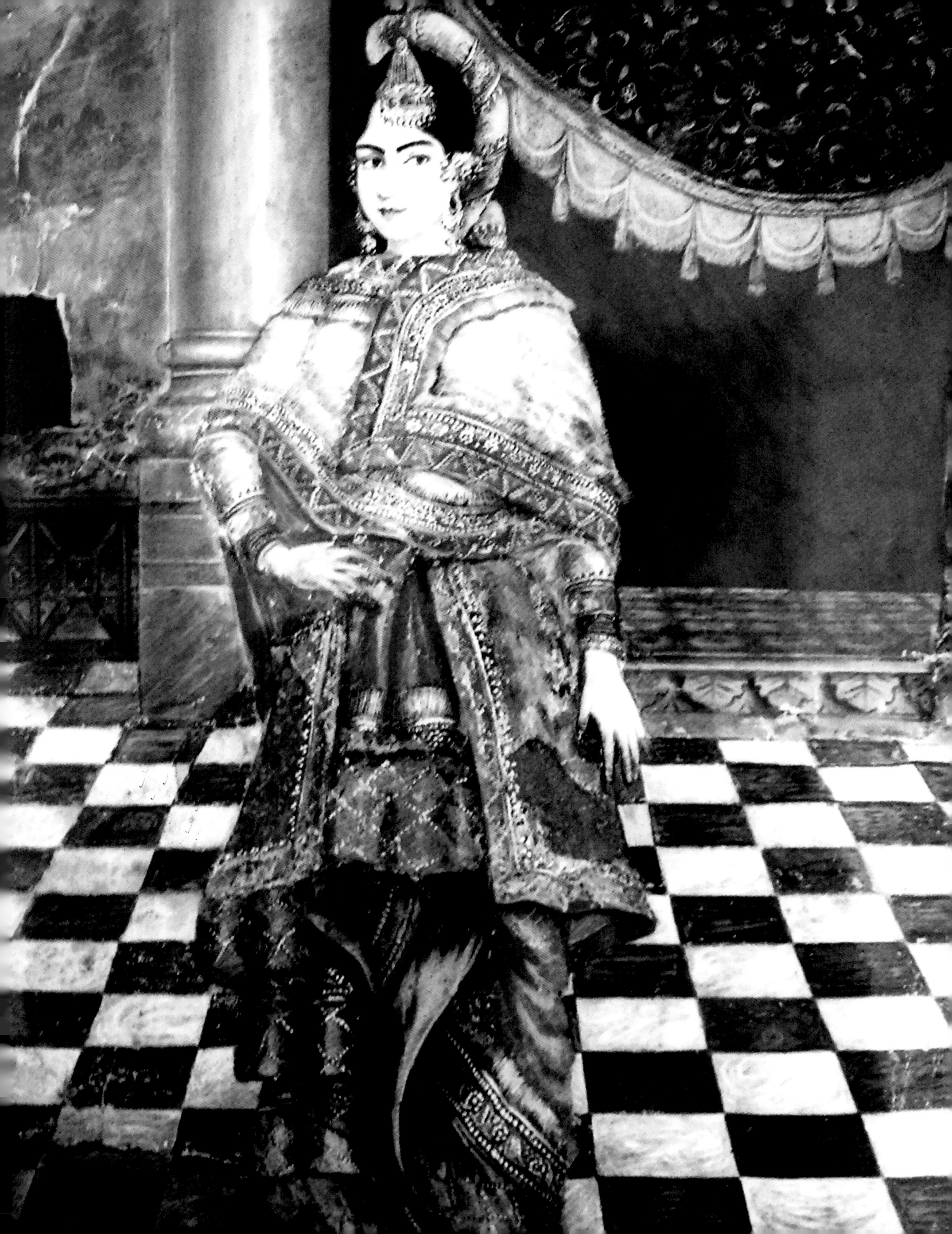

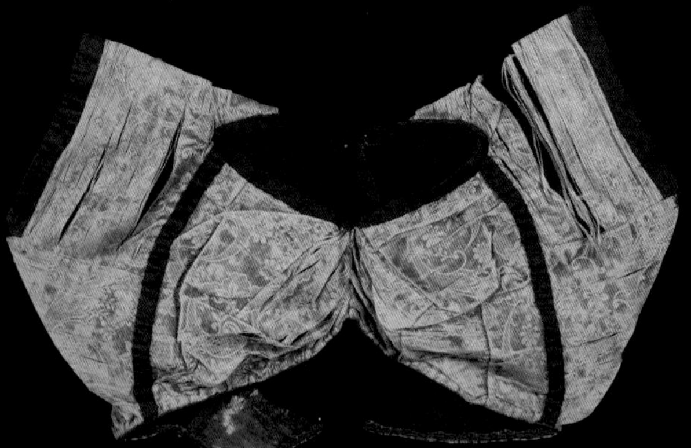

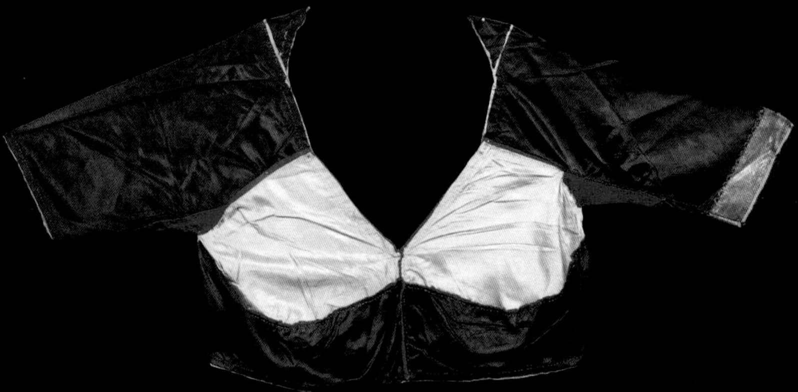

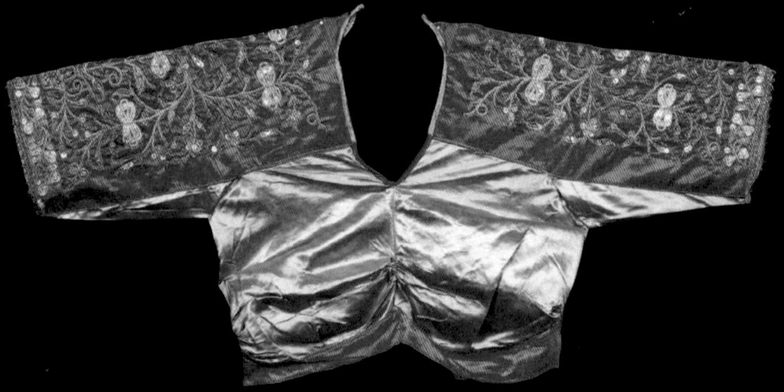

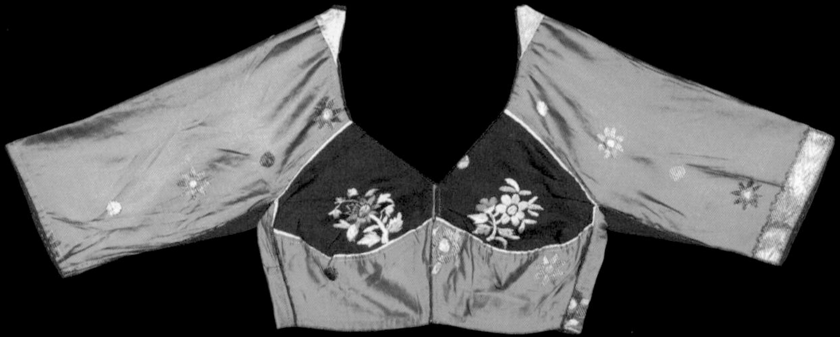

Clockwise from top:

1. This short *choli* is edged with blue piping and fastened at the back with cord strings. Floral motifs have been woven in *tanchoi* silk. The *tanchoi* weaving is said to be of Chinese origin, brought by three Parsi Jokhi brothers (tan - three, Choi - brothers) to India.
2. This hand-stitched *choli* of atlas silk fastens at the back with tie-cords. Only one sleeve is embellished with pure silver-woven *gota* as the other would be covered with the *sidha* pallav of the sari. Cotton red gussets have been used for durability.
3. This turquoise and maroon hand-stitched *choli* is made of Chinese silk, embroidered floral *buta* and *buti*s in satin stitch, long and short stitch with untwisted *resham* thread.
4. This *choli* is made of hand-woven silk with a satin finish. Sleeves are embroidered with gold **zari** in *jaal* pattern with *phool-patti* motif in *ari* work. This silk is also known as *surti gaht* because of its durability like the mountains of the Surat region in Gujarat.

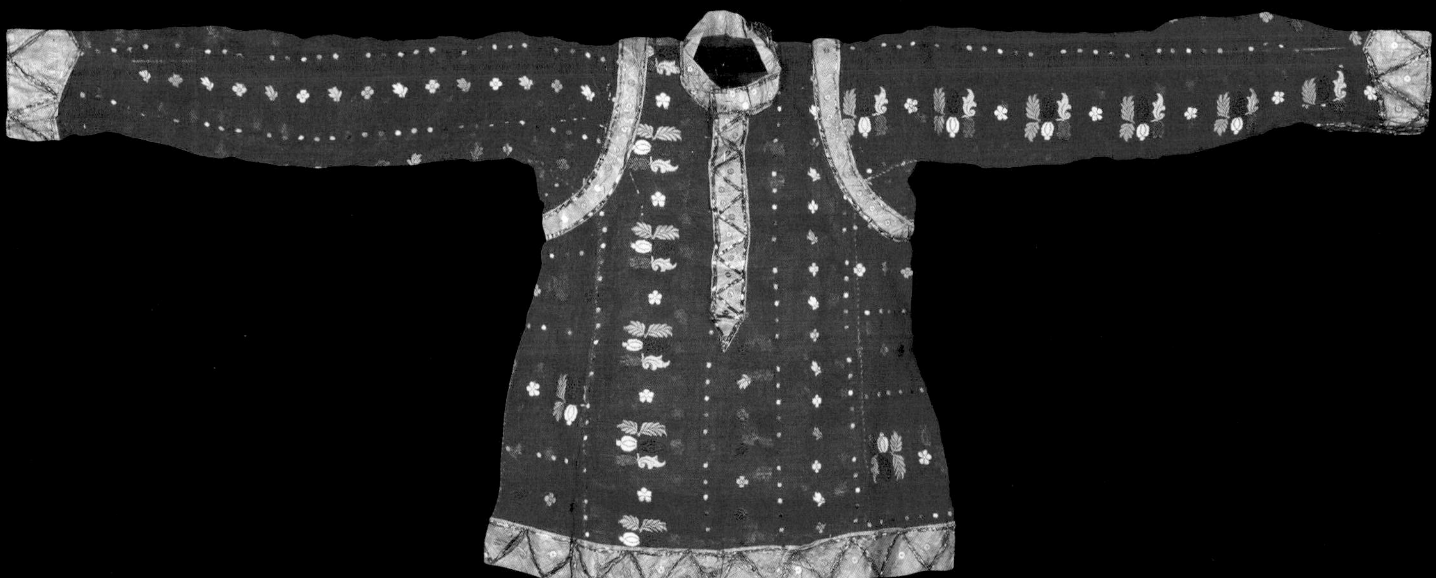

This hand-stitched red **kurti** is in *maldahi* cotton brocade; combination of colours suggests its ceremonial status. The *gota*, and the *salma and sitara* work on bias-cut green silk border is typical of Awadh.

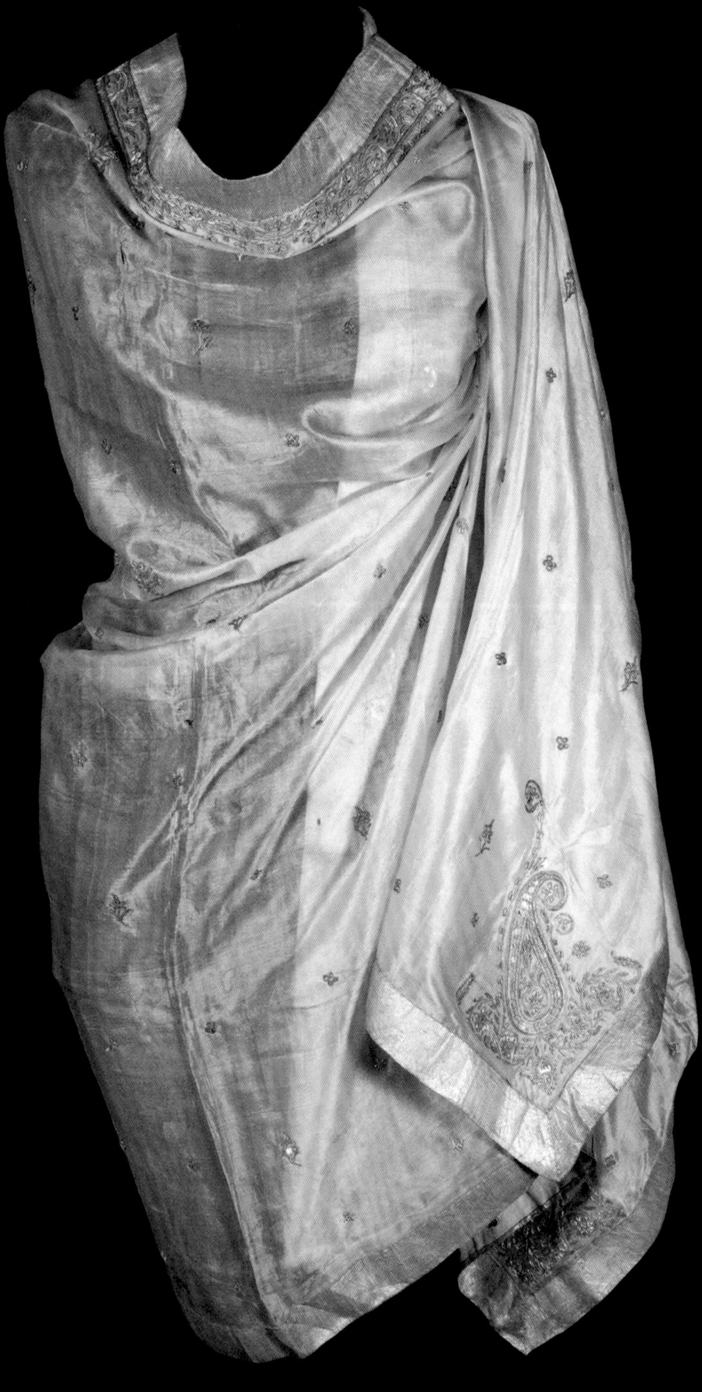

This safflower *odhni* is worn during the *sawan* festival. The *konias* (corners) are richly embroidered with *kalga* motif in pure gold zardozi. The beauty of the border is enhanced by the use of red and green beads giving it a *minakari* look and is edged by a *gota* braid.
Facing page: Detailed embroidery in zardozi work.

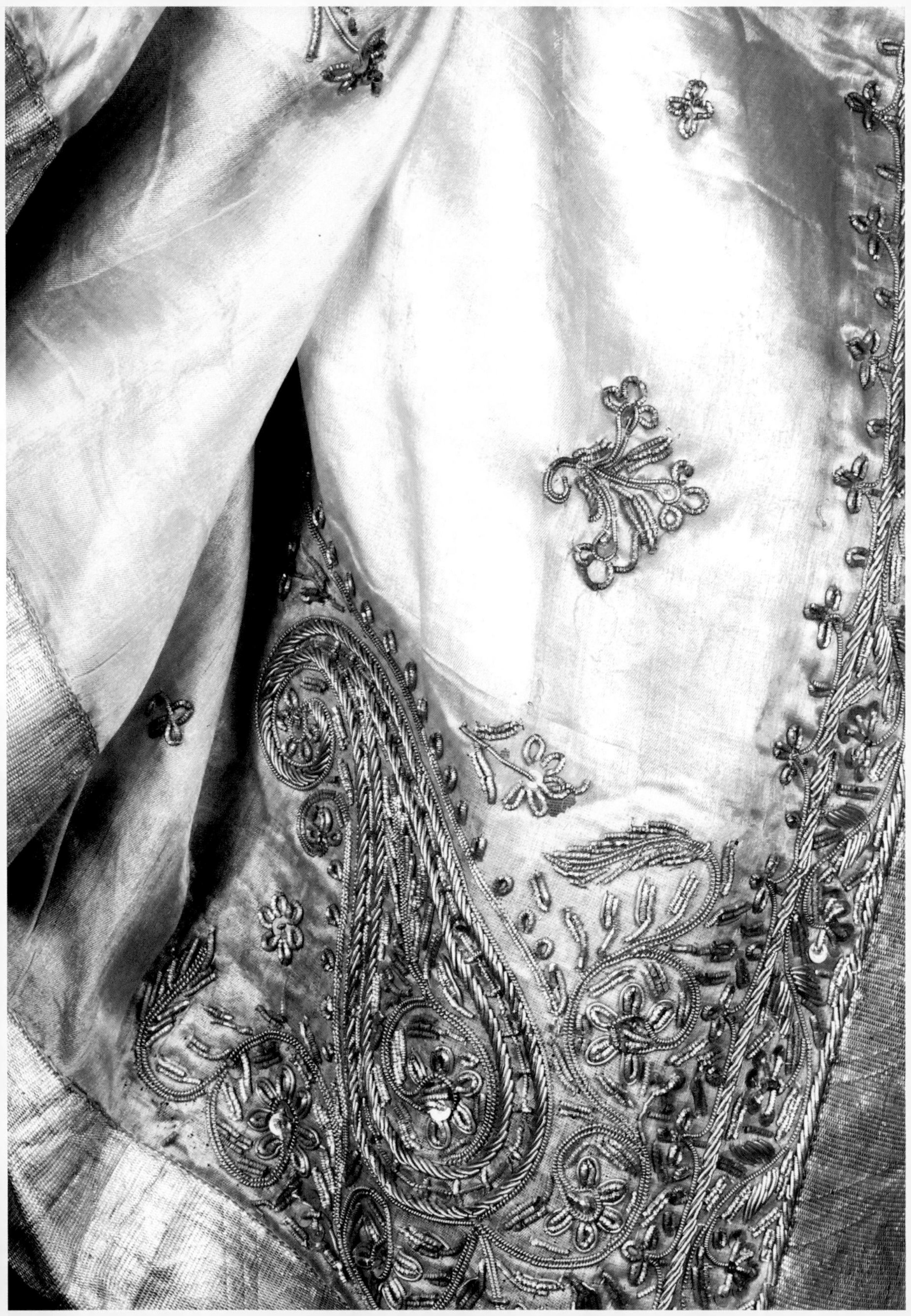

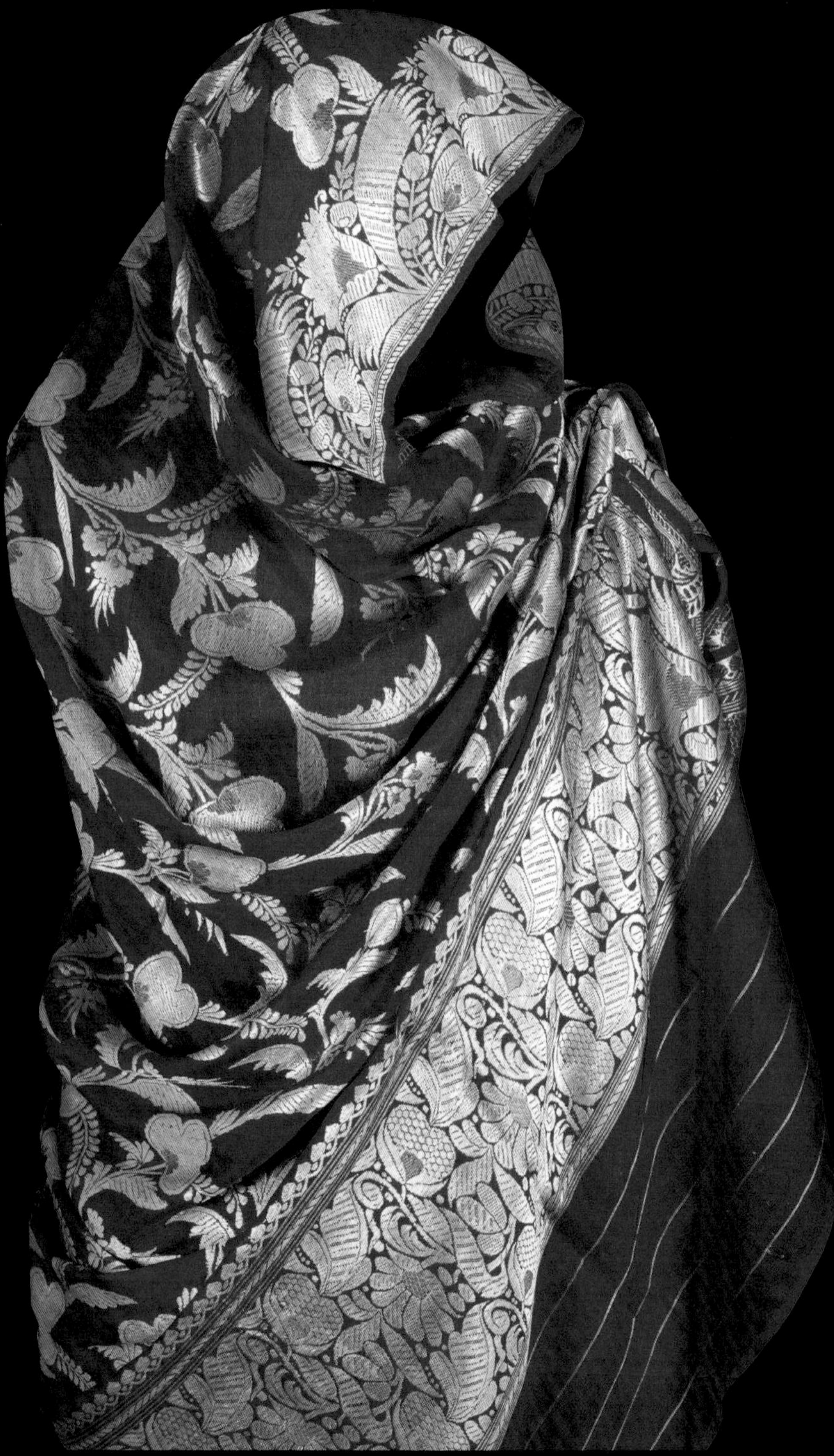

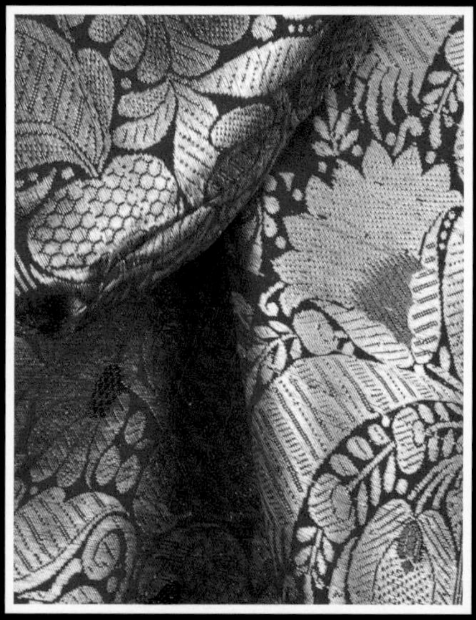

This *gul-e-anari* coloured *odhni* is made of *amru* silk (only silk yarns in warp and weft) brocade from Benares. The weaving in yellow floss *resham* (raw silk thread) gives the richness of gold. The green *resham* used for the motifs giving them the *minakari* (enamel) effect. An unusual pomegranate motif is used with floral pattern. This *odhni* was also used as a *chadariya* for its dimensions. The practice of *purdah* was an accepted way of life for aristocratic and wealthy *taluqdar* (landlord) families of Awadh.

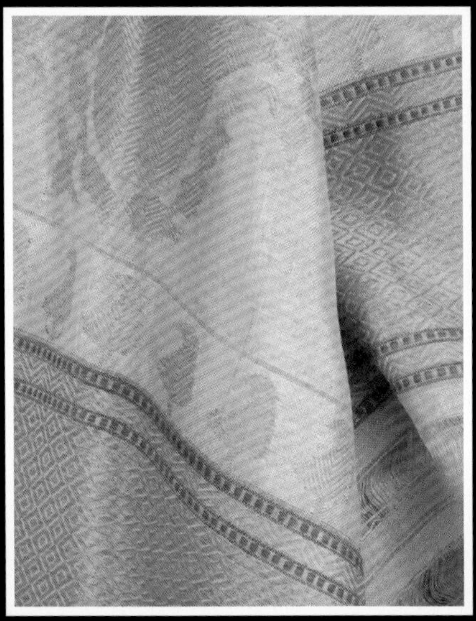

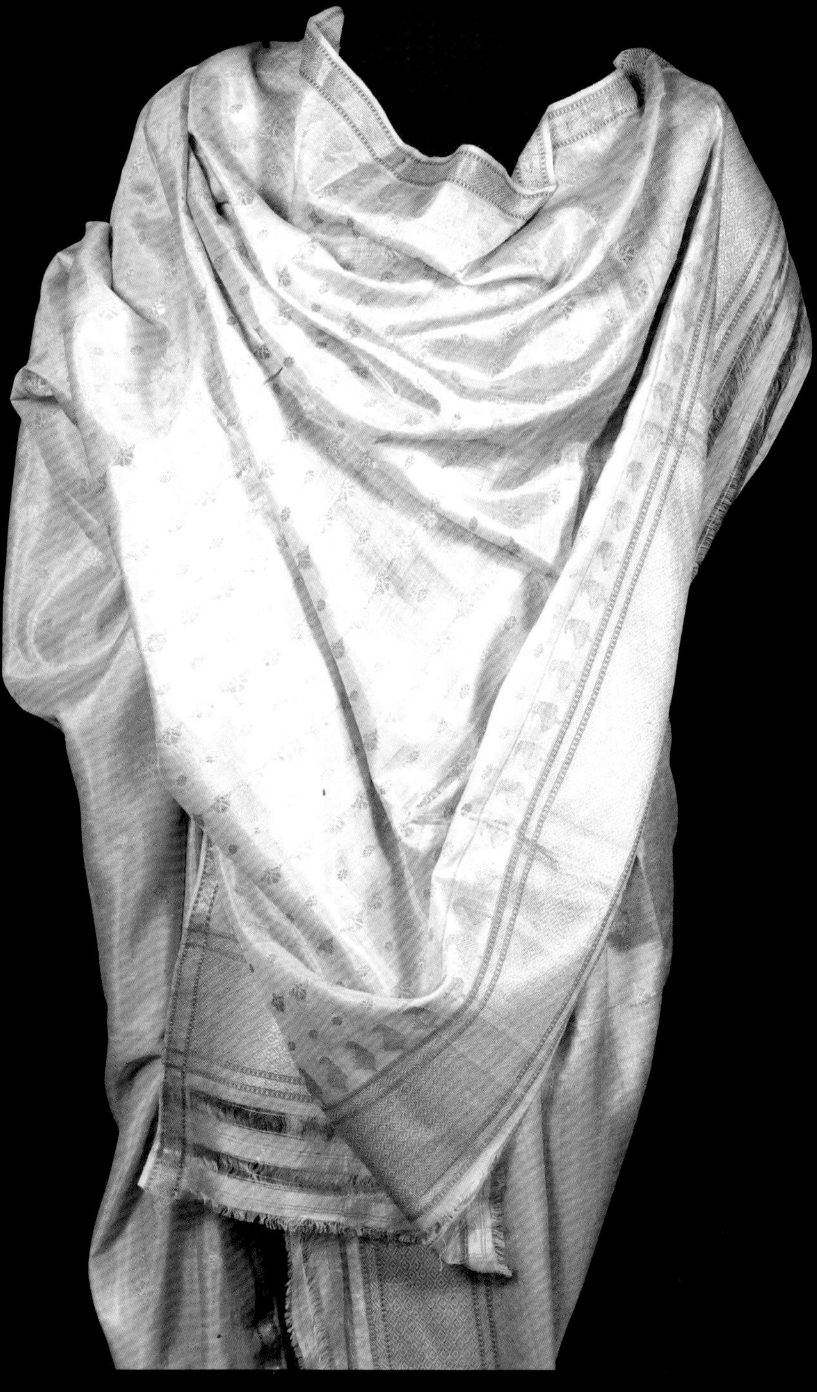

This *odhni* is made of a hand-spun silk-brocade from Banaras. The ground of the *odhni* is dotted with floral *butis* while the pallav and borders are woven with a gold thread in *chashm-e-bulbul* motif. The *pallav* is fuller in *butis* than the rest of the *odhni*. The use of *sindoori* red and gold border with *pista* green of the *odhni* indicates its ceremonial use.

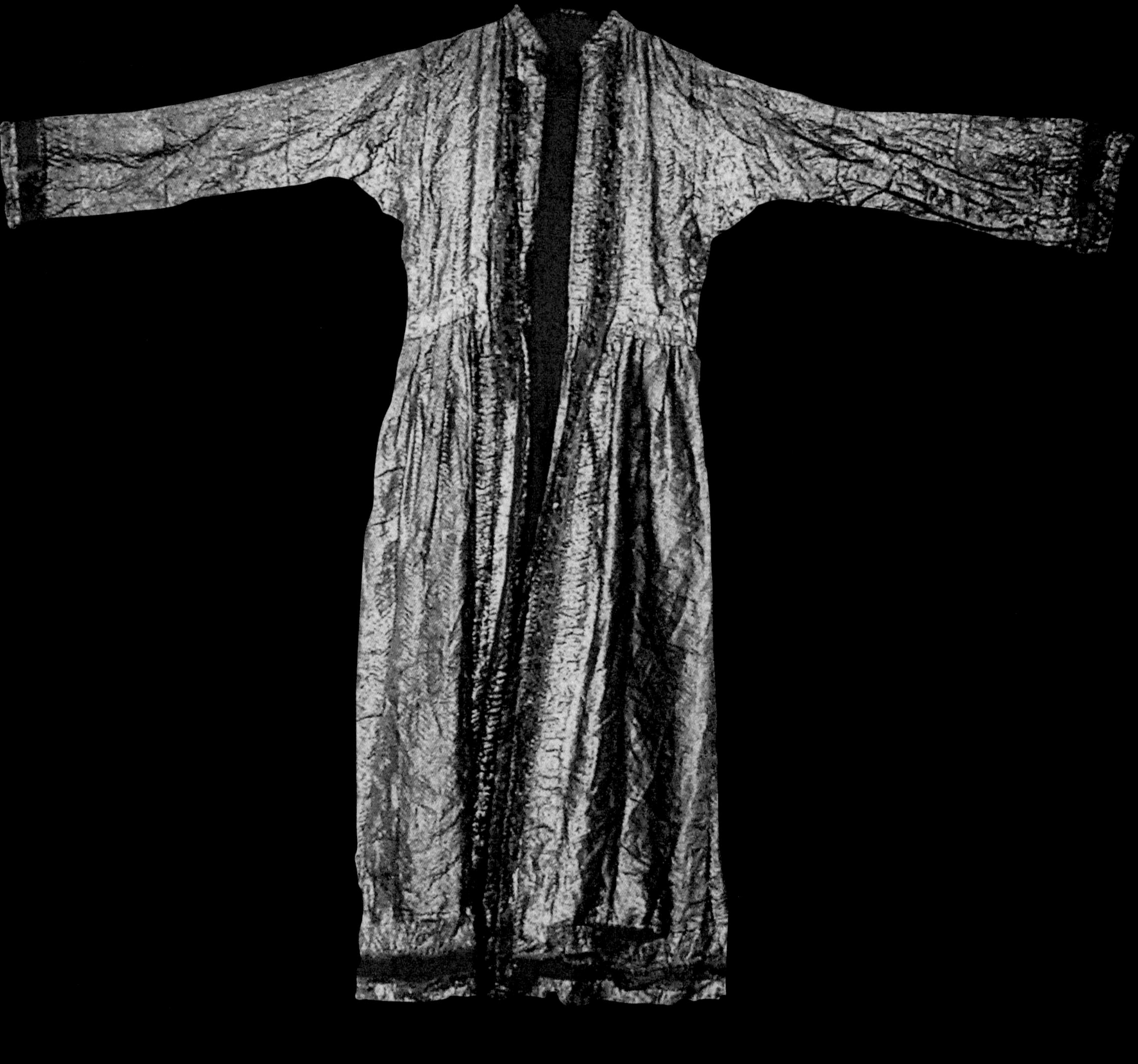

This long sleeved *peshwaz* is made of gold tissue fabric with silk warp and a zari weft. A tight-fitted bodice is joined at the waist with the gathered skirt. Front border, hemline and the sleeve-ends are edged with *sunehri-rupehli kiran* (gold and silver fringed *gota*).

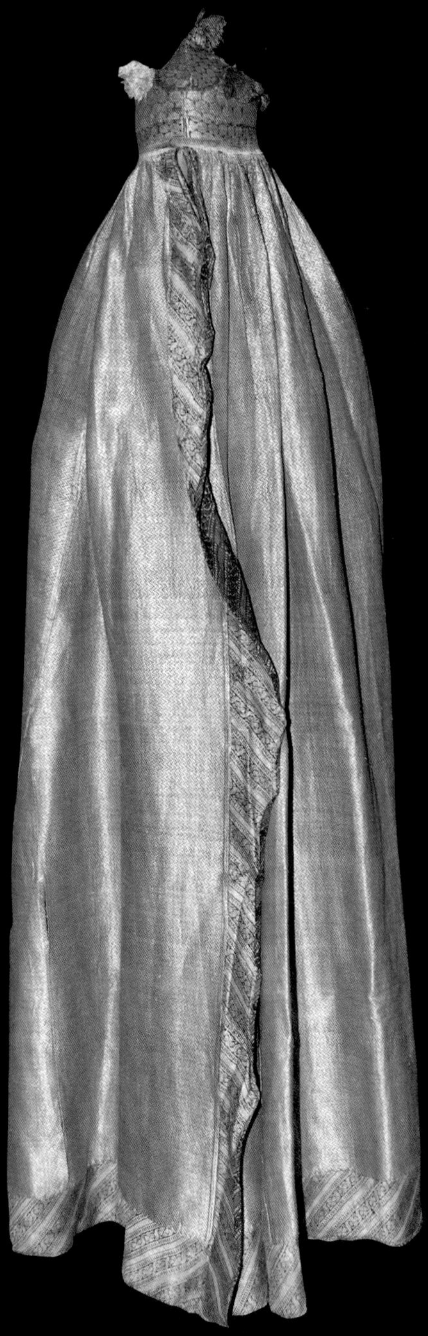

This burqa is a rare piece, possibly designed for a very important occasion. It is made of *kinkhab* brocade in pink and silver threads woven in a zig-zag pattern. Fully gathered at eye level, it leaves only a small opening for the eyes. The head piece, in a complex cut for better fitting, is decorated with *phundnas,* two at each side and one in the centre. The front and hemline are edged with a diagonally-cut broad and multi-coloured brocade border.

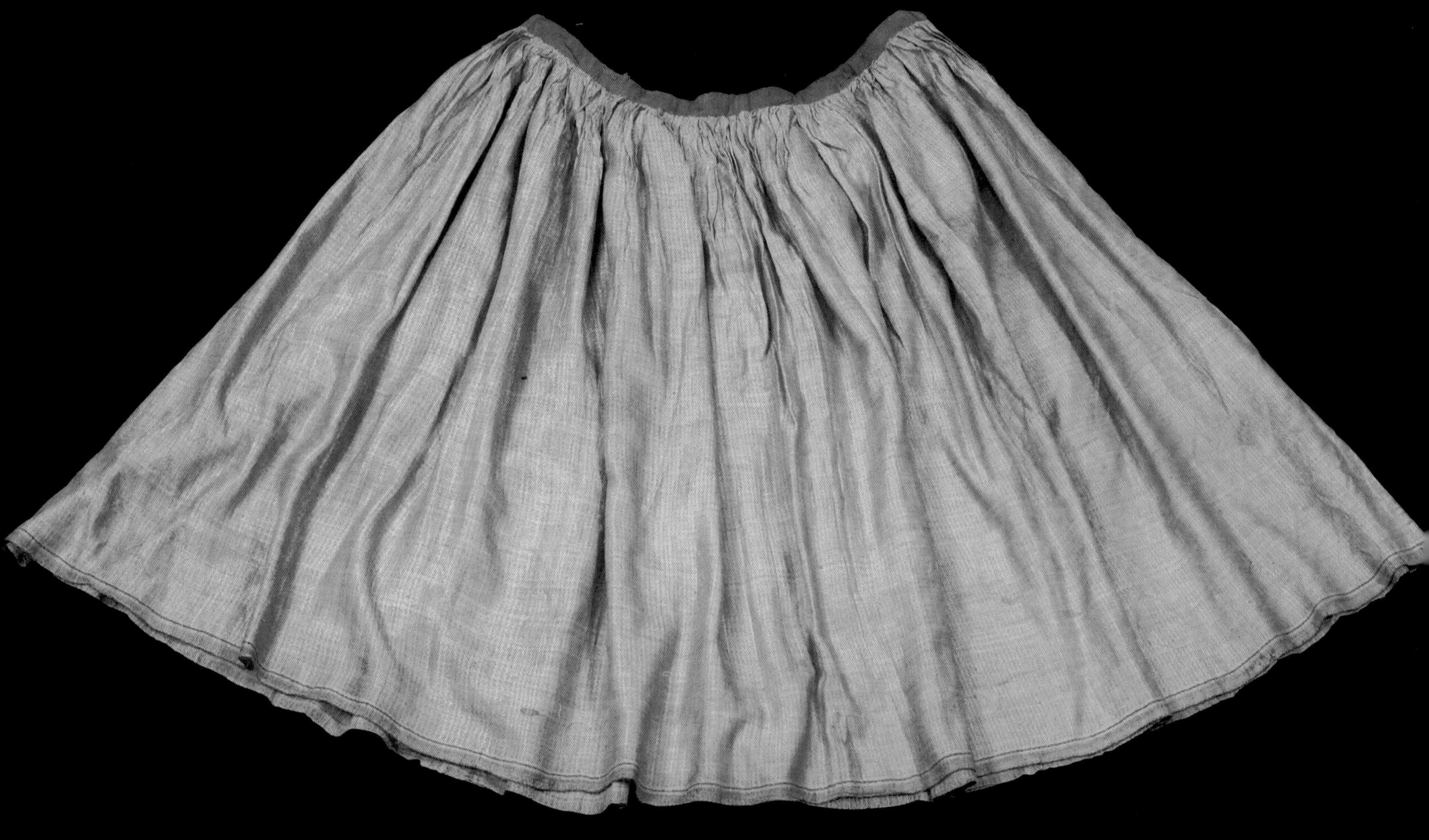

A lehenga made of hand-spun *mashru* fabric with silk warp and cotton weft. It has only one vertical seam and a band at the waist which holds the drawstring, also called *izarband*.

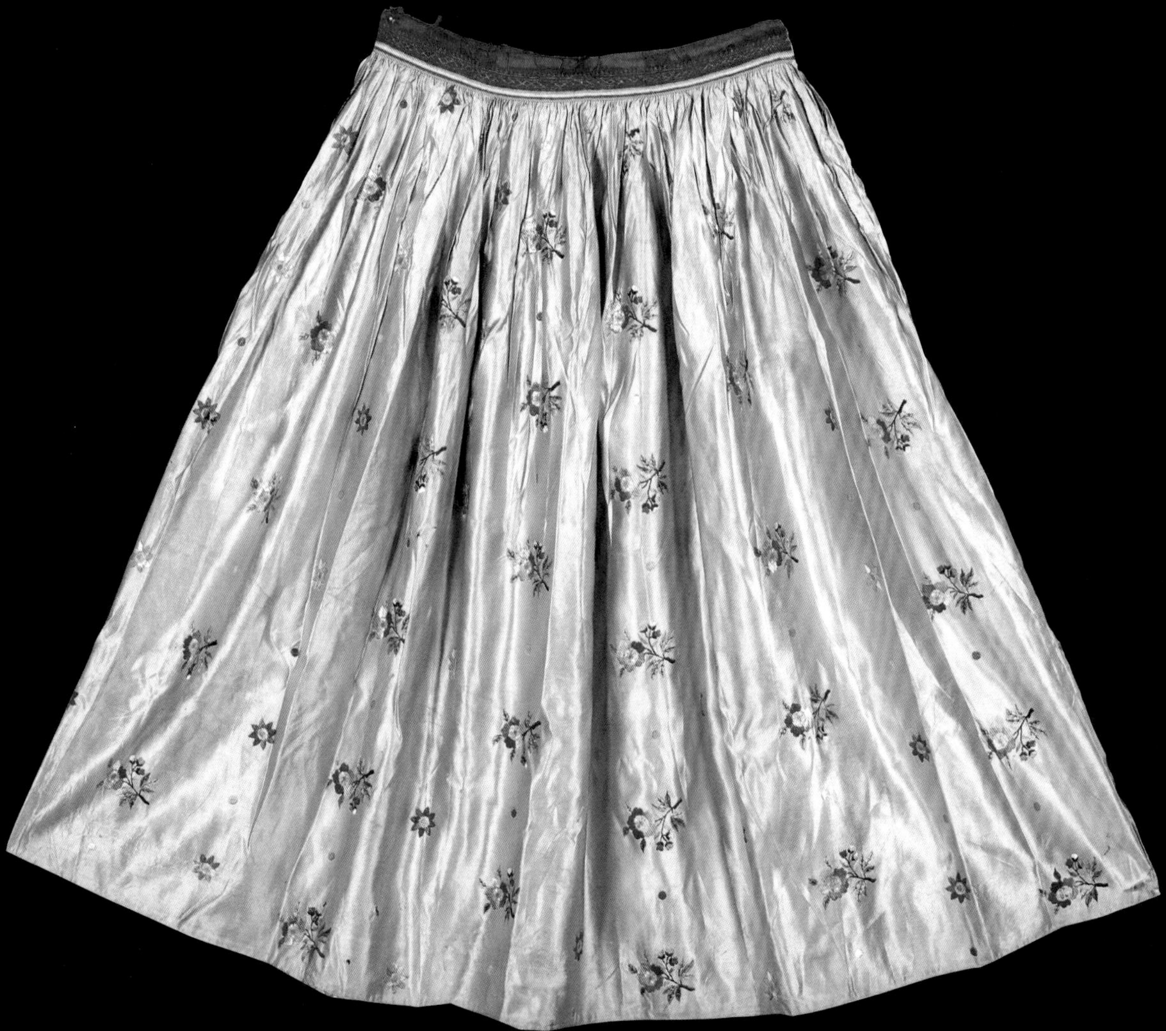

This lehenga is in satin silk embroidered with an untwisted *kaccha* (raw) silk thread. The *nefa* is intricately hand decorated.

This *bafta* brocade wedding *lehenga* is made of silk and pure gold zari. The skirt is gathered to a waistband to hold the draw-string. A *chasak* enriched with *zardozi* on velvet and a *gota* band in *chashm-e-bulbul*, is stitched a little above the hemline. The combination of *buti*s and *butas* scattered on the plain ground, and the zardozi work enriched with *salma, sitara,* and *gota* gives it a ceremonial look. The deep red colour symbolizes good luck, health and prosperity.

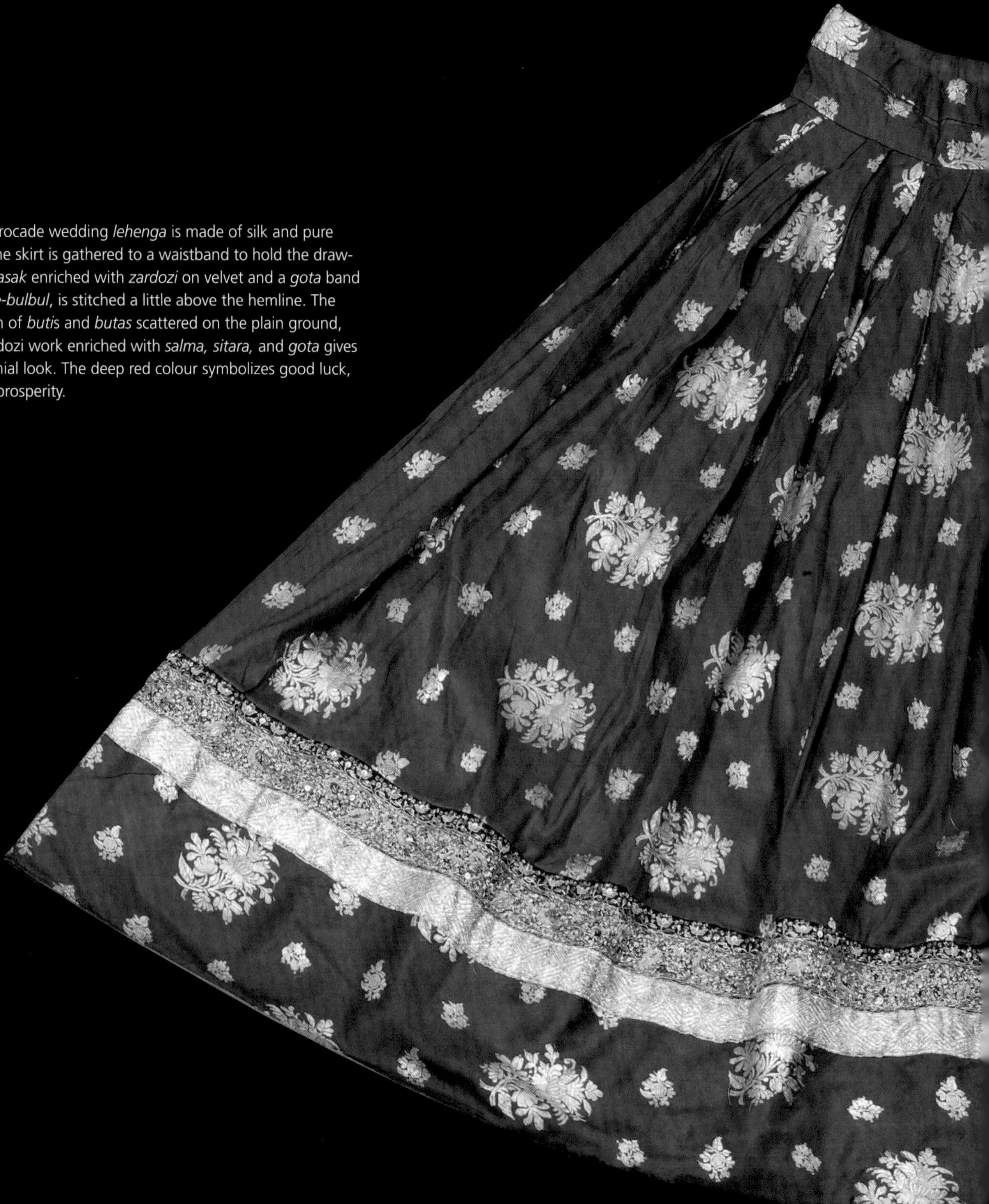

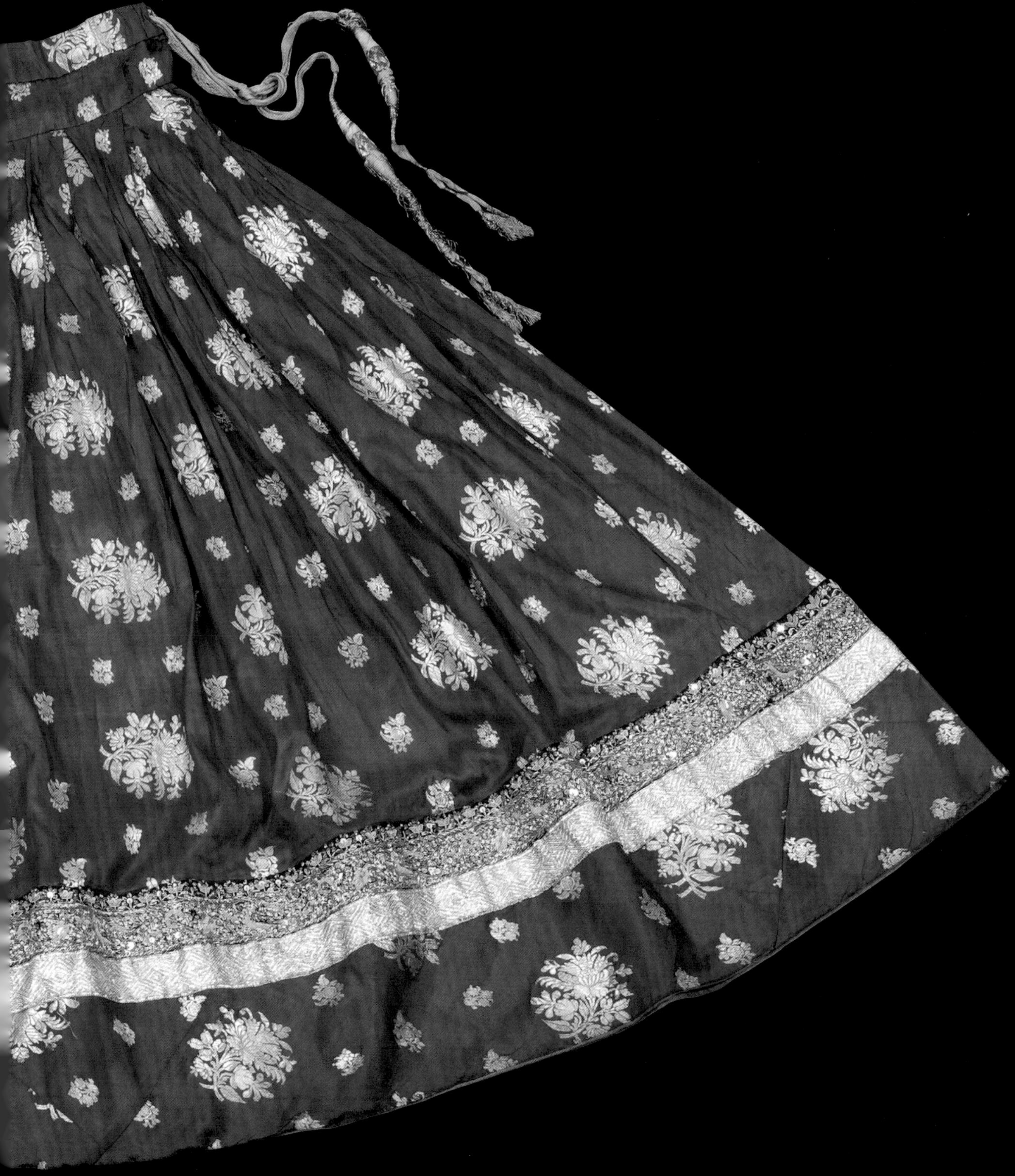

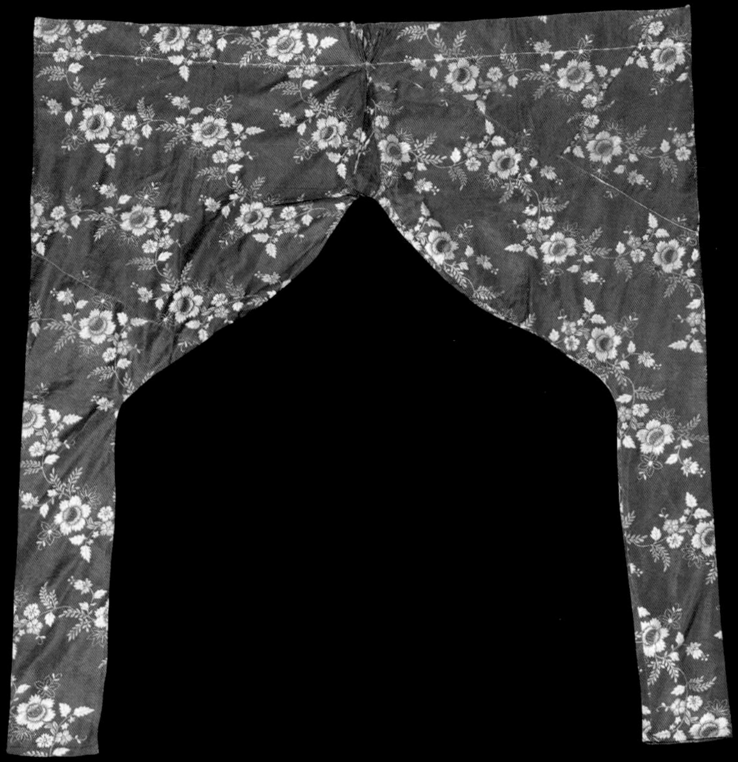

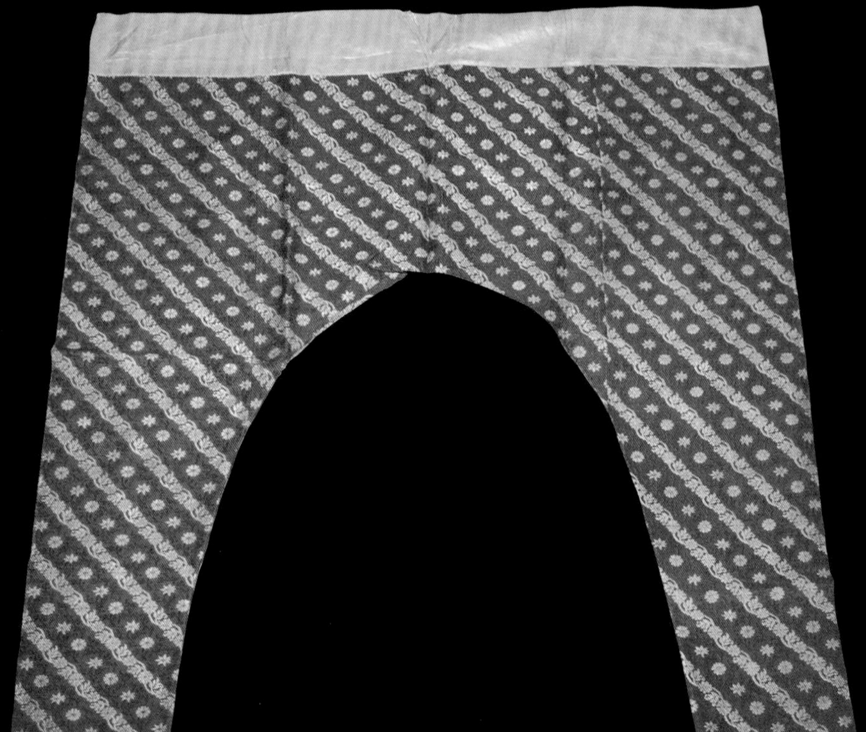

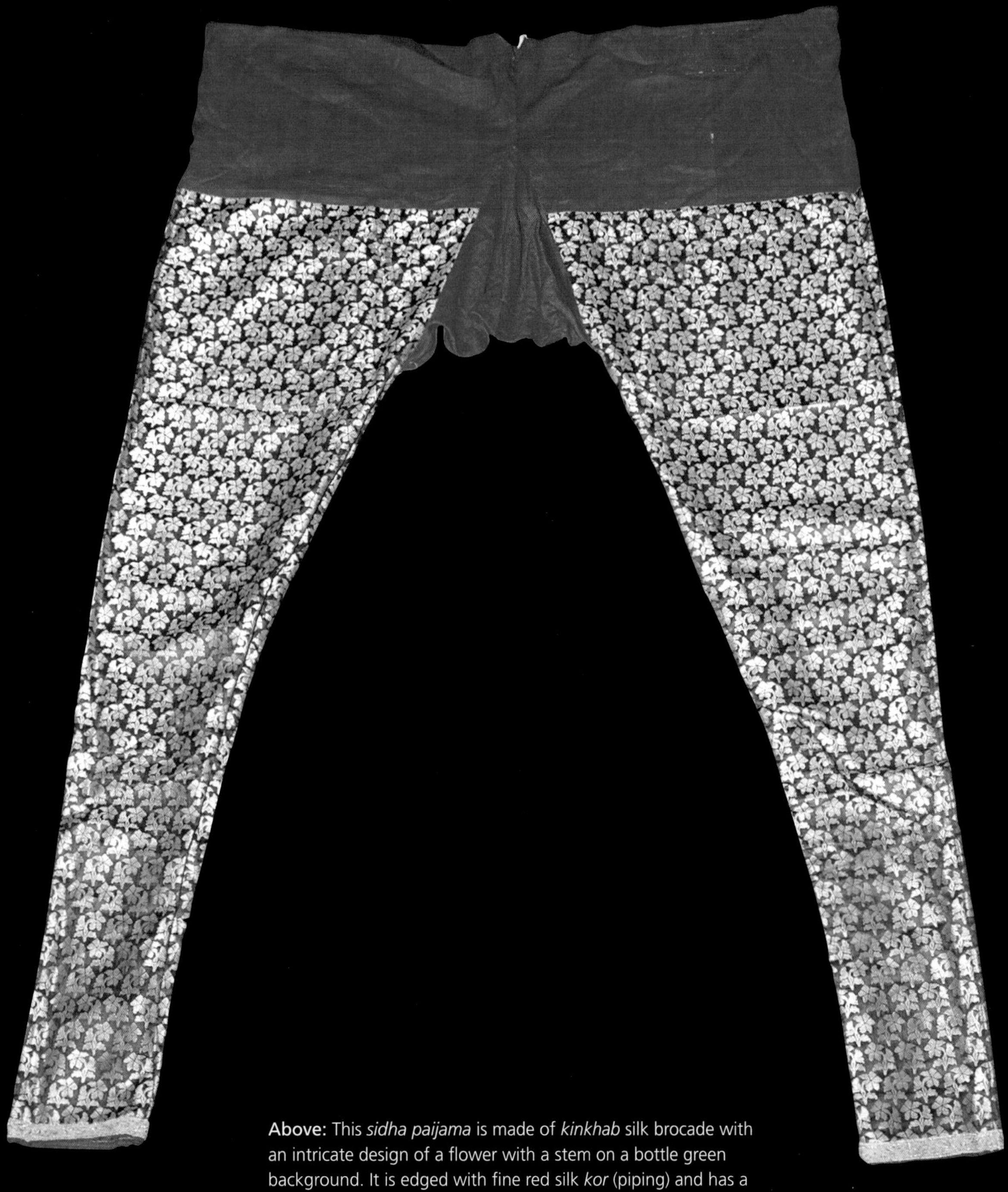

Above: This *sidha paijama* is made of *kinkhab* silk brocade with an intricate design of a flower with a stem on a bottle green background. It is edged with fine red silk *kor* (piping) and has a decorated *mohri* with zardozi work. At the waist, there is a red cotton *nefa* to hold a drawstring or *izarband*.
Facing page, Above: This aureb-cut churidar paijama is made of satin finish *atlas* fabric with woven floral motifs. The centre of each flower is filled with contrasting red colour. The excess length of the paijama falls into folds and appears like a set of bangles resting on the ankle (hence 'churidar'; 'churi': bangle, 'dar').
Facing page, Below: This *gul-e-anari* straight-cut *paijama* is woven in silk brocade with flowers set in diagonal lines. A matching yellow *nefa* (waistband) is sewn to the waist for holding the drawstring or *izarband*. The *mohri* is decorated with a floral border in *minakari* pattern.

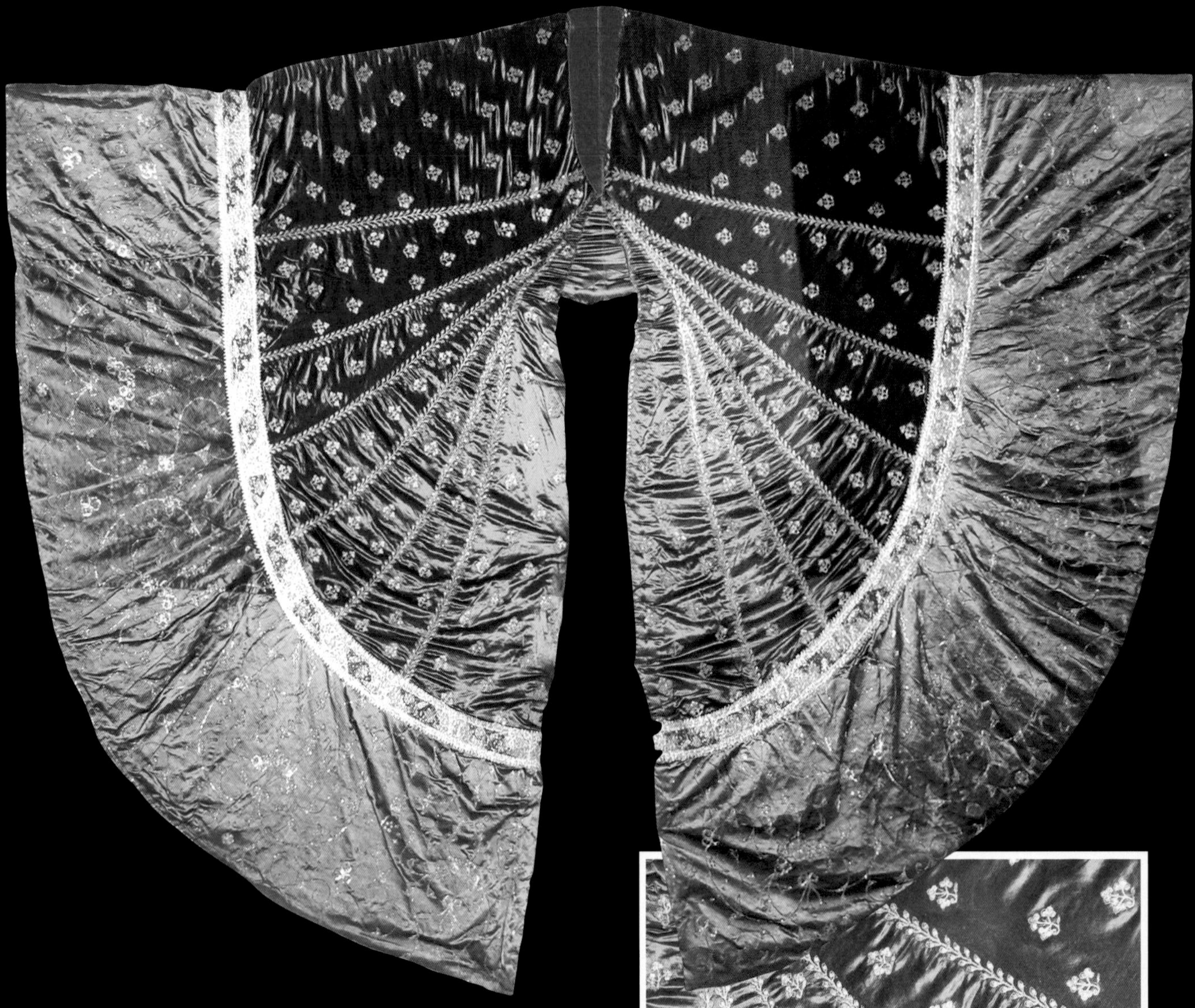

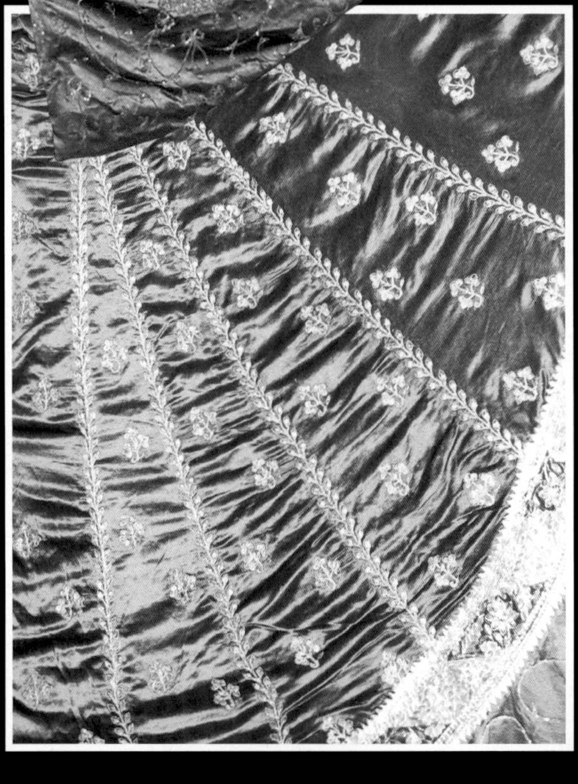

Above: Blue *farshi* paijama of satin silk is embroidered with *gold* zari. The joining seams in *paat* are decorated with *bel* motif, while the rest is covered with small *butis*. The *butis* are embroidered with inverted *katoris* (silver metallic discs).
Inset: *Jaal* of trailing flowers decorates the *gote* of the paijama in *ari* work. The seam that joins both the upper and lower sections is embellished with a decorative diagonally-cut band of alternating light blue and pink silk stripes and edged with *gokuru gota*.

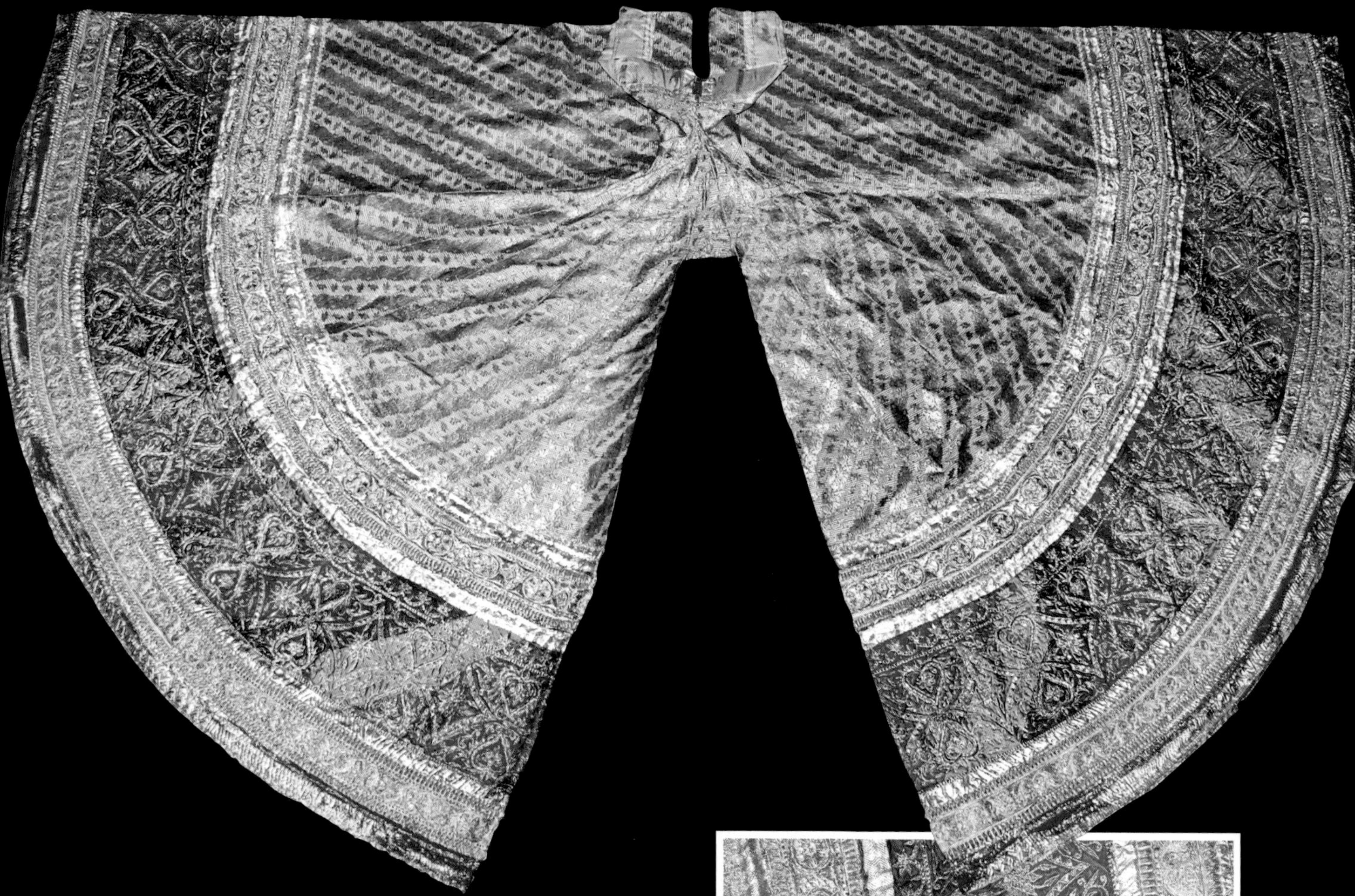

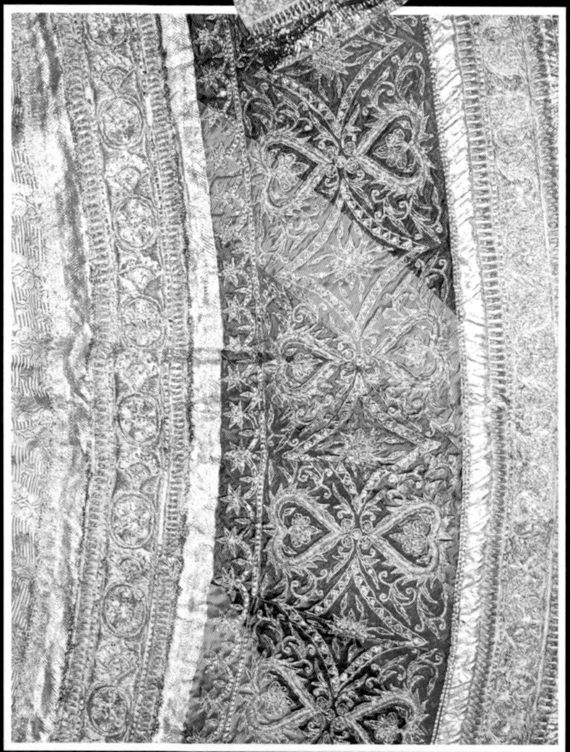

Above: The *paat* of this *kalidar* paijama is made of green and gold brocade panels and the *gote* is made of green, purple, turquoise and *gul-e-anari* diagonal stripes, embroidered with fine zardozi, encased within two composite bands of silver embossed *gota* and embellished with *salma sitara*.
Inset: Detail.

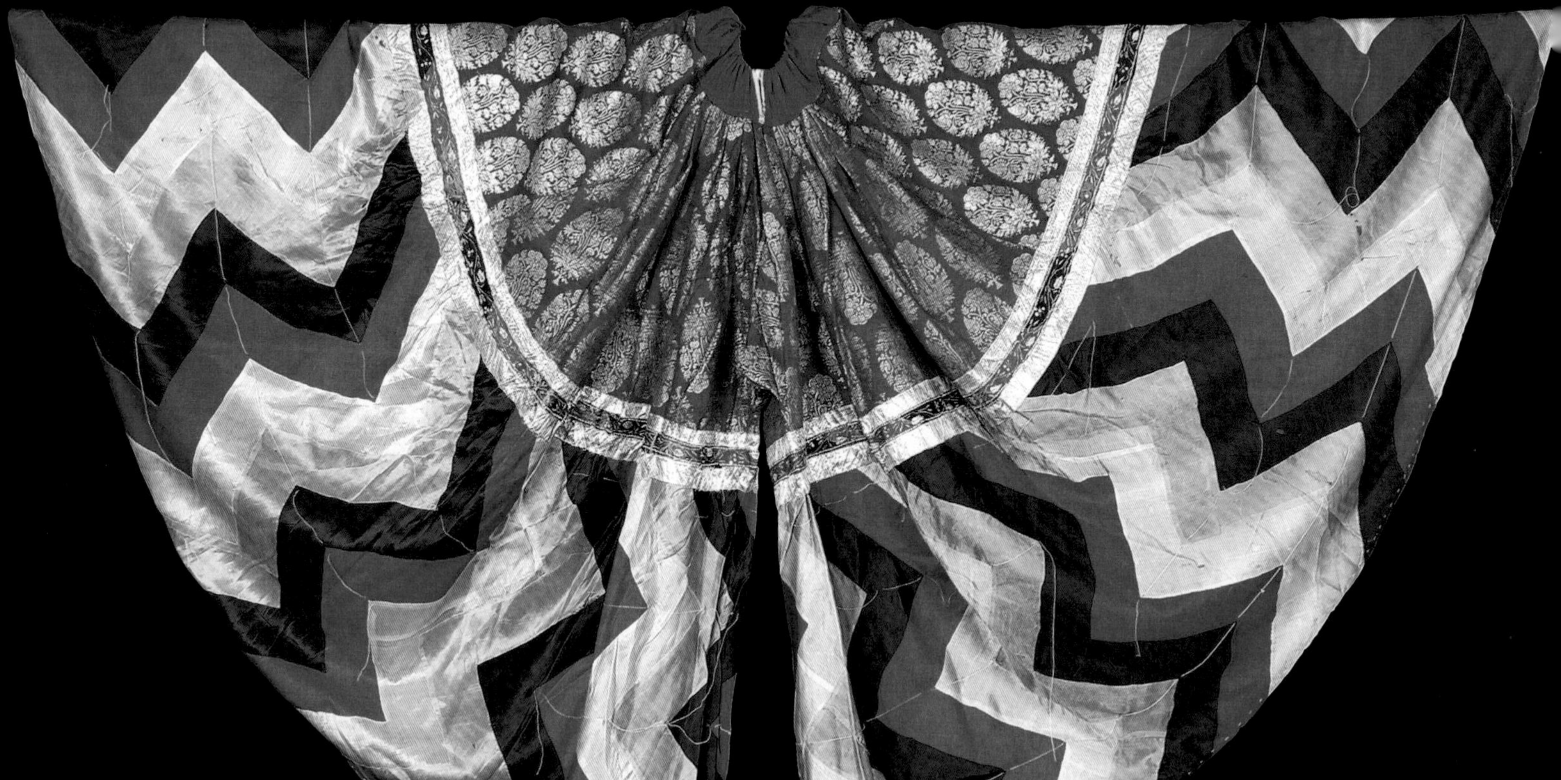

Above: The *paat* of this *bar ka paijama* is made of hand-spun silk, brocaded in gold with a stylized tree-of-life motif across the garment. The *gote* is made of multi-coloured silk fabric in *chatta-patti* work. A *chasak* of zardozi and embossed *gota* separates the upper section from the lower. Embellishment at the joints is referred to as '*dhanak*' or '*chasak*'.

Facing page: Typical colours of Awadh in zigzag pattern.

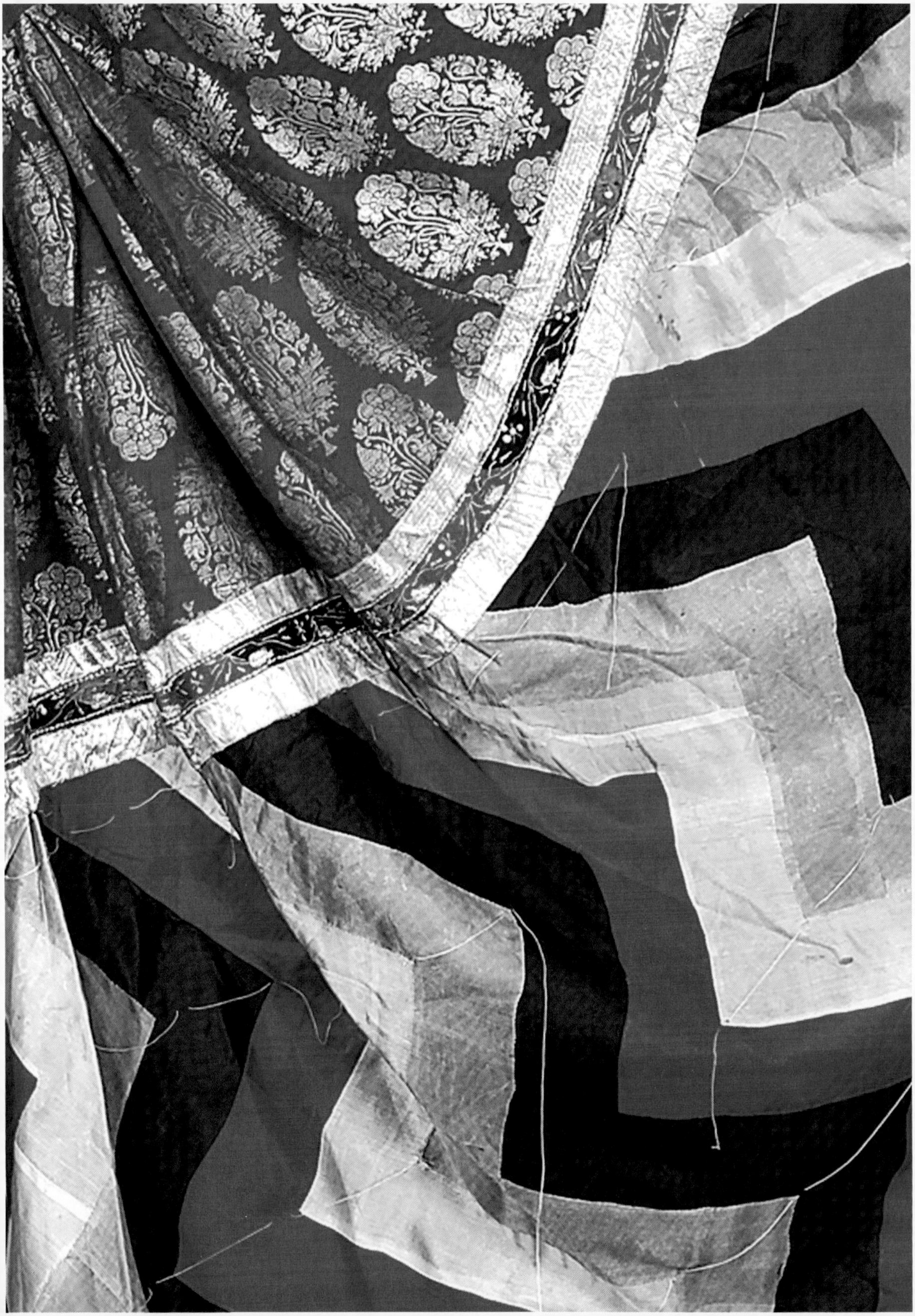

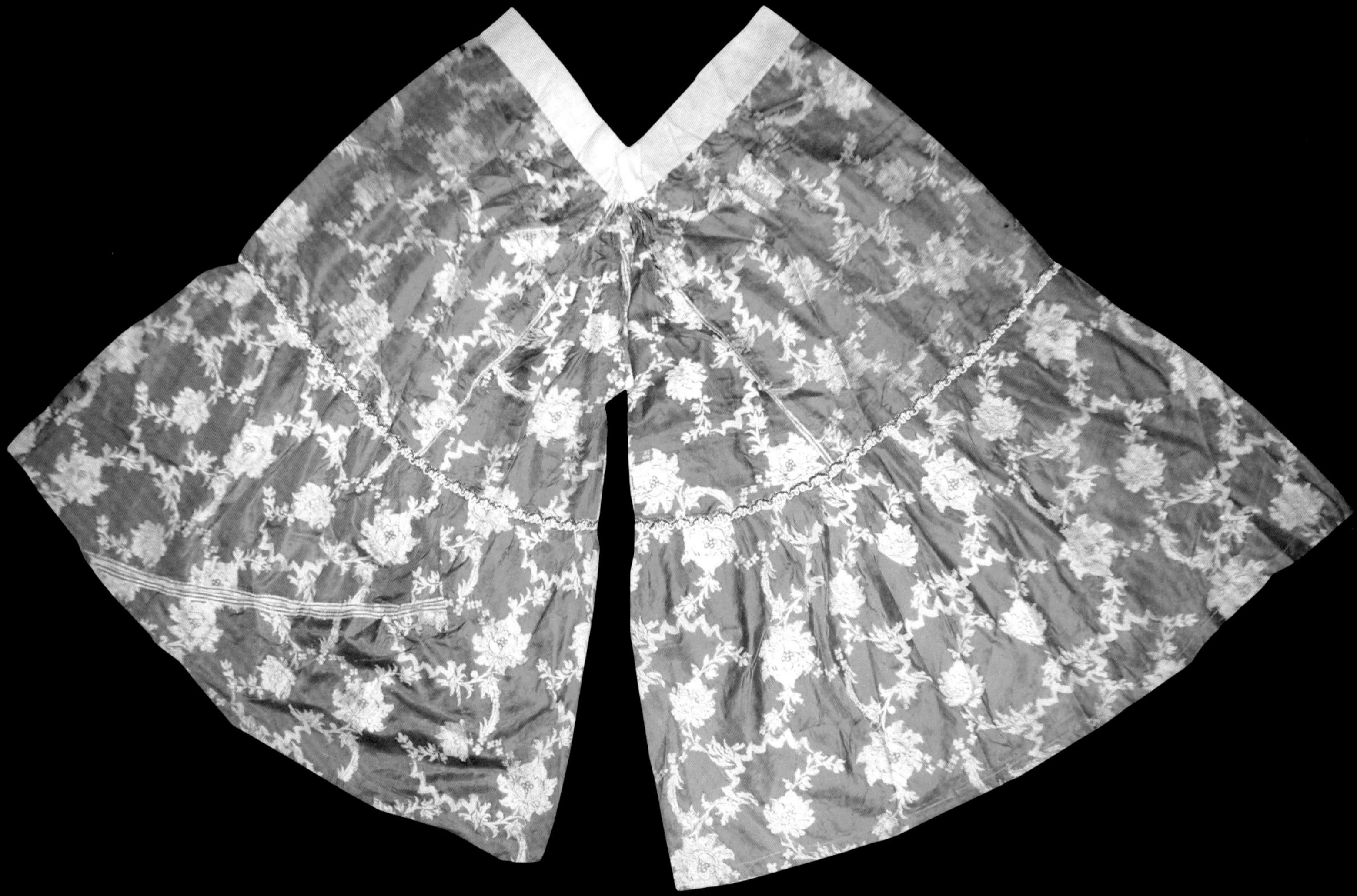

The floral motif *jaal* in yellow in this gharara is brocaded in cotton where as the main ground is in turquoise blue silk. The *nefa*, in matching yellow silk, and the two sections of gharara are joined and decorated with a band of silver and pink braided *gota* ribbon.

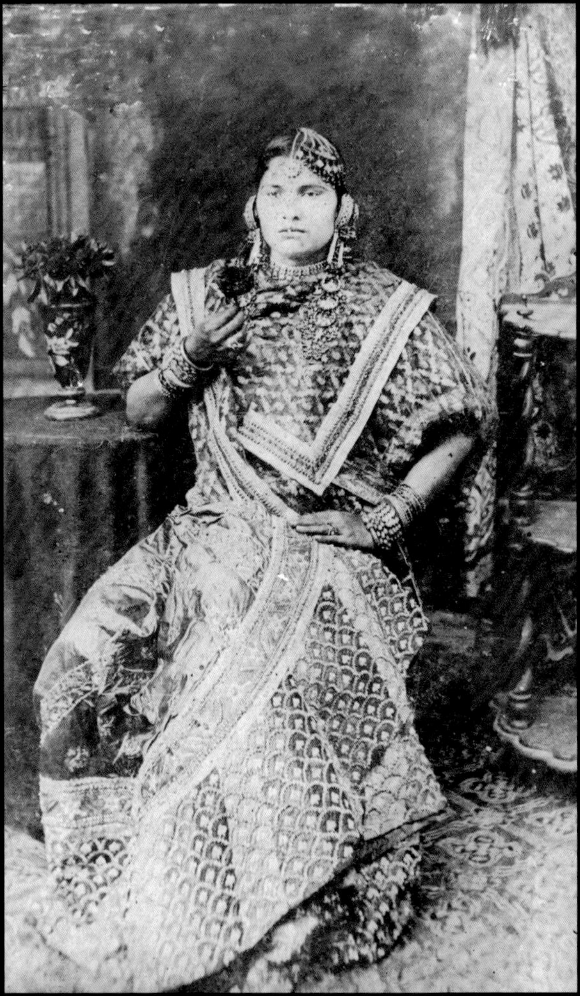

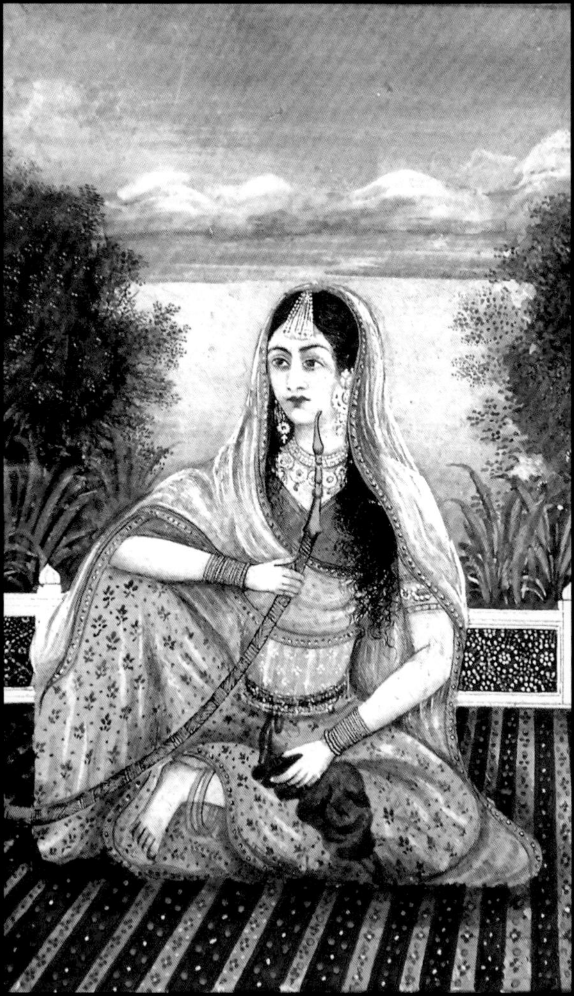

Above: The courtesan is wearing a lehenga, short choli and a *jamdani odhni* with floral *buti*s. The *odhni* has been decorated with a red and green border giving it a *minakari* effect. *Jhumer* is worn like a *tika* in the front instead of on the left side of the head. She is wearing a pair of *paijeb*, bangles, a *bajuband,* a necklace and earrings.

Left: Courtesan Bashti Jaan is wearing an elaborate *farshi paijama* decorated in *chatta-patti* work in a *mahepusht* (fish scales) design. The *gote* and *paat* are joined with a zardozi border. *Odhni* is embroidered all over in *gota* work in a *jaal* pattern. She is wearing typical ornaments of a courtesan, *jhumar, tika* and *nath*.

Influence of Courtesans on Women's Apparel

'The brightness of her plump tapering arms gave to the sleeves of her tunic the appearance of a Moonlit valley; men lost their reason at sight of her bodice gilded with lace, fitting tightly and faultlessly over her bosom. The knot of her trouser strings was voluptuously set like an embossed seal upon her navel. The wide seam of her drawers which held its fastening strings was an alley wherein imagination toiled in vain to find any trace of the waist that was harboured there' (Dar 1969).

Having more than one wife and a large harem was an indicator of prosperity and prestige for the nawabs. The increasing role of the courtesans forced begums to change their dressing style which became more feminine and seductive in appeal. The courtesans wore tight-fitting *peshwaz* with churidar paijama and transparent *odhni*s to enhance their sensuality while performing at *mujra*s. Initially the *peshwaz* was a long gown having a bodice and a lower garment similar to the lehenga, gathered at the waist. The courtesans made these *peshwaz* more sensuous, with a tight-fitting bodice and a skirt of aureb-cut which gave a swirling effect when dancing. They wore a cap similar to *nukkadar*, often worn in a coquettish manner—a little tipped to one side.

Begums began wearing tight-fitted *shaluka*s, farshi paijamas and zari-woven, richly embroidered *odhni*s made of materials such as tissue, muslin and net. Women's costumes, thus, became significantly more sensuous, elaborate and luxurious.

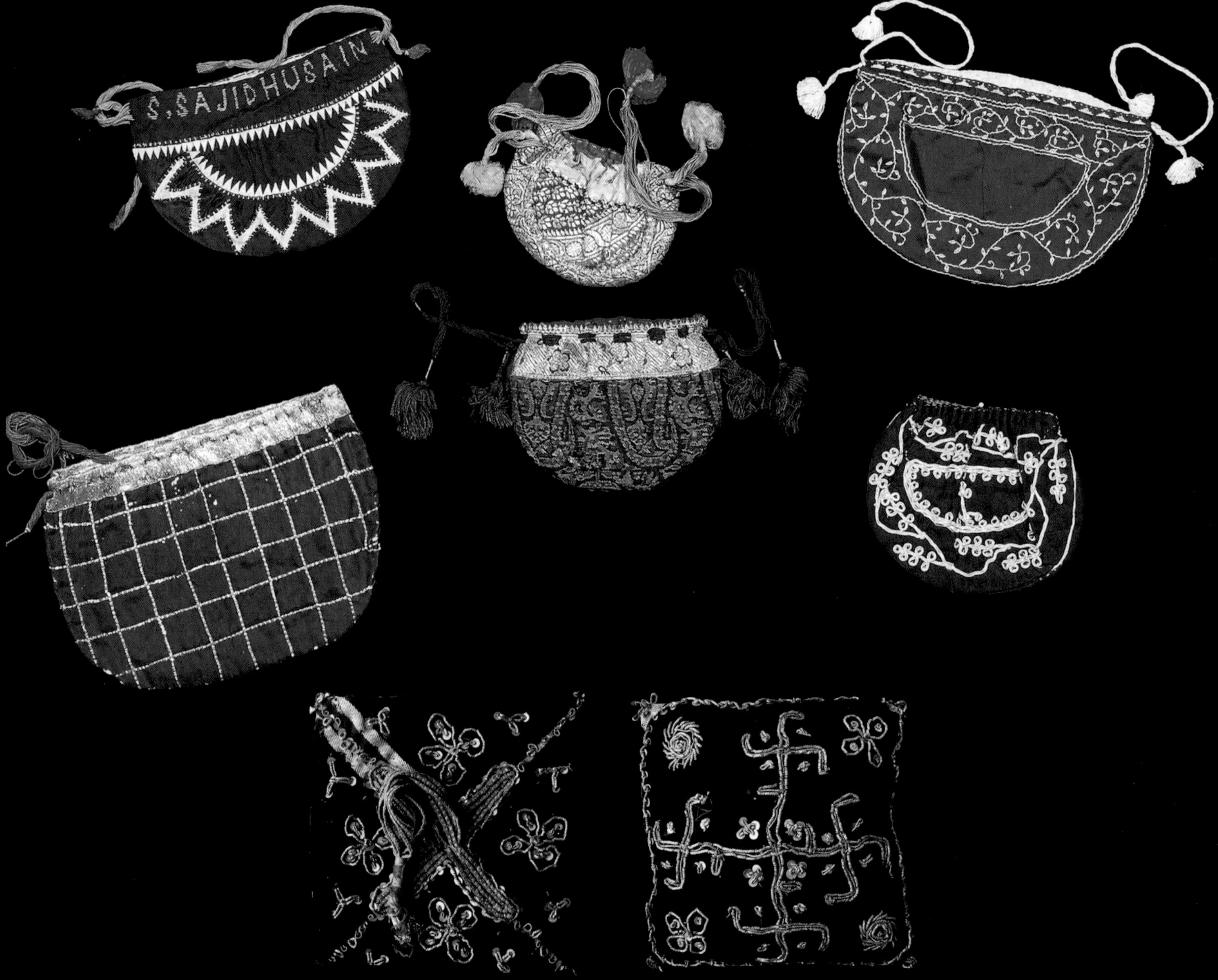

Since *batuiyas* were used for a variety of occasions across seasons, that these demanded, be made in a range of materials. Cotton for summers, silk and *jamawars* for winters. They were also embellished with different kinds of ornamentations and fastened using variety of strings. Purple was a very popular colour with the nawabs and begums of Awadh as it denotes aristocracy.

First row (left to right) : 1. Silk *batua* adorned with zig-zag pattern in yellow silk outlined with metal wire. The half-moon design is created in *daant* (teeth) motif by using yellow silk. The embroidered name suggests its use by a man. 2. *Batua* made of silk brocade and embellished with sequins. The strings with bright-coloured pom-poms make it suitable for special occasion. 3. Purple *batua* embroidered with white resham in floral creeper design with matching strings.
Second row (left to right): 4. Silk *batua* with geometrical squares embroidered in zari. Red contrasting cotton string is passed through the gold *gota*. 5. This *jamawar* black *batua* has red cotton lining and a zari border in *minakari* work. The blue-coloured silk strings are inserted for the fastening. 6. Lower round shaped part is *cur in aureb* while central part has been cut straight. The stylized flowers are attached by stitching.
Last row: 7. This ***batua*** has a very unique design, cut in four pieces and then joined with two strings. It is made of black velvet and then decorated with *kalabattun, salma and sitara.* On its back there are *sathias* suggesting it to be suitable for some religious ceremony.

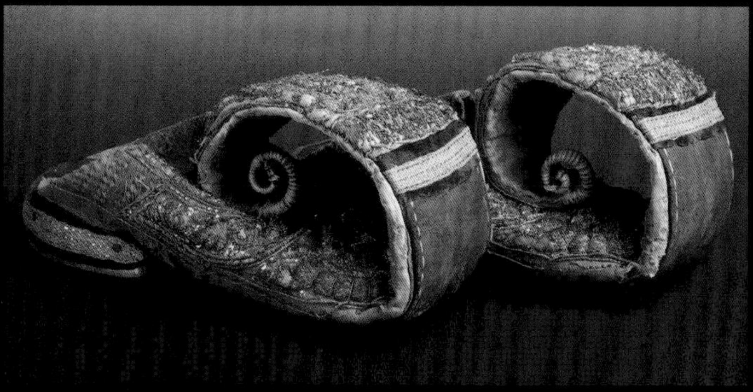

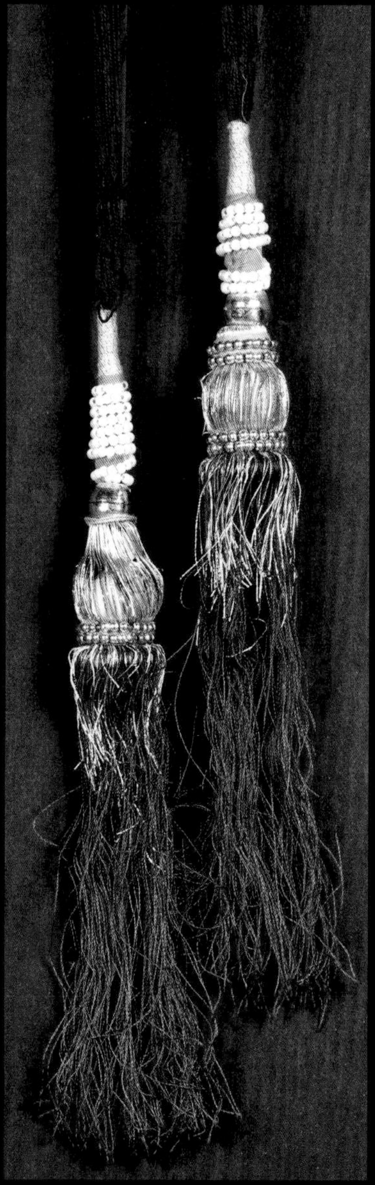

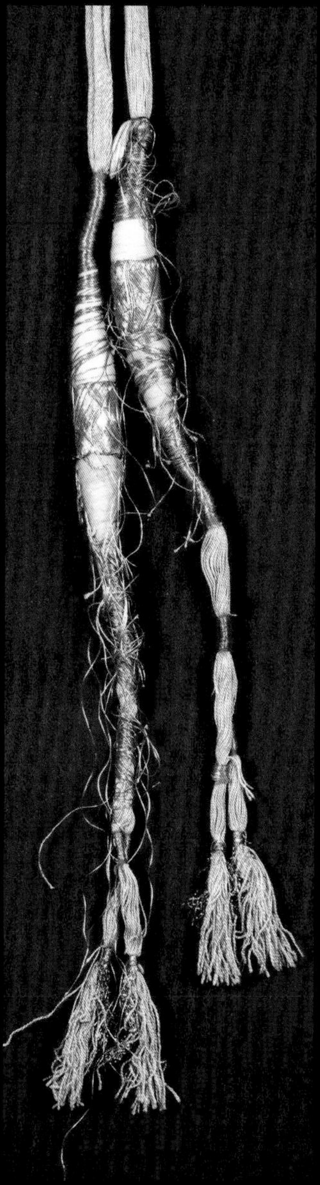

Above: The upper part of this pair of *ghatela* shoes are made of silk and the sole is made of leather. They are intricately embroidered with *kalabattun* and velvet stripes.
Right: A *paranda* is a women's hair-braid ornament. The term possibly originates from the Persian word *parand,* meaning 'winged creature or bird'. When worn by women, it sways from side to side possibly giving it its name. This *paranda* is made of cotton threads, embellished with pearls, zari bands and tasselled with silk threads to make them festive.
Extreme right: The decorative *nada/izarband* (drawstring) made of *kalabattun* is used to hold the lower garment, lehenga or a paijama, at the waist.

CONTRIBUTION OF THE NAWABS TO TEXTILES AND ORNAMENTATION

The nawabs were connoisseurs of art and they patronized the most precious textiles and ornamentations, which then became instrumental in creating the *nazakat* and *nafasat* characteristic of the period. During the period of the nawabs, traditional Indian textiles achieved their beauty from the variety of materials used; like *kinkhwab*, *mulmul*, *jamdani*, *jamavar*, to the variety of embroidery, from *chikankari*, appliqué-work and zardozi. Ornamentations with the use of *kalabattun*, *badla*-work (silver or gilt flat-wire embroidery), silver *tilla* embroidery, *sitara*-work (sequins work), mukaish-work (tiny dots embroidered with *badla*), the technique of *verek*-work (applying gold and silver leaf to a hand-block printed onto the fabric), *gota*-work and *kinari* (edging with a tasselled border) contributed immensely to embellish the garments of this period.

TEXTILES

MULMUL

Mulmul was the preferred textile of the nawabs, as it was fine and well-suited to the climate. The beauty of this textile was such to even attract the attention of poets. Amir Khusrau, the fourteenth-century poet, was so struck by the beauty and sensuousness of these gossamer fabrics that he wrote (Yafa 2006):

'One would compare it with a drop of water if that drop fell against nature, from the fount of the sun. It is so transparent and light that it looks as if one is in no dress at all but has only smeared the body with pure water.'

Fine muslins could only be woven during the rains and specifically in the morning hours when the moisture in the air enables the thread to be easily pulled and then woven. The quality of the cotton was determined by the tendency of the fibres to expand with moisture in the air, the sizing done on the yarns and the inherent design of the pit looms. Teenage girls were engaged to spin on these fine threads with their delicate hands. They were given poetic names, representing the quality or particular use of the material. Generally, they were called by names like *mulmul khas* (the finest sort), *jhuna* (not very fine), *ab-i-rawan* (running water), *shabnam* (evening dew), *albaillee* (unique), *tanzeb* (that adorns the body), *nayansukh* (pleasing to the eye), *seerbund* (used for turbans) and *jamdani* (figured cloth).

Although muslin was earlier produced in Dacca (in present-day Bangladesh), as the demand grew in Awadh during the Nawabi Era, muslins began to be woven in the neighbouring villages of Lucknow. In particular, muslins with damasked patterns were made at Banaras and Rampur; Jais in the Rai Bareilly district and Mamudi in Hardoi district. Varieties such as *sharbati*, *adhi* and *tarandam* were plain muslin and were produced at Mahmudnagar. Striped muslins (*doria*) were made in Mau in the Azamgarh district. The nawabs thus contributed to the textile by adding more variety to it.

JAMDANI

'These fabrics are remarkable for their fineness of texture, intricacy and flawless executions of their patterns, the charm and high artistic values of which have given Awadh a pride of place among the famous seats of the art productions in the world.'

– Pande (1968).

Jamdani is a textured weave where extra wefts are used to create patterns, while muslin is a plain weave. C.A. Silberrad (1898) has described elaborately the manufacturing process involved in the Tanda *jamdani*:

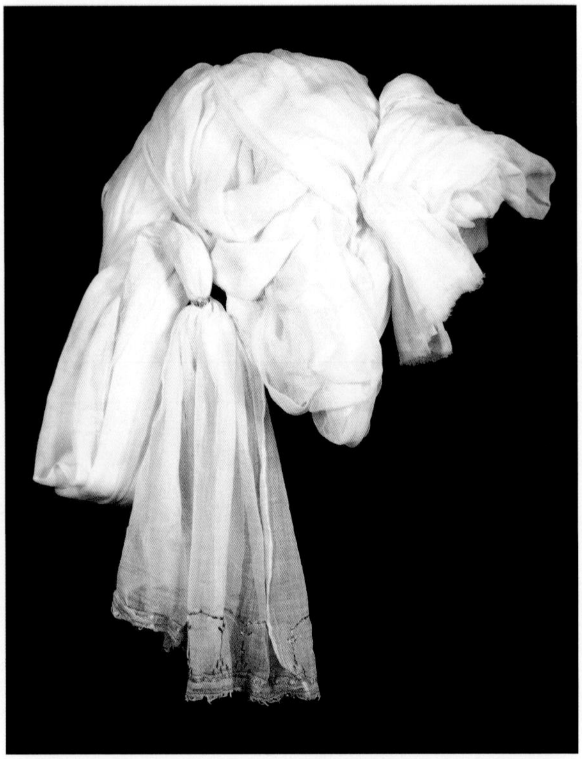

'The body of the fabric is fine muslin, quite similar to "tanzeb". The pattern is interwoven while on the loom, being made up by a series of weft threads of suitable length. Between each pair of weft threads a pair of threads of the figure to be woven is put in, the heddles being raised or depressed after one has been inserted.... The figures are made from memory or from a pattern drawn on paper.'

Earlier *jamdani* was produced in Dacca, Nadia in East Bengal (now Bangladesh), Gwalior and Madhya Pradesh. The nawabs of Awadh developed a fondness for the *jamdani* and, under their patronage, during the eighteenth century; *jamdani* came to be produced in Nawabganj in Barabanki district, Biswari in Sitapur district, and in Baiswara, Kheri, Hardoi and Jais in Rae Bareli district. 'Bhika was the master artisan from Jais, who had presented a kurta and pagri of finest work to Asaf-ud-Daula (1775-1797), interwoven with his name and praises. Unlike Dacca jamdani, where small pieces of cut threads were inserted between the threads of the warp, the weavers of Awadh *jamdani* used small bobbins containing threads (Pande, 1968).' White-on-white patterning of Awadh *jamdanis* also made them different from the Dacca *jamdanis*, where coloured and metallic threads were used.

The most important centre for Awadh *jamdani* became Tanda, in the Faizabad district, during the time of Sadat Ali Khan (1798-1814) and it was considered the most delicate form of *jamdani*. The weaving in Awadh was done by both Muslim and Hindus. Muslim weavers were known as *julaha*, while Hindus were called *katwa* or *koris*. The fabric lengths (*than*) that were produced were used for making *chogas*, *angarkhas*, kurtas and *chapkans*.

Below, Left: This rare hand-stitched *jamdani angarkha* was made at Tanda near Faizabad. The motif was woven using a thicker yarn giving it a three-dimensional effect. The yarns of varying densities created the effect of light and shadow.
Below, Right: This *chapkan* in *jamdani* is woven in a typical motif of *bel-patti adibel* (floral motif in diagonal lines) with *guldaudi* and other floral motifs running between the diagonal lines.
Facing page: The nawabs patronized *mulmul* as Persians believed all gods wore white. This *sarkar-e-ala* variety of *mulmul* is so fine that it can be passed through a ring.

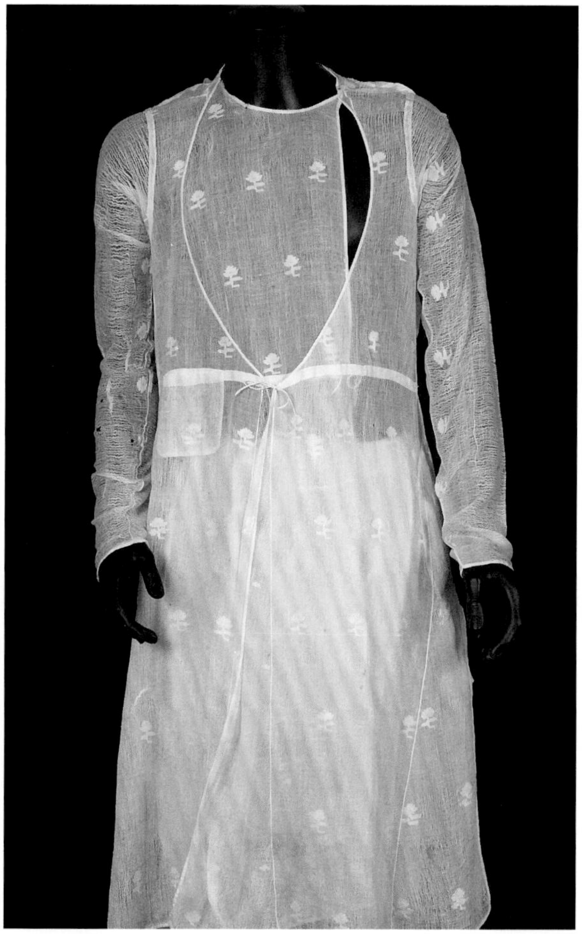

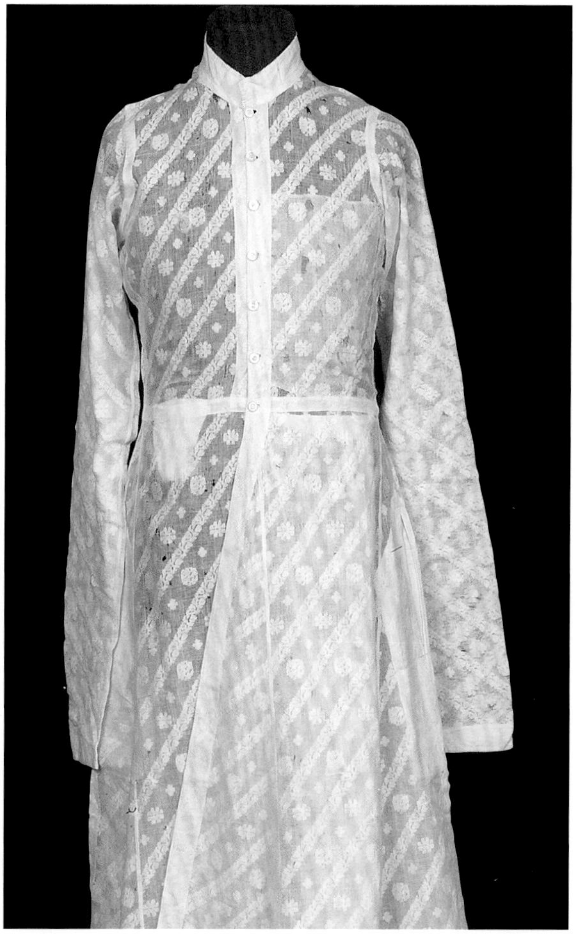

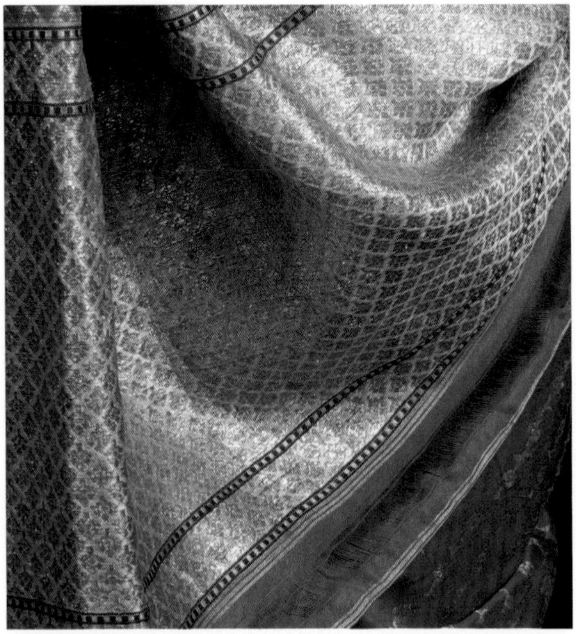

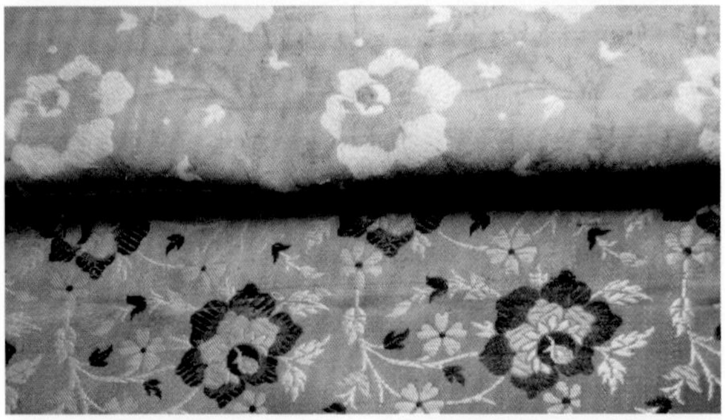

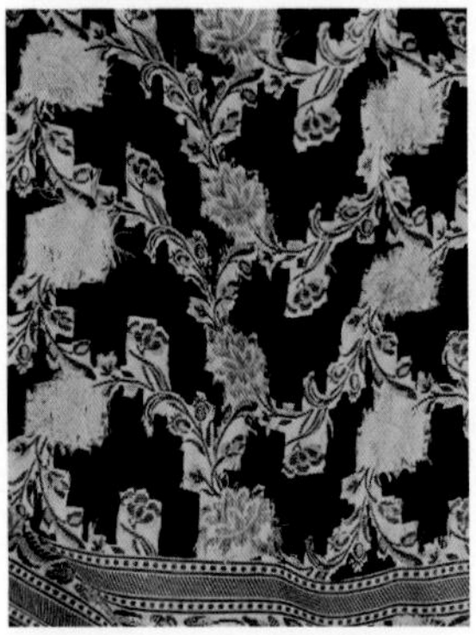

Topmost: *Pallav* of a hand-spun sari in *kinkhab* brocade. *Kinkhab* brocades were made of different thicknesses known as *ekpara, dopara, tinpara, chaupara*, *chhapara* and *satpara*. These grades were determined on the basis of the number of **zari** threads repeated in a given space. The '*ekpara*' represented ten **zari** threads in an inch.
Centre: The inside surface of a *tanchoi* is very smooth as compared to cut-work brocade as the floats are woven across the back.
Above: In this black, gold and silver cut-work brocade sari, the extra thread on the inside is cut for a clear and neat finish.

In Awadh *jamdanis*, the garment was decorated with small floral *butis* or bunches of stylized floral patterns or diagonally arranged *bel-patti* to produce a delicate and sophisticated effect. *Buti* is a single motif and is called *buta* when the motif happens to be large. The various flowers and fruits depicted were *chameli buti* (jasmine), *guldaudi buti* (chrysanthemum), *genda buti* (marigold), *turanj or kairi* (shape of a green mango with a light curve at the tip) and paan *buti* (heart-shaped or like the betel leaf). In accordance with the layout and design, these muslins were known by different names – *butidar* (when flowers were scattered all over), *tercha* (when they were grouped in diagonal lines) and *jaal* (when a running floral pattern covering the entire surface like a net). The crown motif was particularly characteristic while animal figures were rarely made.

The most sought-after *jamdanis* were known as *pench*, *juhi* (flower motif) and *khada bel barik* (fine diagonal lines), whereas the *khada bel* (straight line), *marqa* and *chand-tara* (moon and star) *butis* were considered to be of inferior quality.

BROCADES

It was in the brocades that the distinctive Awadhi Ganga-Jamuni effect was most discernible, through the simultaneous use of gold and silver threads. Silk and zari brocades were the most attractive and beautiful among fabrics, which also indicate the higher status of the wearer. Brocade is a term that applies to elaborately and intricately woven patterns in silk and cotton. Zari thread making and zari cloth weaving date back hundreds of years. The artisans were brought to Banaras from Surat during Mughal period. Shantilal Zariwala of Surat,a silk weaver says, 'One of the reasons for the development of the zari industry in Surat could be the humid climate here because of the Tapti River and the city's proximity to the Arabian Sea.' He also explains that the humid atmosphere ensures that the core yarn filament used in the zari sticks together.

The nawabs of Awadh showed a preference for the brocades of Banaras for their *chogas* and *angarkhas* and patronized these artisans. Sometimes, the *pote* (material) was specifically woven according to the designs of the *chogas*. Banaras silk brocades are mainly of three types: zari, *amru* and *abrawans*. In zari brocades, the silk yarn was interwoven with pure gold and silver threads to make patterns, which thus retain their shine for years. The two types of zari brocades are *kinkhwab*, in which gold and silver threads are more prominent than the silk yarn and *bafta*, in which the silk yarn is more predominant than the gold and silver threads, thus keeping the textile lighter. Other varieties of brocades are woven without any gold or silver. In *amru* brocades, only silk yarns are utilized to weave patterns. The two variations of *amru* are cut-work and *tanchoi*. In cut-work, the floats on the reverse are cut later by hand, whereas in *tanchoi*, a more refined type of workmanship, the floats are woven back into the fabric. In *abrawan*, organza is used in combination with silk yarn to create a stiffer texture.

Brocade weaving involved a well-defined process. The *naksha* (design) was first made on paper, known as *likhai* (writing), and was then woven with a cotton thread on a small wooden frame as a sample. Once the sample was acceptable, the weavers proceeded to the final weaving with zari threads, silk yarn, or both. *Naqshabands* were the pattern makers who translated a design into a system of pattern making that was suitable for *jaala* weaving. They frequently also planned the original sketch of the design. They trace their ancestry to Muhammad Bahud-din au-Naqshaband (1389), the founder of the Naqshabandiyya Sufi sect from Bokhara. Even today, the *naqshabands* of Banaras observe the annual day of the pir.

The main motifs used in Banaras brocades were classified as *butidar* (with small, single flower pattern), *phulwar* (floral motifs), *tasvir* (portrait or picture), geometrical and *shikargah* (hunting scenes). Patterns with flowering stems were called *adibel* (diagonal lines), *gende ki bel* (marigold flowers), *khajuri bel* (date-like) and *dohri bel* (with double lines).

The weavers experimented with newer shades like *sultani surkh* (scarlet), *pyazi* (onion coloured), *karaundia* (light crimson), *nibu* (lemon yellow), *kapasi* (pale yellow), *gandhaki* (sulphur yellow), *mungia* (olive green) and *lajwardi* (lapis lazuli) for rendering the effect of *minakari* (enamel), in addition to the main colours (red, maroon, yellow, orange, blue).

Mainaphal and *maldahi* were types of cotton brocade when coloured *butis* were brocaded on a coloured base. *Maldahi* derives its name from a place called Malda near Banaras. *Jamdani* is also a kind of brocade.

MAKHMAL (VELVET)

Makhmal or velvet, one of the most beautiful and luxurious fabrics, was used profusely by the nawabs in Lucknow. *Makhmal* is Arabic in origin and was brought

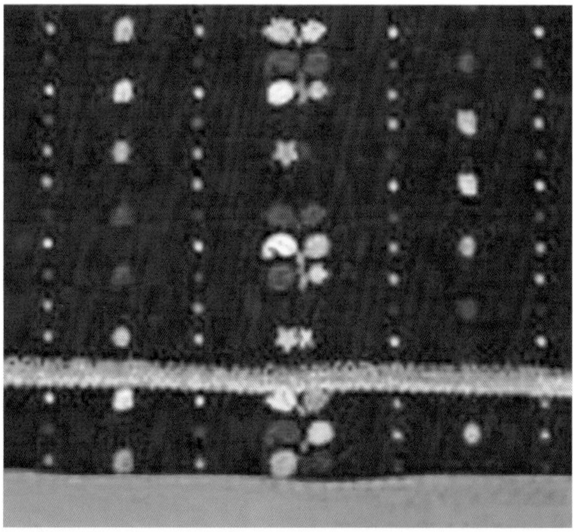

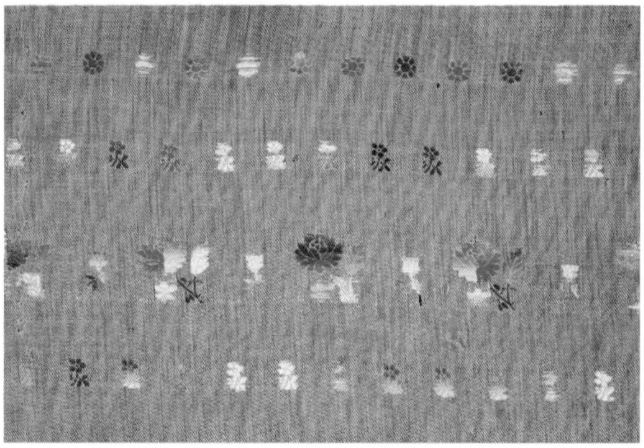

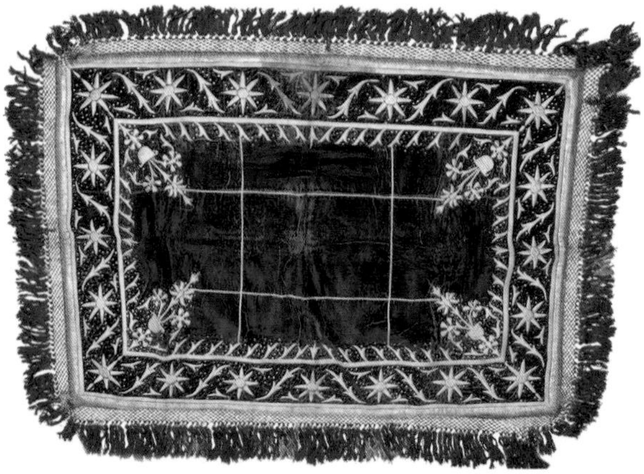

Topmost: Vibrant colours have been used in this *maldahi* cotton brocade on purple background to enhance the richness of the design.
Centre: Cotton brocade *maldahi* with multi-coloured floral *butis* on ochre field.
Below: This heavy velvet *takht-posh* (bedcover) is embroidered in gold zardozi with contrasting blue border edged with tassels. A *gamla-buti* motif decorates the corners and small metal discs are used to give a shimmering effect.

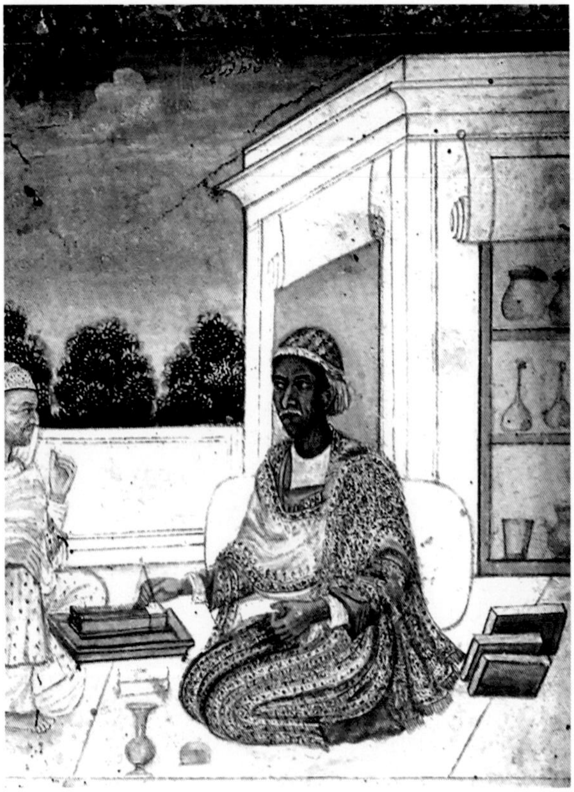

Calligraphist Hafiz Nurullah wearing *jamawar choga* and an intricately woven multi-coloured *jamawar* shawl.

to India by Arab traders. Earlier, it was mainly used for tents, canopies, carpets and saddles. In Awadh, *makhmal* was used abundantly in ceremonial costumes and for special occasions.

Unlike the brocade, *makhmal* offered a plain background to the artisans to show their workmanship, and the zardoz artisans enriched them with gold, silver, pearls and precious stones to render exquisite pieces of work.

JAMAVAR

Jamavar weaving holds the pride for being one of the best forms of the weaving art. Originally, the word *jamavar* referred to the 3 ¾ yard woven fabric lengths used for making *jamas* (long coats)—*jama* meaning robe and *var* meaning yard. The nawabs were fond of this art that has its origins in the fifteenth century when Zain-ul-abidin ruled Kashmir, and reached its zenith during the Mughal period. Emperor Akbar started the practice of wearing it as a shawl in winters.

Jamavar shawls were made from the fine yarns spun from the wool of the Capra hircus goat found in Kashmir. First, the wool was cleaned, spun into yarn by women and then sold to the dyers. It was woven with a twill-tapestry technique by using wooden spools known as *tojli* or *kanni*. These wooden spools wrapped around a specific number of warp threads and interlocked whenever a change of colour was required. In this technique only weft threads formed the pattern and several *kannis* of different colours were used for a single weft line of the fabric, running across horizontally. The number of spools used depended on the complexity of the design, varying from 400 to 1,500.

The process involved in the making of a *jamavar* shawl is best explained by Meera Kumar: 'Once the warp was laid, it would take anywhere between 18 months to three years to weave a *jamavar* depending upon the intricacy of the design. To prevent yarn breakage for these long sessions on the warp, warp dressers starched the threads with a thin paste of rice flour to prevent them from fraying and breaking on the loom. This was later washed out and the waters of Jhelum were said to have a special effect on the fabric imparting a unique softness to the finished product (The Taj Magazine, 2006).'

A vast variety of colours were used for weaving. Up to fifty colours could be used to make a single shawl. The most popular colours were *zard* (yellow), *safed* (white), *firozi* (turquoise), *ingari* (green), *uda* (purple), *gul-e-anar* (pomegranate crimson), orange, saffron and *kirmiz* (scarlet). Most of the colours were produced by vegetable dyes. To produce *mushki* (black) colour iron fillings were used, which was also responsible for the early damage of the shawl cloth.

The typical design of the *jamavar* shawls consisted of patterned borders, running along the four sides and two broad ones at both ends. Usually there were a row of *kairis* at the base borders and the surface was intricately filled with numerous smaller motifs and scrolling vines. Tree-of-life motif, small flowering plants and animal motifs were also popular. According to Paisley Museum, the *turanj* or *kairi* pattern can be traced back to ancient Babylon, where a tear-drop shape was used as a symbol to represent the growing shoot of a date palm. The palm provided food, drink, clothing (woven fibres) and shelter, and so became regarded as the 'Tree of Life', with its growing shoot being gradually recognized as a fertility symbol.

As the nineteenth century progressed, designs became even more complex and production was split between two or more looms. The woven pieces were then sewn together by a *rafoogar* (master needle worker) with stitches so fine that the joints were invisible.

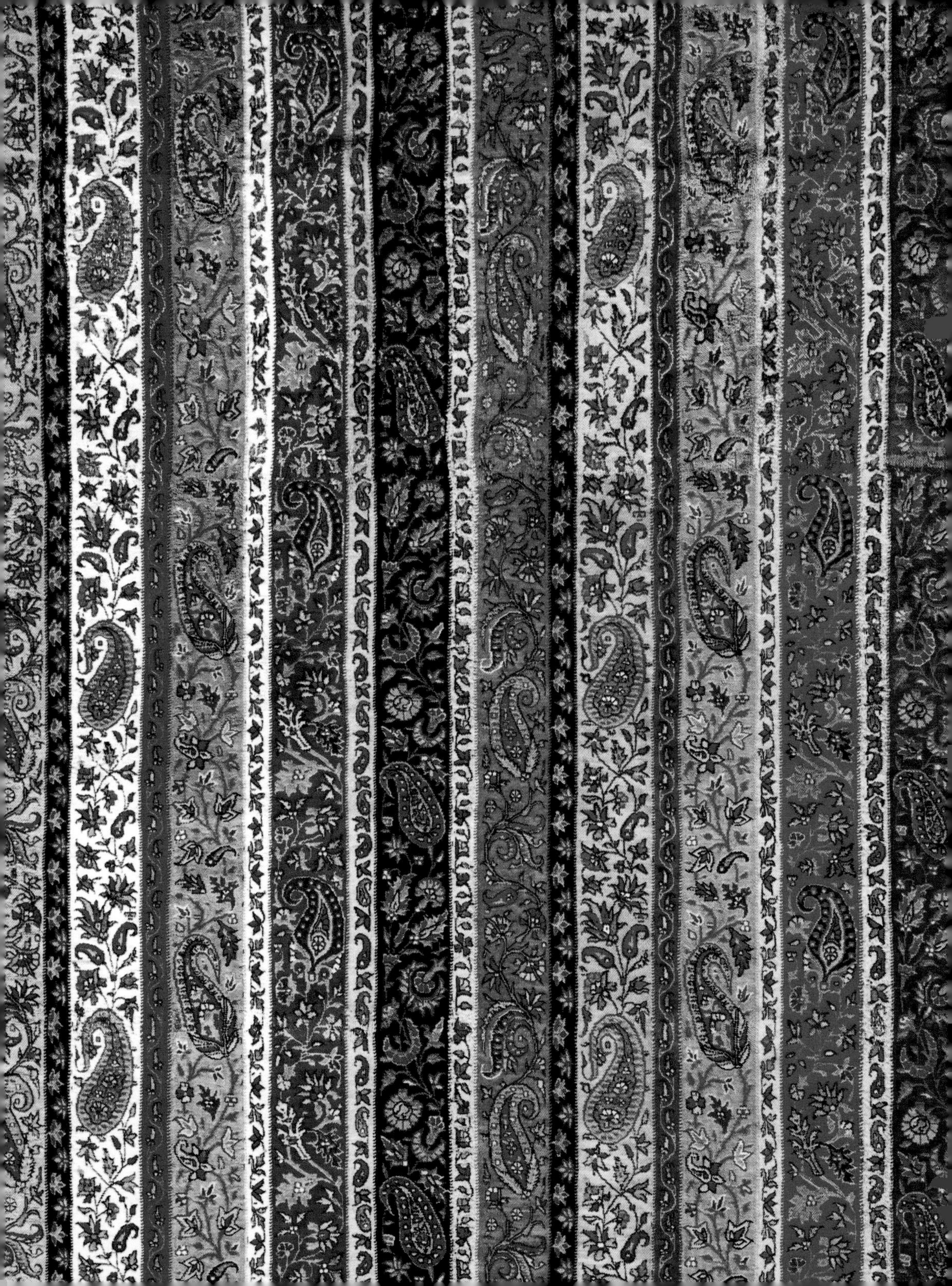

ORNAMENTATIONS

There was no textile centre in Lucknow before the nawabs: brocades were produced in Banaras, muslin in Dacca and *jamavar* in Kashmir. In the late eighteenth century, under Nawab Asaf-ud-Daula, when the court of Awadh was flourishing with its capital in Lucknow, many of the master artisans of India came from Bengal, Gujarat, Hyderabad, Rajasthan and Kashmir. It became a centre for creativity and developed its own ornamentation styles. These were unique and of unparalleled beauty. Some of these ornamentations are still in current use.

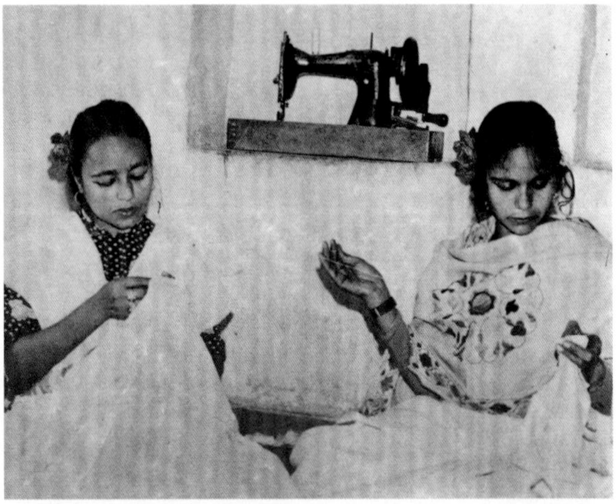

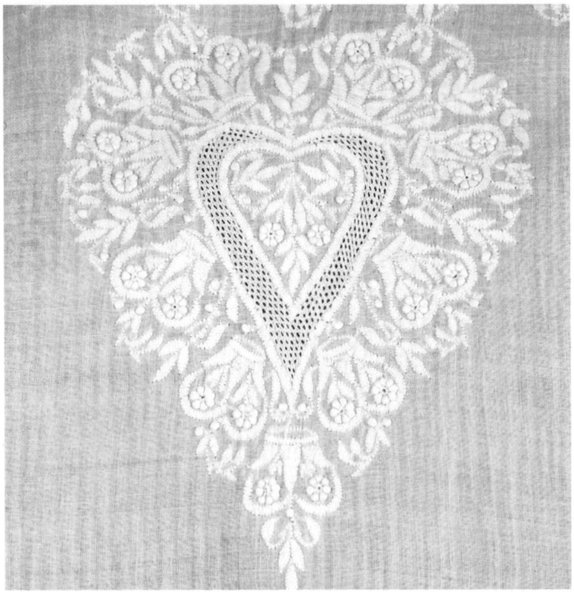

Topmost: Aktar Jahan (left) working on chikan embroidery.
Above: *Pusht* of a *chapkan showing* intricately embroidered *kanta-patti, ghas-patti, jaali* and *phanda* stitches. The crown motif became popular after the nawabs were given the title of King.

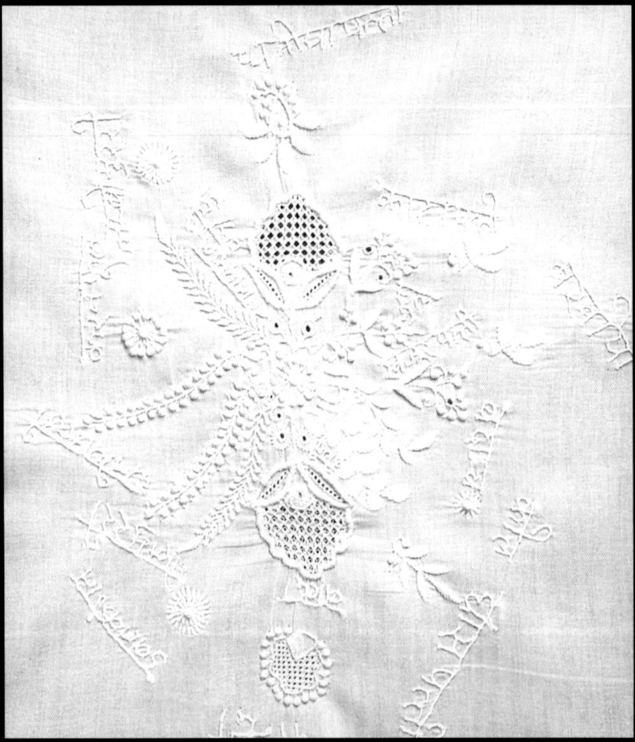

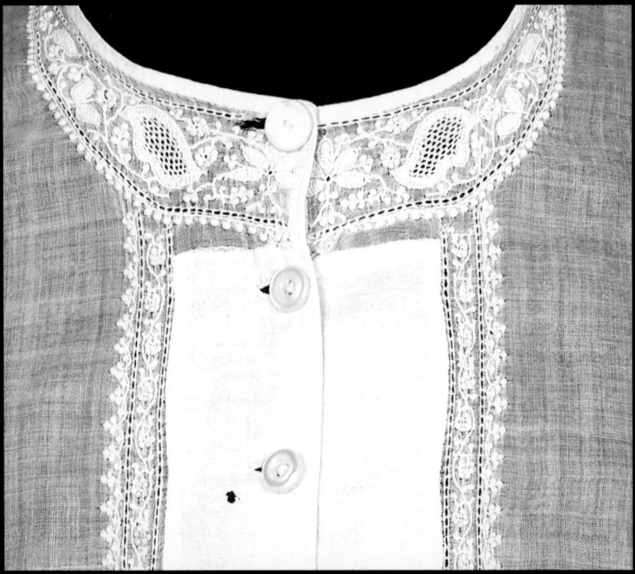

Above: A sample of *chikankari* showing a bouquet of various *chikankari* stitches. The finely embroidered muslin with *chikankari* came to be identified with the nawabi culture.
Below: The delicate *siddhaur* and *hatkati jali* stitch is used to decorate this half-moon design on round neck and *phanda* stitch in *muga paat,* using golden silk from Assam, to highlight the borders. The overall effect is that of gold zari.

Chikankari

The artisans involved in chikan embroidery can be classified as *thappagars* (block-makers), *chhapagirs* (printers), *rangrej* (dyers), *darzis* (tailors), *chuckendoz* (embroiderers) and *dhobis* (washermen). Then there are traders who take care of the marketing of the goods and control the whole process of *chikankari*.

The designing on the fabric is done with the help of wooden blocks. The wood blocks are made of shisham wood (Dalbergia sissoo). The printer then transfers the design on to the cloth; the woodblocks do not have a handle as these are rolled onto the cloth. Then a dye of fugitive colours, *neel* (indigo) or magenta, is made by mixing with gum acacia. Gum acacia is used as a binder because it dissolves easily in water. This is called *likhai* and thereafter the fabric is embroidered. These clothes are steamed over a *bhatti* (clay oven) overnight to take out the indigo or magenta dye. These were then washed in soapy water along the River Gomti. The last step of the process consists in applying starch to these clothes and ironing them.

There are thirty-six stitches of *chikankari* in all and six basic ones, on which the others are based. There are three main categories of basic stitches in *chikankari*; to name them in increasing order of difficulty: flat, *murri* and *jali*. The stitches are sometimes used individually but more often in combination of two or more together to make a full pattern. Each stitch has an individual name, specific number of threads and a specific use. Some stitches are worked from behind the fabric and others from the front. Chikan embroidery is done with a 3.5 cm long needle with a small eye, and a little longer one (5.5 cm) is used for *jali* work or (pulled thread work).

Flat stitches are delicate and are mainly used to provide a subtle background by remaining close to the surface of the fabric. Some stitches are used to create the designs on the front side of the fabric such as the *hool* (eyelet), which is used to form the centre of a flower, and the *zanzeera* (chain stitch), which is used to outline leaves or petals. Additional stitches are used either for background or to complete patterns, such as banarsi and *tepchi* (running stitch), which are often used to create stems for flowers. Other stitches are adopted to create a design from the wrong side of the fabric, such as *bakhiya* (shadow stitch) and *rahet* (stem stitch).

Murri work is characterized by a relief on the surface of the fabric and creates an embossed effect. These stitches give richness to the pattern. One stitch of this kind is known as *phanda* (loop), which is similar to a big French knot. The knots are very minute and spherical not oval shaped as in *murri*. It is done with six threads and on the right side of the fabric. This is one of the most graceful stitches of chikan work. *Mundi murri* is used for making a longish petal, broad on one side and pointed on the other end, tapered towards the stem, while *nukili murri* (pointed leaf), is used to form a petal tapered on both ends – it is worked on the front side of the fabric with nine threads. The *murmora* stitch is used to finish the trailing stem with a small bud. *Kauri* (shell-shaped), *boot patti* (a leaf with a central spine) and *chikan ki ghass* (grass) are used to finish the leaf giving it a spiked look.

Jali work or 'pulled-work' stitch is the most striking stitch of chikan embroidery. For *jali* work only one strand is used while for other stitches up to twelve to fourteen strands can be used. In true *jali* the tar (threads) of the warp and weft are pushed on one side by the needle and held in position by an extremely minute button-holing. It is mainly used for filling the flowers. A blunt needle is used to work smoothly on the reverse side of the fabric. Main types are known as *siddhaur jaali* (diagonal design), *chataya jaali* (square effect), *bangla jaali* (alternates squares of fabric with square holes, worked diagonally) and the more complex *madrazi jaali* where a small cross is seen in each of the holes. A fifth stitch known as *hatkadi* (handcuff) is used to give a straight outline of pulled holes to an edge. This very stitch has two more variations to give an ornamental look, known as *dohri hatkadi* (double) and *maheen hatkadi* (very fine).

The most common motif used is that of a creeper. Among floral motifs, jasmine, rose, flowering stems and the paisley motif are the most popular. Calligraphy, bird motifs and, in later period, coronary motifs were also used. Individual floral motifs are also used to embellish the entire garment or to embellish the corners of the garment.

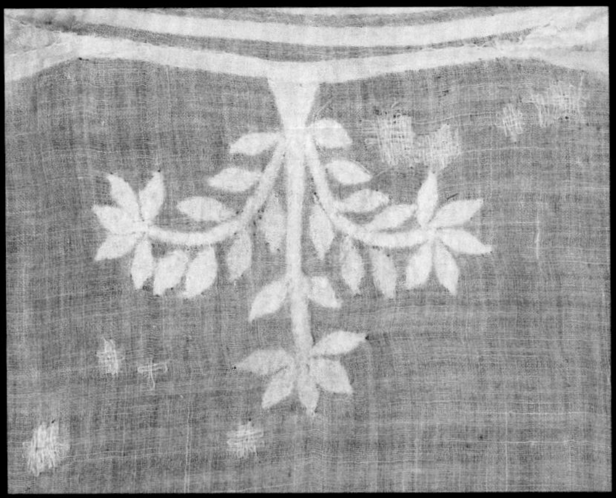

This *phool-patti ka kaam* is also known as *khatao* or reverse applique. The flower and leaf motif applied on the inner-side of the garment embellish the *pusht* of the *angarkha*.

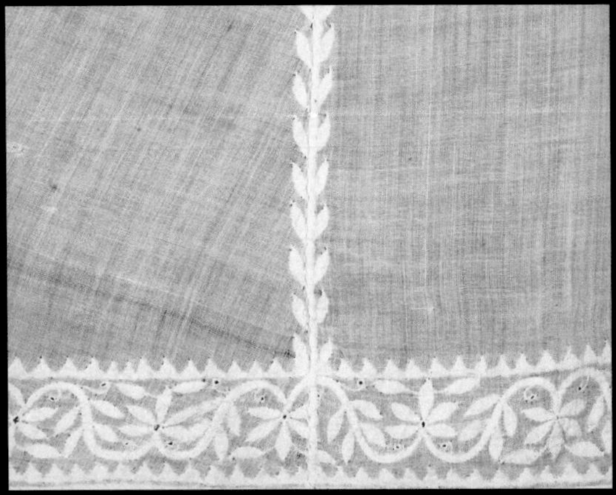

The *kalis* are joined together and the seams are decorated with *daraz ka kaam* with a leaf motif.

CHIKANKARI

Chikankari is the most artistic and delicate type of white-on-white embroidery and provides elegance to the garment by laying special emphasis on the technique, forms and designs. In perfect nawabi *nazakat* and *nafasat*, its charm lies in its minuteness, evenness and its subtle appearance. This craft was used to embellish *chogas*, *angarkhas*, kurtas, topis and *chapkans*.

Historically, *chikankari* was done in Dacca and Calcutta in Bengal. It was brought to Lucknow during the period of luxury and extravagance that characterized the court of Awadh. The *chikankari* of Lucknow became popular and reached its zenith in the nineteenth century.

PHOOL PATTI KA KAAM

As the name suggests, the embroidery motifs are in the shape of flowers and leaves. This is a delicate form of applique work on cotton that flourished in Aligarh under the nawabs. This textile decoration style consists of little pieces of fine muslin fabric that are cut by hand and then delicately folded and stitched onto the fabric to create a variety of beautiful patterns in shapes of *phool patti*. The entire embroidery is done by hand. This work used to adorn the neckline and *pusht* (back) of *angarkhas* of the nawabs and *shalukas* and dupattas worn by the begums. This art is mainly practised by womenfolk, who are referred to as *patti karigars*. In *khatao* work, or reverse applique, the pattern is cut and sewn on the inner side of the garment, creating a smooth finish on the outer side of the garment.

DARAZ KA KAAM (COTTON)

Daraz ka kaam is a unique way of assembling two pieces of a garment through invisible stitches, that are concealed in the *daraz* (fissure) and produce a decorative see-through effect. Tiny pieces of muslin, cut out in different shapes, are applied either on the surface or between the two surfaces and outlined with fine stitches. All this used to be done by hand, including the finishing of edges and joining of the seams. It is visible only when seen against the light. It was through these kinds of touches of detailed workmanship that the nawabi refinement and elegance permeated the atmosphere. Different motifs were used for joining the seams, such as *phool daraz* (flower), *macchli daraz* (fish) and *patti daraz* (leaves).

ZARDOZI

Zardozi, being opulent and luxurious in nature, was greatly adopted and appreciated by the nawabs and reached its highest level of sophistication during the Nawabi period. It is an embroidered extravaganza in gold and silver threads, predominantly produced on *makhmal, kinkwabs* (type of brocade) or precious silks. The word zardozi is derived from two Persian words, *zar* meaning gold and silver threads, and *dozi* meaning embroidery. It is said that Prophet Hazrat Yusuf was the inventor of this regal craft and his anniversary, Huzur ki Miraj, is celebrated by offering prayers and food.

Israr Husain of Lucknow, an artisan of zardozi, has described the workmanship as follows. The first step is to trace a pattern or design on butter paper, which is then transferred on the cloth to be worked upon. Next, the

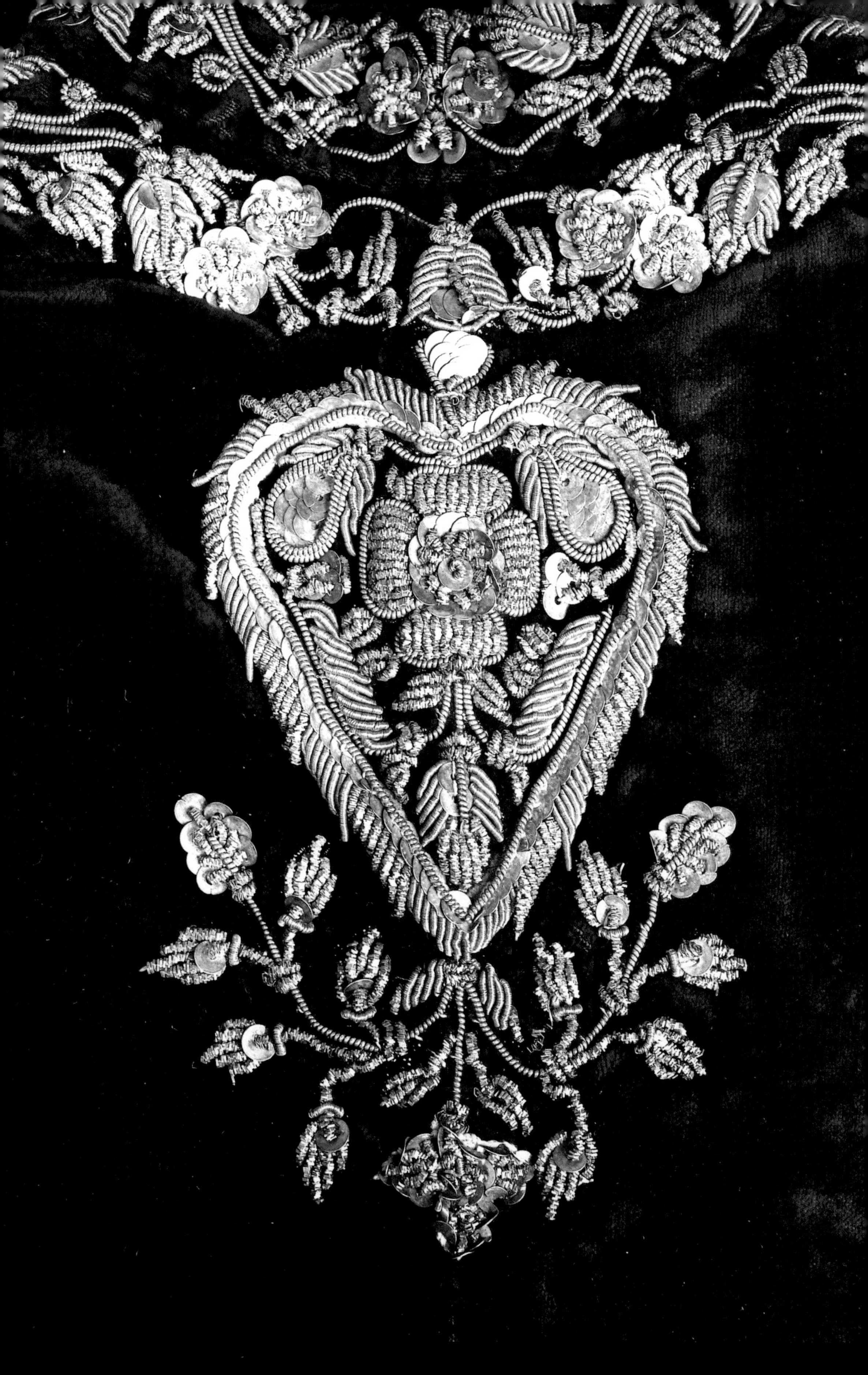

A floral motif is embroidered in pure gold **zari** with *tilla, kasabs, tiki, salma, sitara* and precious stones on purple velvet.

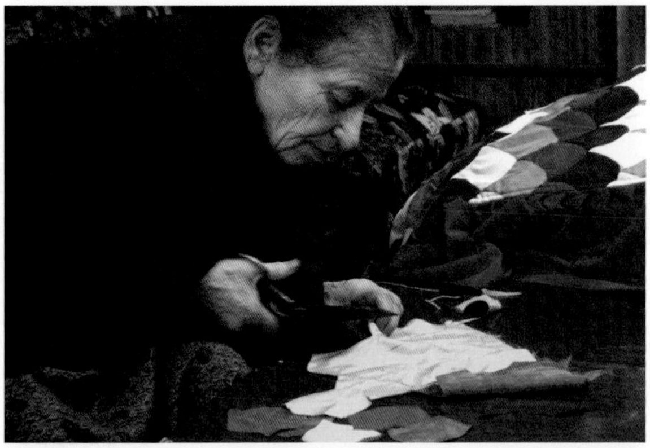

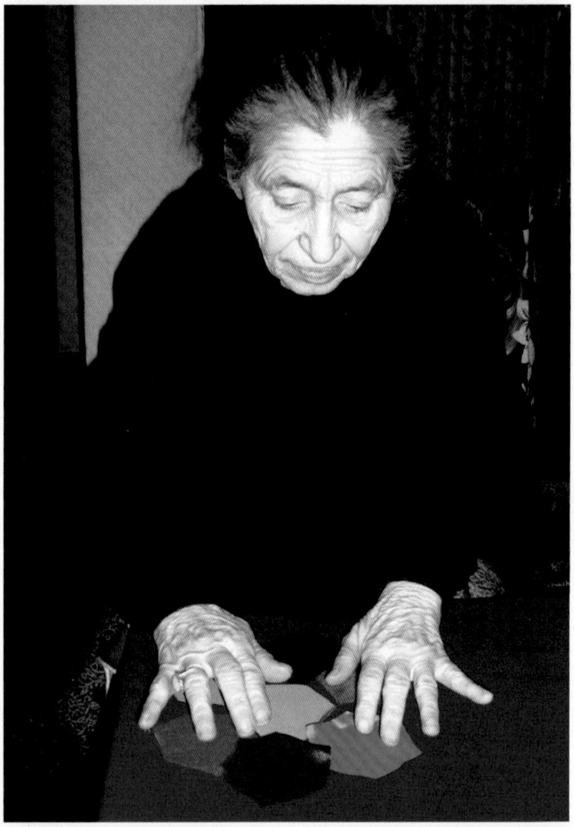

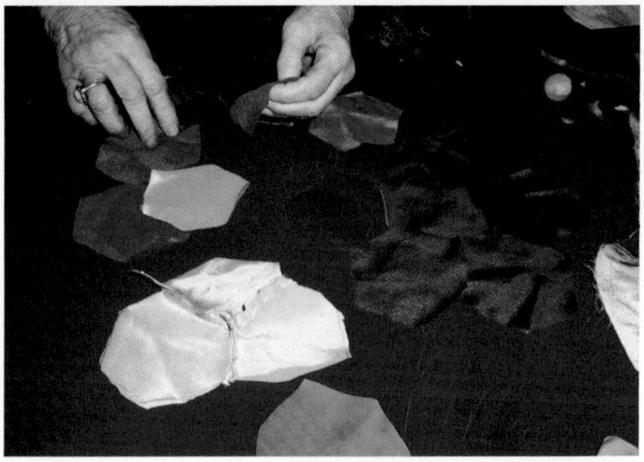

cloth is tightly fixed to an *adda* (wooden frame also known as karchob) with the help of a cord, ready for embroidery. A peculiarity of zardozi is that the embroidery is not done with a needle, but with a *muthia*, which is a crocheted type hook with a wooden, rounded top. A second, more noticeable, characteristic is the rich look derived from the materials used in zardozi: pure gold and pure silver threads of different types like *tilla*, *gird*, *chapta* (flat) and *jhilmil* (offering shimmering effect); *kasabs* (sequins); *tiki* (flat sequins); *katori* (cupshaped sequins); pot (small beads); *surahi* and *kardan* shaped sequins; *kalabutton* and pearls. Zardozi was profusely used for decorating lehengas, dupattas, *farshi* paijamas, gharare, *batua*s, and later also *chapkans*, *achkans*, waistcoats, caps and shoes. The main motifs were buds, flowers, fruits, birds, peacocks and fish.

CHATTA-PATTI OR TUKRI KA KAAM

The most unique and original type of workmanship in Awadh was the *chatta-patti* work. This work was labour-intensive and required large quantities of precious silk. I had the pleasure of interviewing Dr Attia Zaidi, a famous *chatta-patti* artisan of Lucknow. The chief garments upon which such embroidery was done were *kalidar* paijamas and *farshi* paijamas. The finished paijama was called 'tukri ki gote ka paijama'.

The workmanship consisted in sewing various fabrics of varying colours and designs. A pattern was made on a piece of cardboard called *farma* and layers of differently coloured fabrics were cut according to the designs of the *farma*. These pieces were then skilfully sewn together, according to a particular colour scheme. The colours chiefly used were *rani* (pinkish-purple), yellow, *pistai* (pistachio-green), *firozi* (turquoise), *pyazi* (onion-coloured) and *baingani* (violet). Light colours were contrasted with dark colours. Some popular combinations were orange-green, cream-maroon and purple-yellow.

Chatta-patti has a rich repertoire of patterns. The most common was the *mahapusht* (shape of fishscales) as it developed on the emblem of the nawabs of Awadh. The level of complexity in the workmanship depended on the number of angles involved in the pattern. In fact, the most difficult patterns were the *sitare ki gote* (star-shaped) and *ashtpahal* (having eight sides). Other patterns included *chariyon ki gote* (straight vertical lines), *gilloriyon* or *singhare ki gote* (triangular-shaped), *patake ki gote* (square-shaped), *namakpare ki gote* (diamond-shaped), *katari ki gote* (semi-circular shaped), *koni ki gote* (horizontal zig-zag design) and *aari-chariyon ki gote* (diagonal lines).

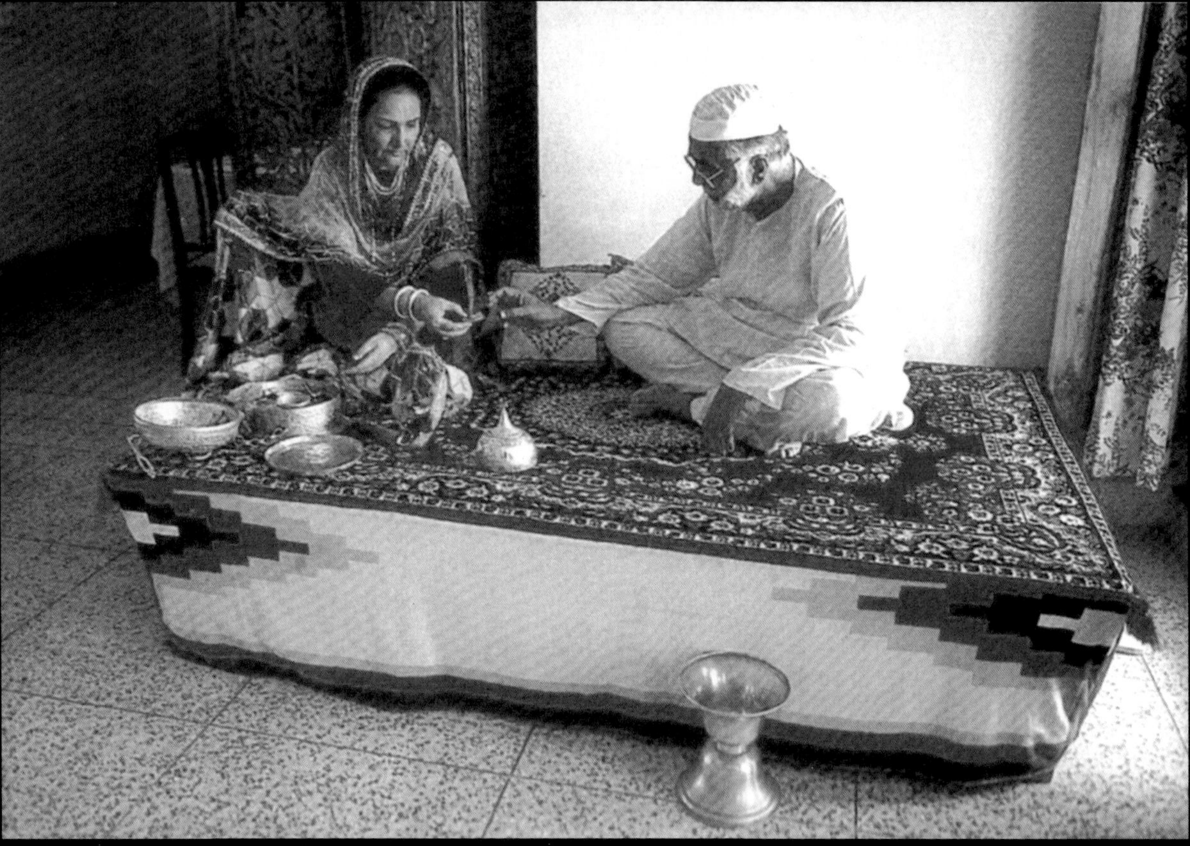

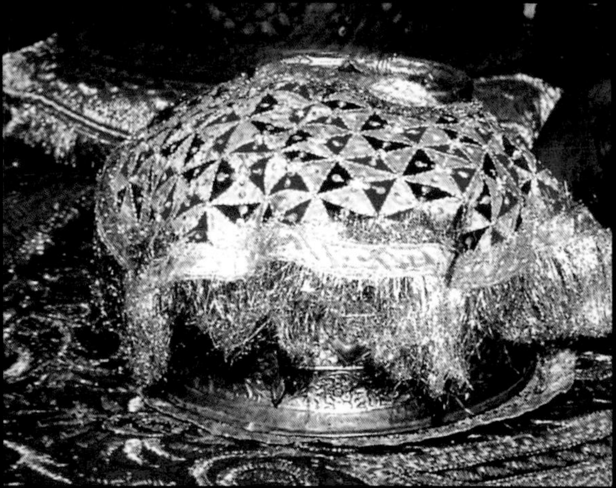

KAMDANI

Kamdani is another rare craft of Awadh and epitomizes the exemplary Lucknavi delicacy of the opulent courts of the nawabs. Using both gold and silver wires together created the beautiful Ganga-Jamuni effect, characteristic of the era. While in brocades this effect is achieved by weaving with gold and silver zari threads, in *kamdani* it is achieved by embroidery with gold and silver wires. Such embroidery was usually produced on silk and cotton.

Pure gold and silver flat wires were used to create small knots or dots called fardi. In the words of Sudipta Dev, 'The *badla* [flattened gold or silver wire] is attached to the thread of a needle. As the needle passes through the cloth, tightened around the finger, the succeeding folds of the wire on the cloth make the knot or *buti*. A minimum of three folds are needed for *teen sui ki fardi* [three-thread knots]. By increasing the number of wire folds, the size of the knots also increases … the folds are rubbed with a cowrie (shell) in order to deeply embed it in the cloth (Marg, 2003).'

The main stitches used were *karanphool* (straight-line flower), *mundaphool* (flower with petals) and *patta* (leaf) and the popular motifs were floral *buti*s, peepal or paan and *amiya* or *kairi*. This craft is mainly done on white chiffon and, once completed, it can be dyed in any colour desired without losing the shine of the *badla*. The chunnis of cotton, and later of net and chiffon, were sprinkled with *fardi buti*s that created a shimmering effect of star-lit night. The minute *fardi buti*s were joined to form elaborate motifs.

GOTA KA KAAM

This craft had its origin in Rajasthan and the artisans were given patronage in the court of the nawabs. A *gota* is a ribbon in which gold or silver thread forms the weft and silk or cotton thread the warp. With a slight hemming or simple running stitch, *gota* work involves placing woven ribbon onto the garment to create different surface textures. This can be plain or can be pressed with a hot wooden block to produce crimples, giving a sense of movement to the surface. The pressings are of various designs. Different names are given according to the width of the *gota*. A two-inch broad *gota* is called *lachka* and when it is pressed with a hot wooden block, it is known to be pattha; thin *gota* is

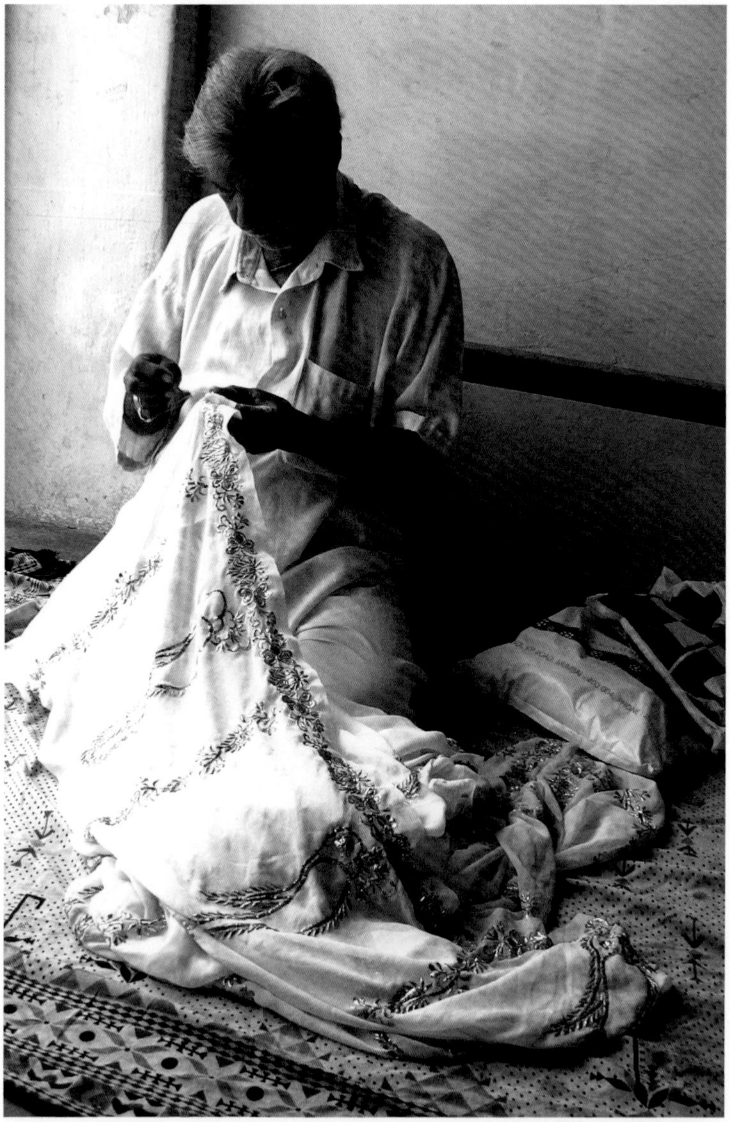

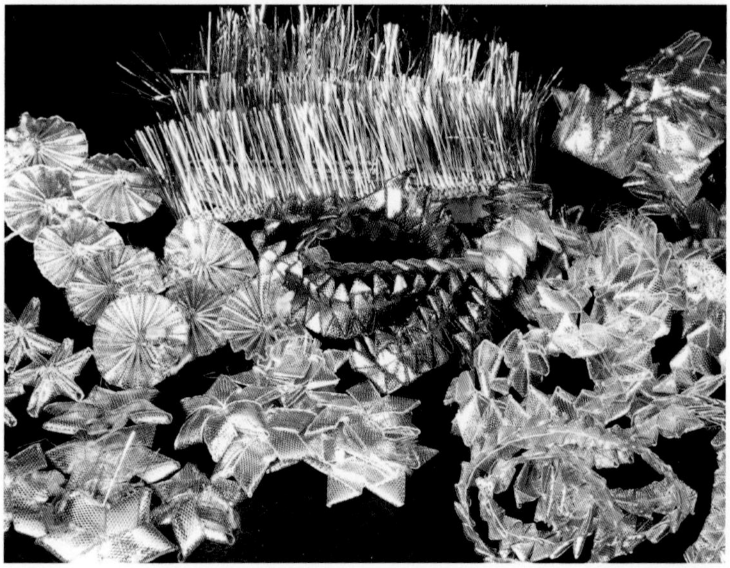

Above: An artisan of *kamdani*. **Right:** A variety of embellishments made with *gota*. *Kiran* (fringe) is used only to embellish the edges, similar to tassels.

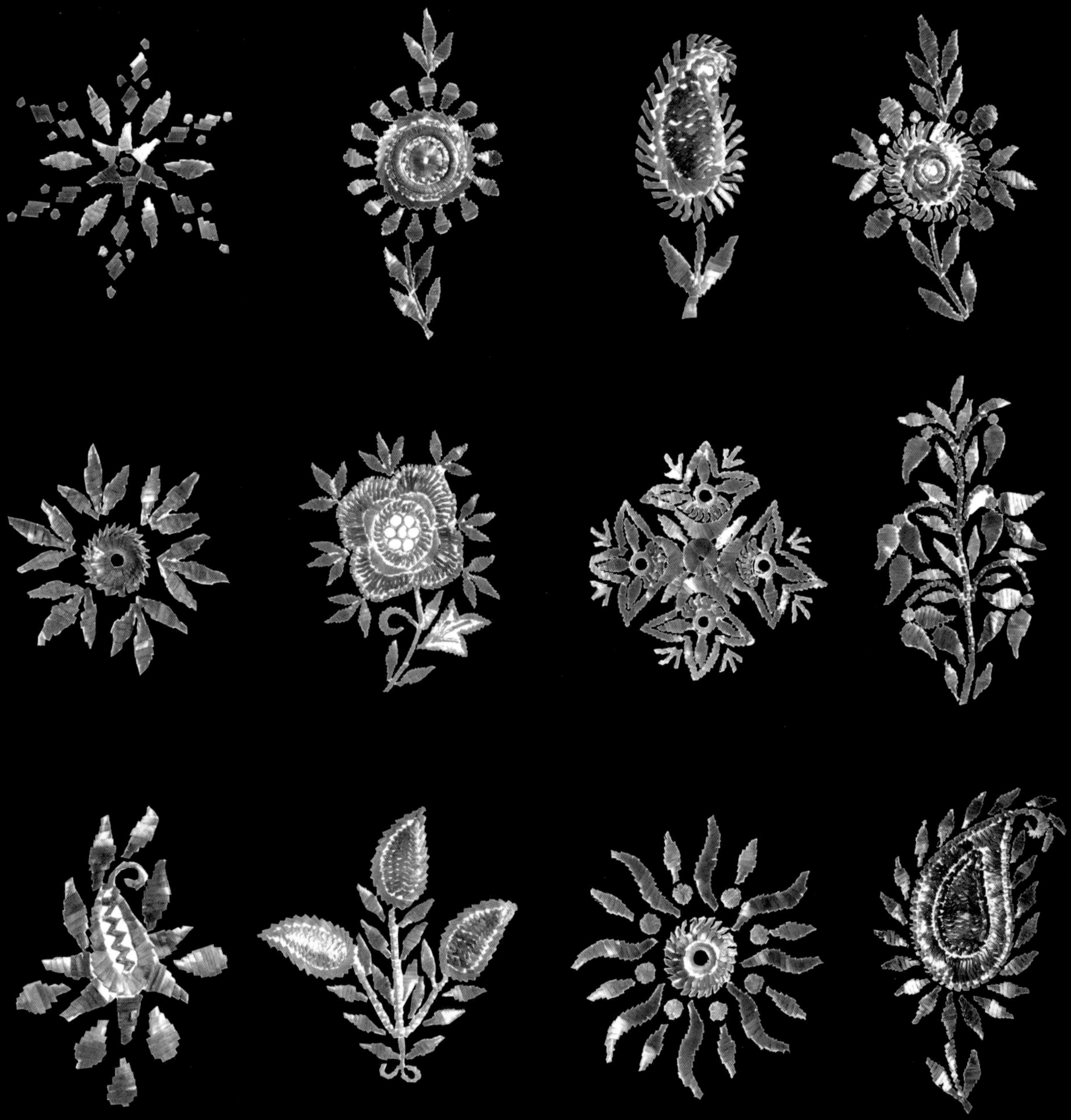

First row: *Sitara* (star motif), *phool* (flower motif), *amiya* (raw mango motif), *phool* (flower motif).
Second row: Variation of *sitara* motif, *phool* motif, *guldasta* (bunch of flowers) motif, tree of life motif.
Third row: Flower bud motif, trifoglio motif, *suraj* (sun) motif, *juhi kali* (jasmine bud) motif.

called *dhanak* or *dhanush*, meaning rainbow; hoof-shaped is *chutki*; pointed *gota* is *champa*; and one with diagonal lines is *uttudar*; *bankuri* is a thin *gota*, used to embellish the borders of chunnis. It was used in various forms and shapes to make motifs and created sheer magic on dupattas, *farshi* paijamas, *kalidar* paijamas and lehengas. This made these garments perfect for festive and formal wear. *Kinari/kiran*, or edging, is the fringed or tasselled border used to add a beautiful finish.

VEREK KA KAAM

The popularity of *verek ka kaam* (a technique of printing) reflects the luxurious lifestyle of the nawabs. In this technique, engraved hand-blocks were dipped in a resinous substance and then stamped on to the fabric. The pattern is then sprinkled with gold, silver or mica, which adheres to the area with resin on it to produce a rich surface. Further lustre is given to the fabric by buffing it on a stone. Gold and silver were used to add a rich effect to the garments of nawabs. This technique was brought to Awadh from Rajputana region (present-day Rajasthan).

BLOCK PRINTING

The textile hand printing industry of Awadh is over 300 years old with its centre in Farrukhabad. Although established much earlier it flourished under the patronage of the nawabs. A number of wooden blocks, depending on the complexity of the design, are needed to complete one design. These blocks are made of shisham and come from the neighbouring city of Lucknow. The blocks are kept in oil for a few days to increase their softness.

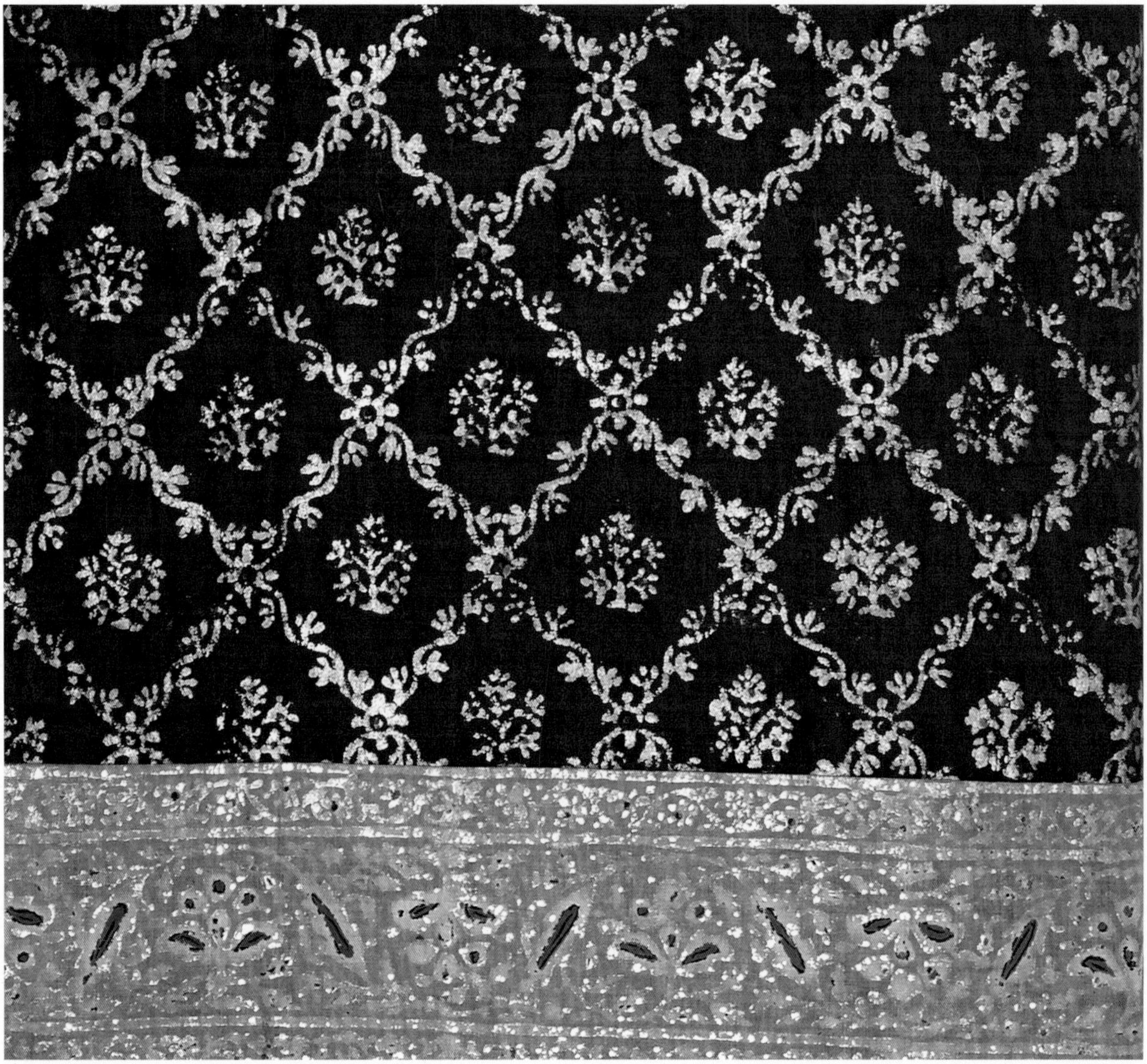

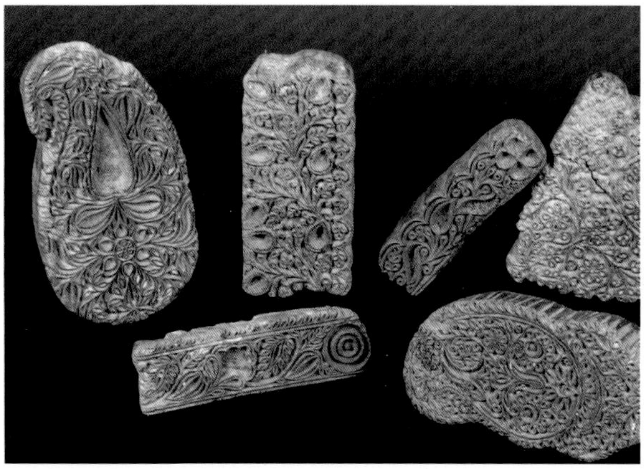

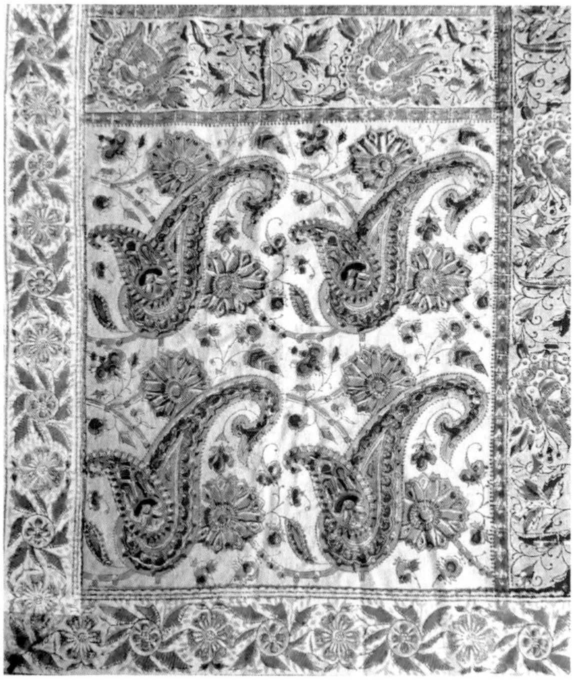

Above: Wooden blocks used for block-printing.
Right: *Turanj/kairi* motif is seen in the block printed fabrics of Jehangirabad (Lucknow), known for toned down colours and bold lines in the Indo-Persian tradition. The ideal seasons for block printing are the dry months. Excellence is achieved only if the block is freshly and perfectly chiseled.
Facing page: Fabric is hand-spun and block printed with a resin to which silver leaf is applied. The border is in contrasting green colour. The floral diagonal grid holds a *buta* with matching green dots in the centre of the flowers.

The first step in the process of transferring the design on to the fabric involves making an outline called *raek*. The block makers from Philakuva in Uttar Pradesh specialize in making blocks with engraved brass wires into the grooves, that are used for outlining the design. The design is traced on the fabric with the aid of a small *tipni* (iron needle). Through a process called *dattai*, different colours are then printed over the outline in sequential order. Once the design is complete, the textile is dipped in diluted sulfuric acid for fixing the colour. Finally, the textile is washed in running water.

During the nawabi period, block printing was mainly employed on hand-spun cotton, silk and *mashru* fabrics and it was used for quilted *angarkhas*, *dagla*, *mirzai*, quilt covers and curtains. It was known as Lakhnavi fard. The traditional prints of Lucknow were *kairi* (mango) called *kehri* or *turanj* in Awadh, *bicchu, phool, chena-patti, bajra* and *jamavar*. Animal, bird and human figures, along with the floral and the geometric patterns were other designs.

DYEING

Doshe nazuk par dupatta is kadar rukta na tha,
Kal jo rangne me zara gahra gulabi ho gaya.
(The veil was unable to rest on my delicate shoulders,
For yesterday it was dyed to a deeper pink than usual.)

The Awadh region has always been famed for its dyes. Dyeing is the process by which a fabric is immersed in a solution, mixed with colours extracted from vegetable, animal and mineral sources, in order to dye it. Begums and other women dyed their chunnis in various colours for festive occasions. Excellence in dyeing was achieved by a dyer from Fatehganj, who was capable of dyeing two sides of cloth in two different colours. Gama was another master dyer at the time of Nasir-ud-Din Haider. The use of *jhamak* or *bukka* (mica flakes), mixed with colours, added extraordinary beauty to the chunnis and saris.

A technique of tie-and-dye called *lahariya* (diagonal lines of alternate colour) was also used for dyeing chunnis. Compared to other regions, Awadh developed its own method. Firstly, the dampened chunnis were folded in various layers and spread horizontally on wooden planks. Then *fitas* (cotton ribbons) of various colours and widths were applied on the chunnis. This process involves two dyers simultaneously: one holds it tight with the index finger and thumb on both sides and the second person presses the *fitas* with the finger. In this way the colour penetrates all the folds of the chunni and creates the coloured diagonal designs. Latif, a famous dyer of Lucknow, told me that the secret of the vibrancy of colours resulted from the use of alum as a mordant in dyeing textiles.

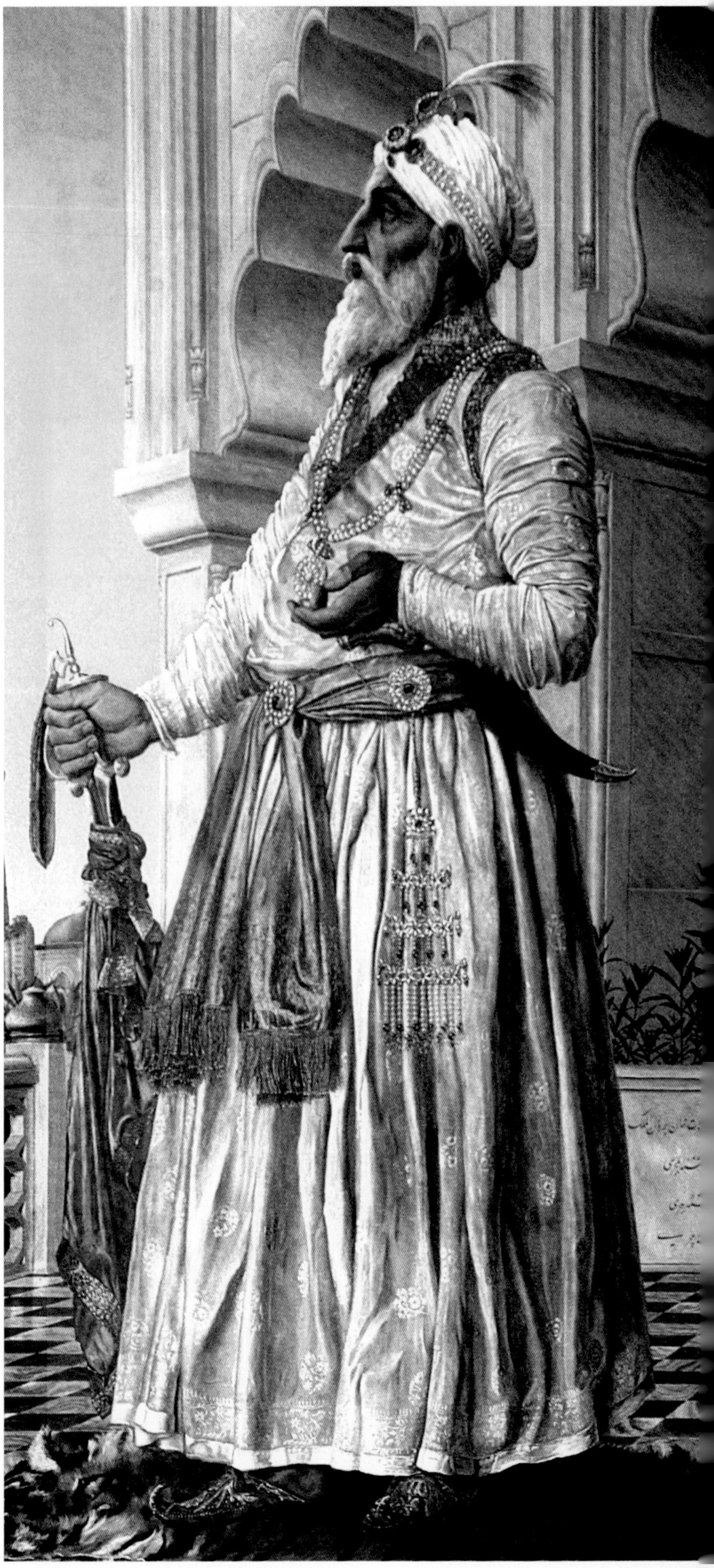

SHAHAN-E-AWADH: Rulers of Awadh

The grandeur and splendour of the Nawabi Era is evident from the elaborate costumes worn. The beginning of the era included three nawabs: Nawab Sadat Khan Burhan-ul-Mulk, Nawab Safdar Jung and Nawab Shuja-ud-Daula. They continued with the Mughal legacy of opulence in the costume, but later they developed new patterns. It was reflected in the volume of expensive material used, such as Dacca muslins, *jamdani*, brocades and *jamavar* wool cloth. A variety of embroidery techniques and ornamentation with real gold and silver threads demonstrated the increasing prosperity and lavish lifestyle of the nawabs. With the increasing influence of the new British materials, new elements of designs, motifs and details were incorporated. The chronological order of the nawabs is based on the data from State Museum Lucknow.

Nawab Sadat Khan Burhan-ul-Mulk (r. 1722-1739) followed the latest fashions of the Delhi Court without bringing in any significant change. The pagri, *jama* (long dress), paijama, *kafsh* (high-heeled shoes) and a *patka* (sash) round the waist were the main garments of men. The *patkas* were worn in Mughal courts for tucking in the weapons and arms which left free the hands. The matching fringed *patka* is held with a jewel piece. He is wearing a long white muslin *jama* embroidered in *chikankari*, over an inner dress brocaded with gold zari. A ring behind the ruby studded sarpesh of the pagri holds a feather plume. Wearing necklaces of precious stones and pearls, plumes in a turban indicated royal status in Mughal India, so in Awadh. He is holding a dagger, a mark of nobility, and a scabbard enclosed in a rich embroidered silk cover. His turquoise-green shoes are embroidered in zardozi work and have upturned toes. A beautiful beaded tassel fringe is hanging from the sheath of the *kutar* (dagger), the symbol of armed authority.

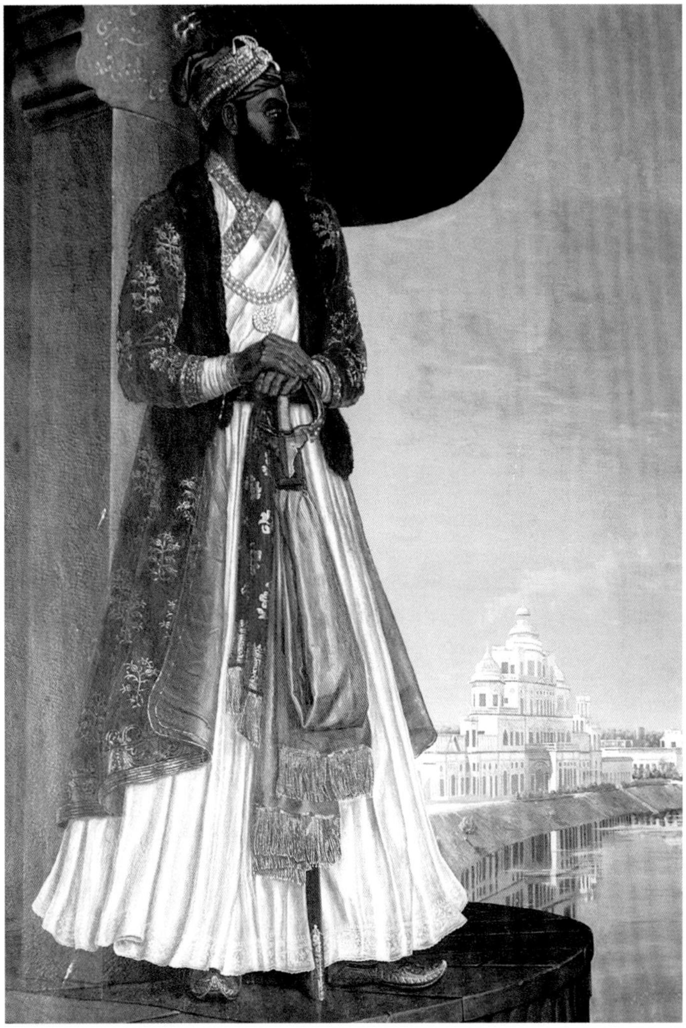

Nawab Safdar Jung (above) (r:1739-1753) is wearing an ankle-length muslin *jama* with front panels crossed over each other. The sleeves are rouched. The border of the *jama* is beautifully embroidered in *chikankari*. He is wearing a silk -brocaded *nima-jama* (short coat), richly embroidered in *zardozi*. The cotton lining is in a lighter shade of the outer green garment. This opulent *nima-jama* was an addition to the earlier nawabi costume consisting of *jama*, paijama, pagri and *patka*. It is interesting to note that the pagri, *patka* and *nima-jama* are in the same colour scheme making it an elegant outfit. The pagri is more elaborate with a gold band and a pearl string over it. A fur stole is added for the winter season. A stole of rich brocade with gold tassel fringes hangs close to scabbard. The nawab's gold-embroidered shoes are without heels and have upturned toes.

Nawab Shuja-ud-Daula (below) (r: 1753-1775) is wearing a flower-patterned heavy silk brocade *jama* with a matching *nima-jama* and a fur stole. The woven red flowers with blue outlines give impression of *minakari*. The *jama* is enriched with heavy gold embroidery border and a contrasting green piping. The shoulders are decorated with supplementary fur which was an important element in the costumes worn at court. The *patka* is in gold brocade with gold bullion fringes. The red sleeve border recalls the colour of the feather of the cap. This kind of *jama* is less voluminous and of shorter length, suitably worn with leather boots. The turban is no longer a pagri but seems more of a cap with fur band, bejewelled with a sarpesh. The green velvet sheath, embellished with zardozi work matches the green piping of the dress.

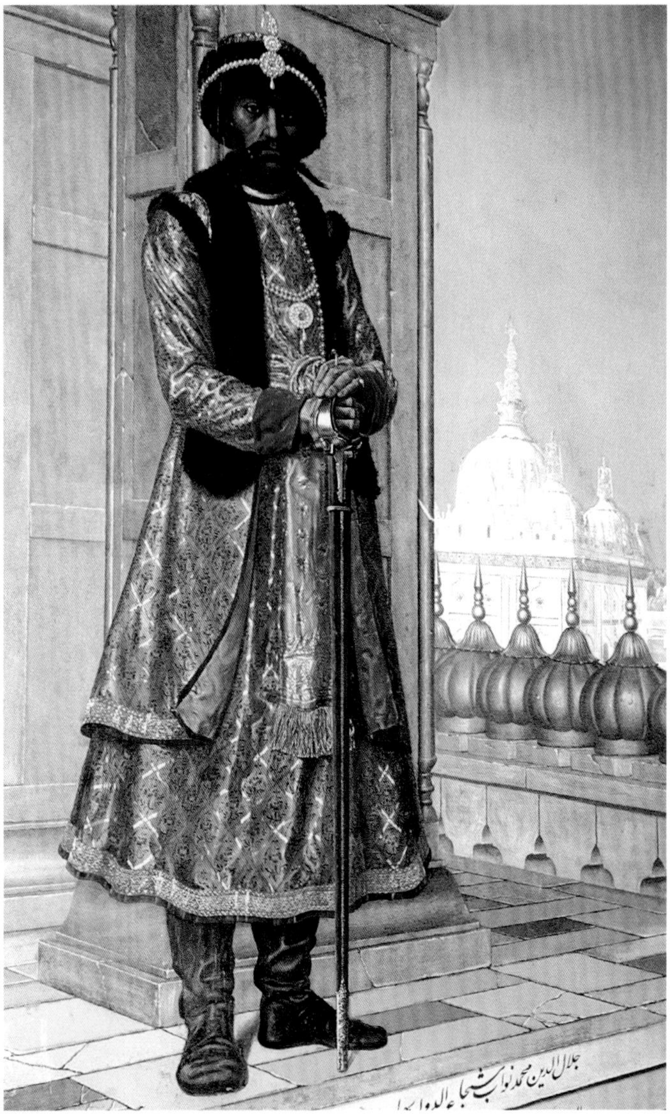

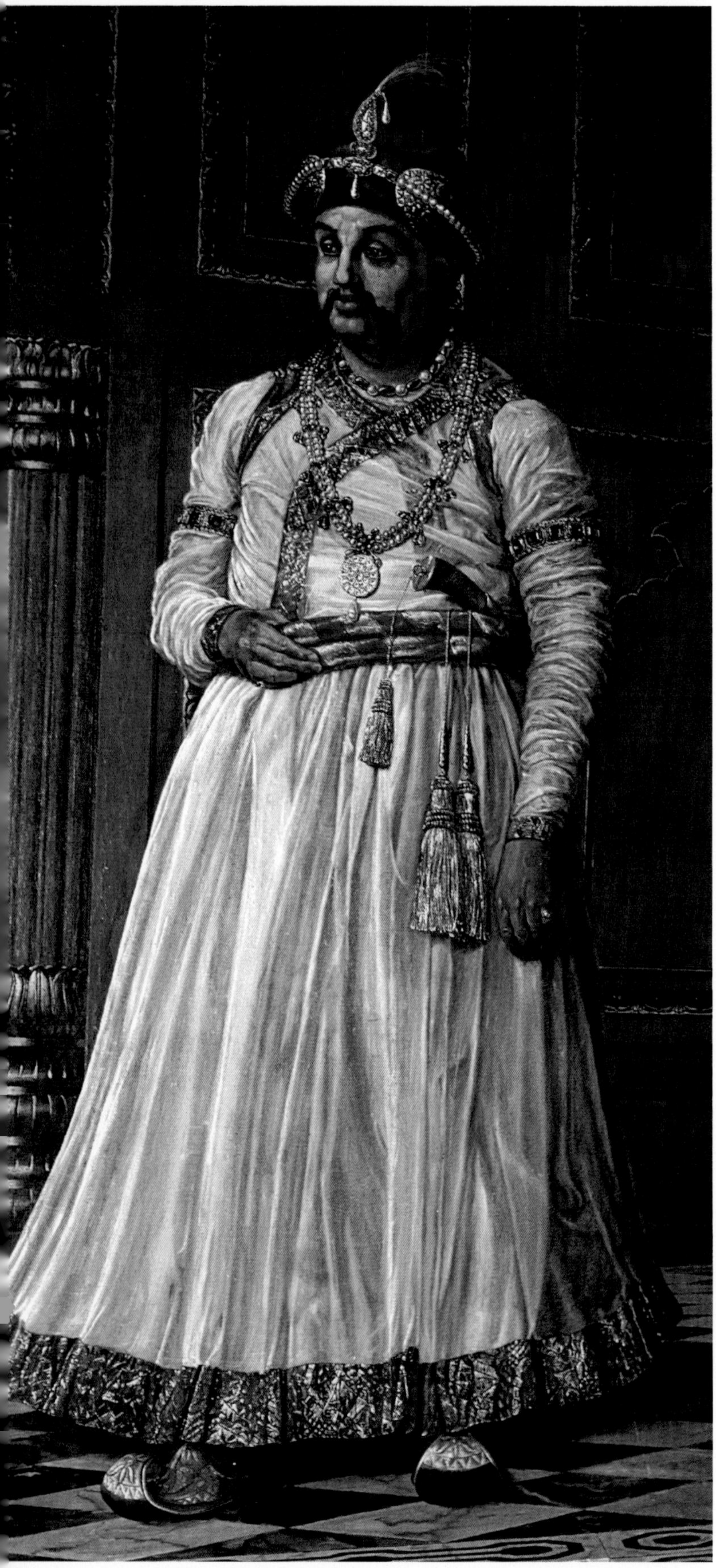

Nawab Asaf-ud-Daula (r: 1775-1797) is wearing a *jama* made of *sarkars-e-ala* muslin of very light texture and edged with pattha *gota* at border and *lachka gota* at sleeve borders. The sophisticated technique of crinkling and rouching, known as *chunnat*, was used for the sleeves. This *chunnat* was done with the help of a certain stone. The woven brocade *patka* is replaced by red and yellow silk strips of fabric entwined together like a rope. He is wearing armbands made of precious stones, in addition to necklaces and sarpesh. Gold bullion tassels hang from the metal scabbard. He is wearing intricately embroidered *kafsh*.

Nawab Wazir Ali Khan (r: 1797-1798) is wearing a greenish-blue ankle-length *angarkha* worn for the first time in Awadh. By the early 1800s, the *angarkha* started gaining popularity over the *jama*. It is made of velvet and ornately embroidered in zardozi with *kalabattun* and edged with contrasting red piping. A sash is added to the outfit with the *patka* similar to the ones worn by his ancestors. The pink-coloured wide paijamas are visible below. The richly embroidered saddlecloth and the jewels worn by the horse are examples of the growing nawabi extravagance.

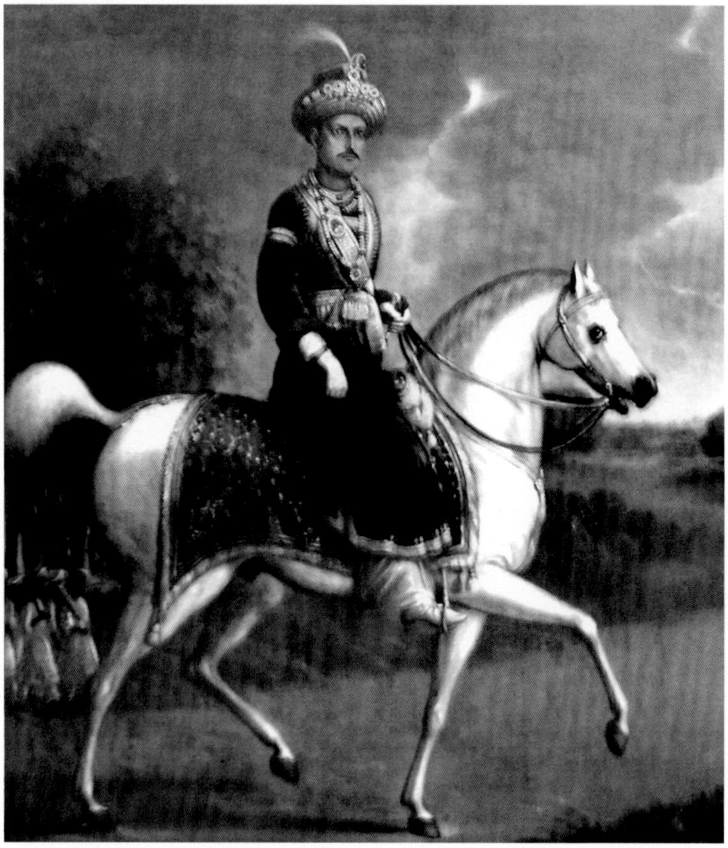

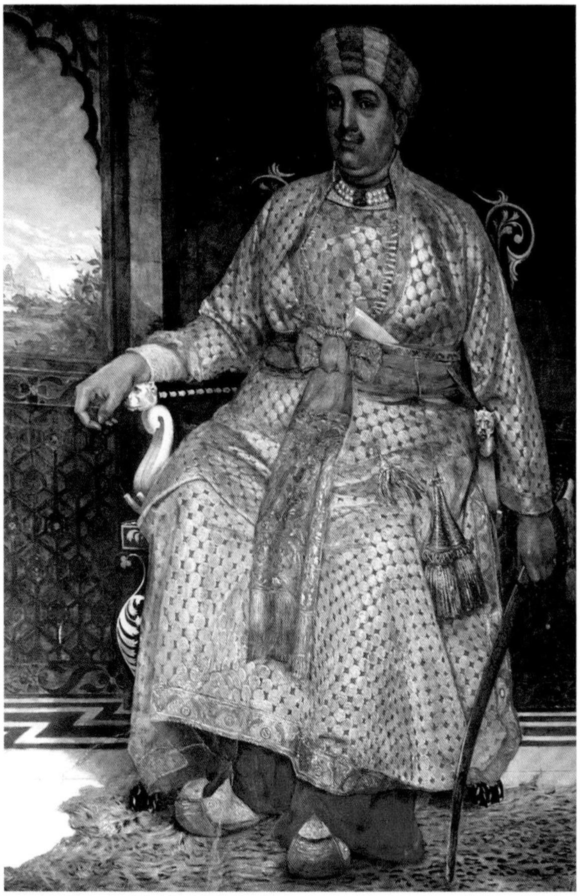

King Ghazi-ud-Din (below) (r: 1819-1827) is wearing the traditional *jama*, worn with a wide *patka* and *arz ka* paijamas. European influence became visible in the costumes after the British turned the nawabs into 'kings'. The pagri was replaced by the crown. The crown is lined with a high red velvet cap and a plume in the centre. It consists of a 12-point diadem covered with diamonds and with a big ruby in the centre. Another important addition in their costume is a full-length blue velvet coat, and an ermine cape with three rows of sealskin spots on the cape designating the rank of an Earl.

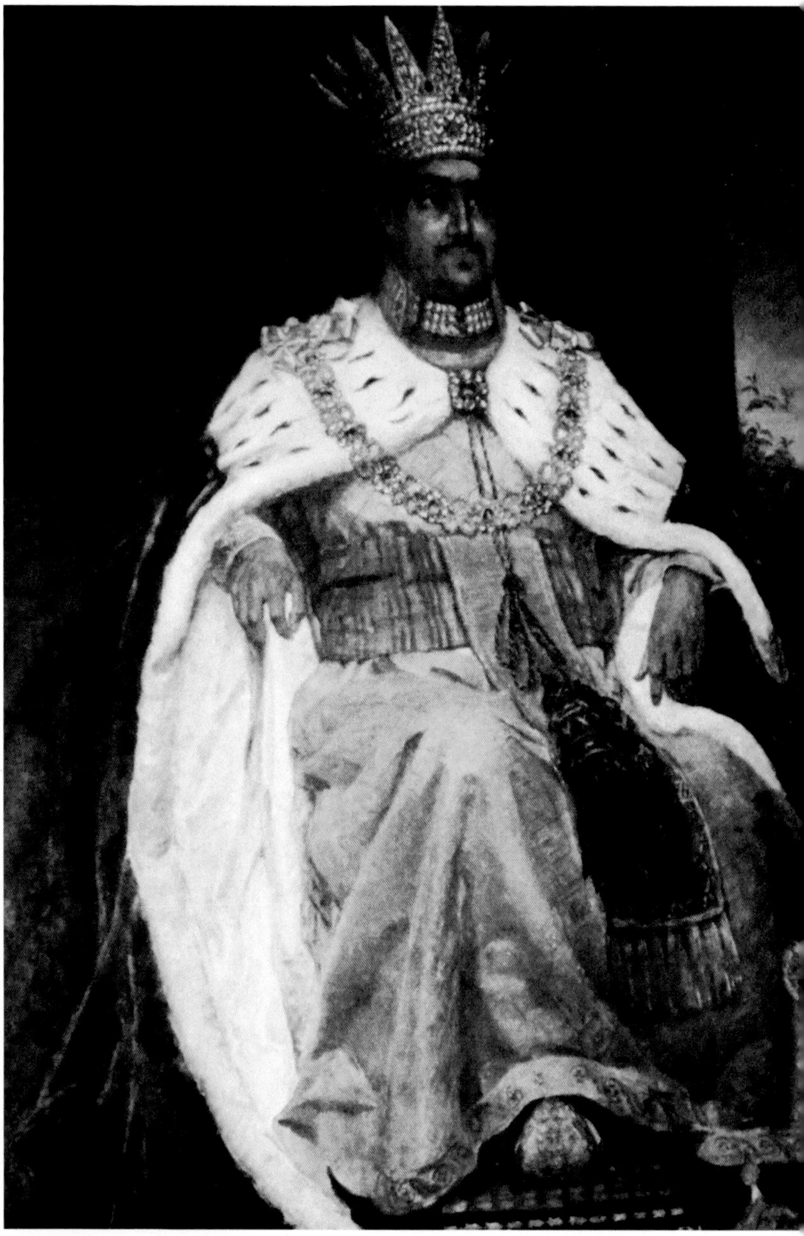

Nawab Sadat Ali Khan (above) (r: 1798-1819) is wearing a voluminous *angarkha* in gold and red brocade, over a fine *jamdani* kurta or *nima* with long wide red silk trailing flared paijamas. The *angarkha* has a raised collar with circular neck opening, embroidered in zardozi work. A high collar to the *angarkha* is a new introduction. The front is decorated with a series of stylised jasmine buds in gold zari. The gold zari border, embroidered with fish motif (emblem of the court of Awadh), embellish the front, sleeves, slits and hem. The *patka* of contrasting green brocade is densely patterned with floral motifs and tied with a bow in the front. He introduced shimla cap. He is not wearing long necklaces like his ancestors. The shoes are embellished in matching red and gold combination. The metal scabbard is intricately decorated in enamel work without any cloth covering. The *patka* is tied in a fashionable style in a bow design.

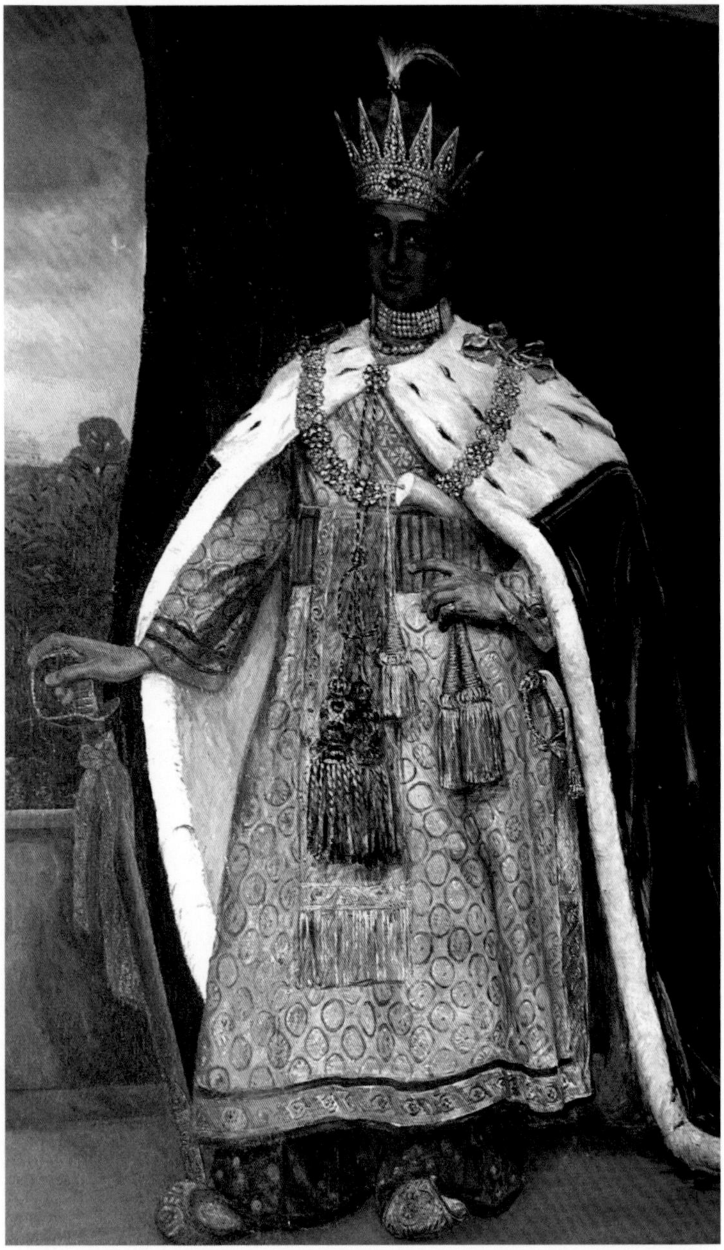

King Nasir-ud-Din Haider (r: 1827-1837) like his predecessor, continued wearing the crown and the cape over his sumptuous silk brocade *angarkha* with round *asharfi* motifs and wide, flared paijamas. A wide *patka* holds the dagger sheath with gold tasselled cords. The style of ornaments also changed considerably and started resembling to European broaches and necklaces with stone encrusted ribbons studded with precious stones and ribbons. More decorative fringes, made of gold, silver and silk, as were in vogue in Europe at the time, were added to the nawabs' apparel. They continued to wear their upturned *kafsh*.

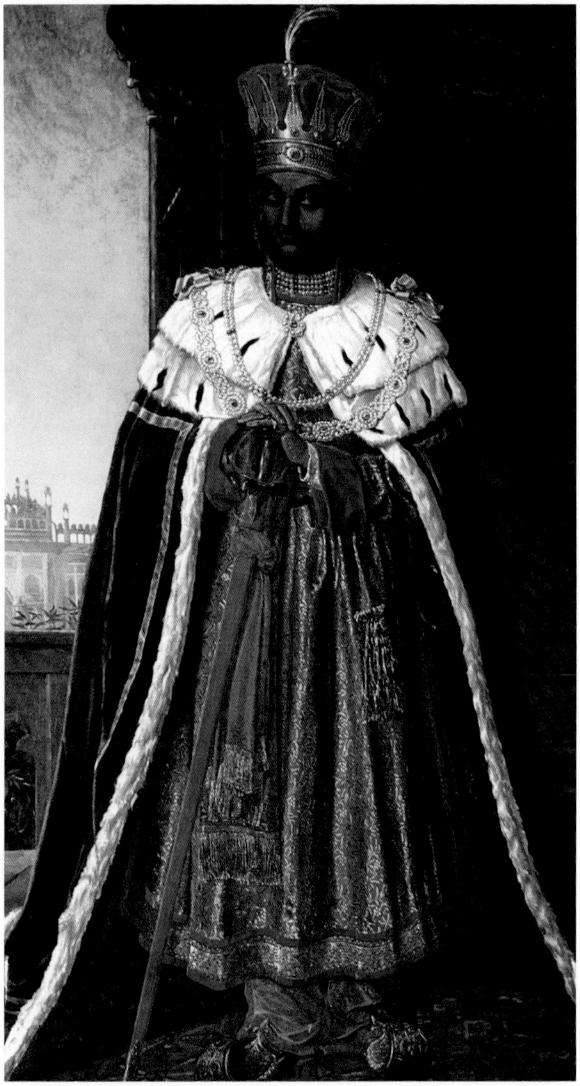

King Muhammad Ali Shah (r: 1837-1842) is wearing gold brocade *angarkha* edged with double red piping over an inner garment of muslin. The paijama in grey silk is flared and of full length. The sword has red scabbard and gilt mountings, while a gold silk stole is hangs with bullion tassel. He is wearing a magnificent pearl necklace in addition to one worn by his ancestors. He is wearing the velvet coat with ermine cape only with two rows of sealskin spots denoting the rank of a baron and not of an earl as his predecessors.

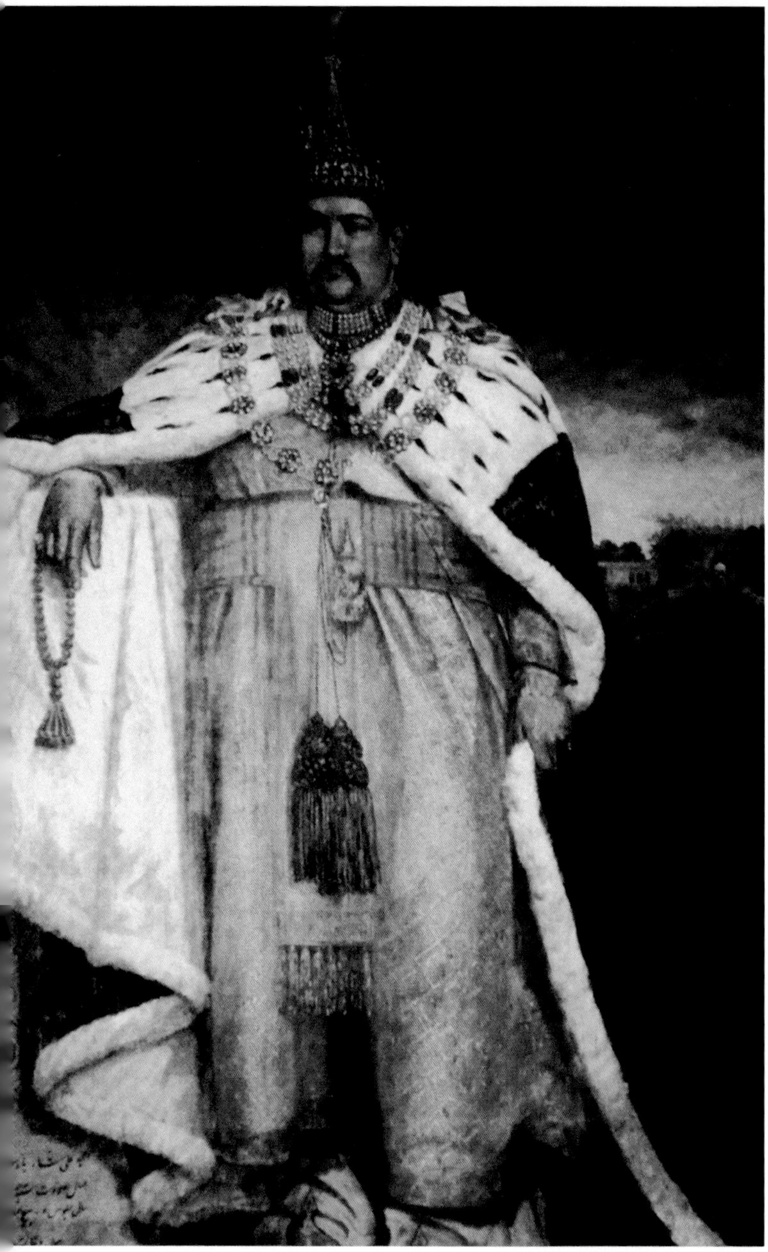

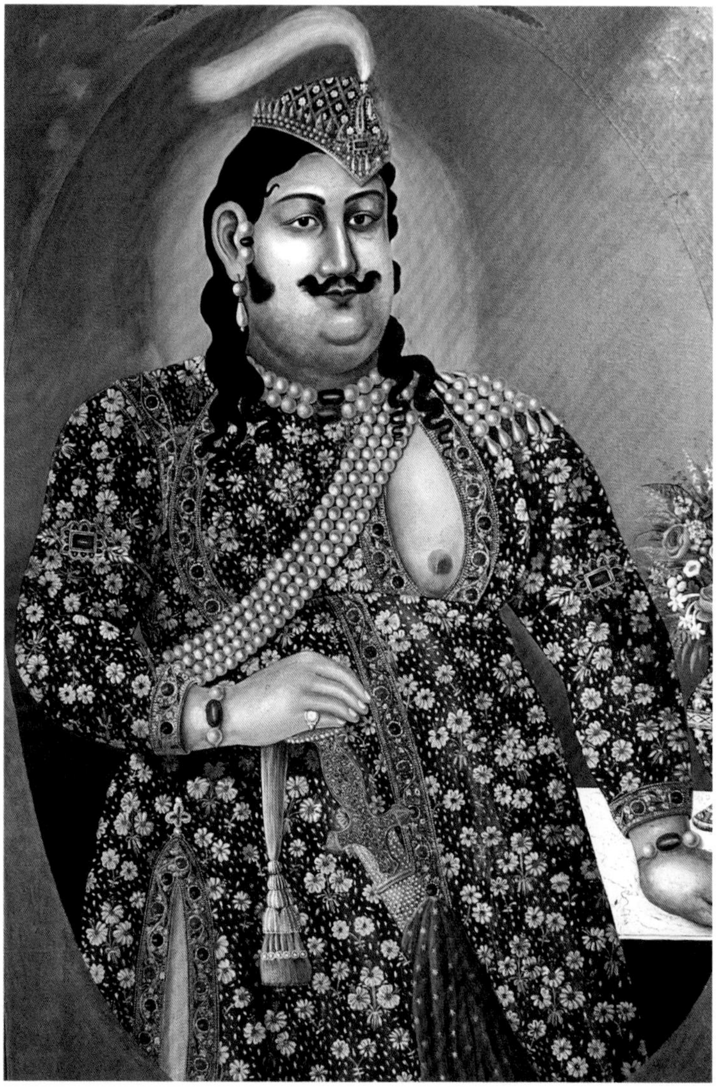

King Amjad Ali Shah (r: 1842-1847) is wearing his traditional *angarkha* made of *kinkhab* silk brocade, edged with red *kor*, matching *patka* with cream-coloured silk wide paijamas. He is wearing three elaborate necklaces of precious stones and pearls. Such necklaces were worn to symbolize the exalted rank. They were common amongst nineteenth century royals of India.

King Wajid Ali Shah (r: 1847-1856) is wearing the traditional *angarkha* with paijama, without the cape worn by his predecessors. Wajid Ali wore the *angarkha* without a vest, thus revealing part of his bare torso. His style caught on and became very fashionable in the Awadh Court. He also introduced a new kind of cap known as *alampasand* or *jhula*, which, however, did not become as popular and disappeared soon after his own exile.

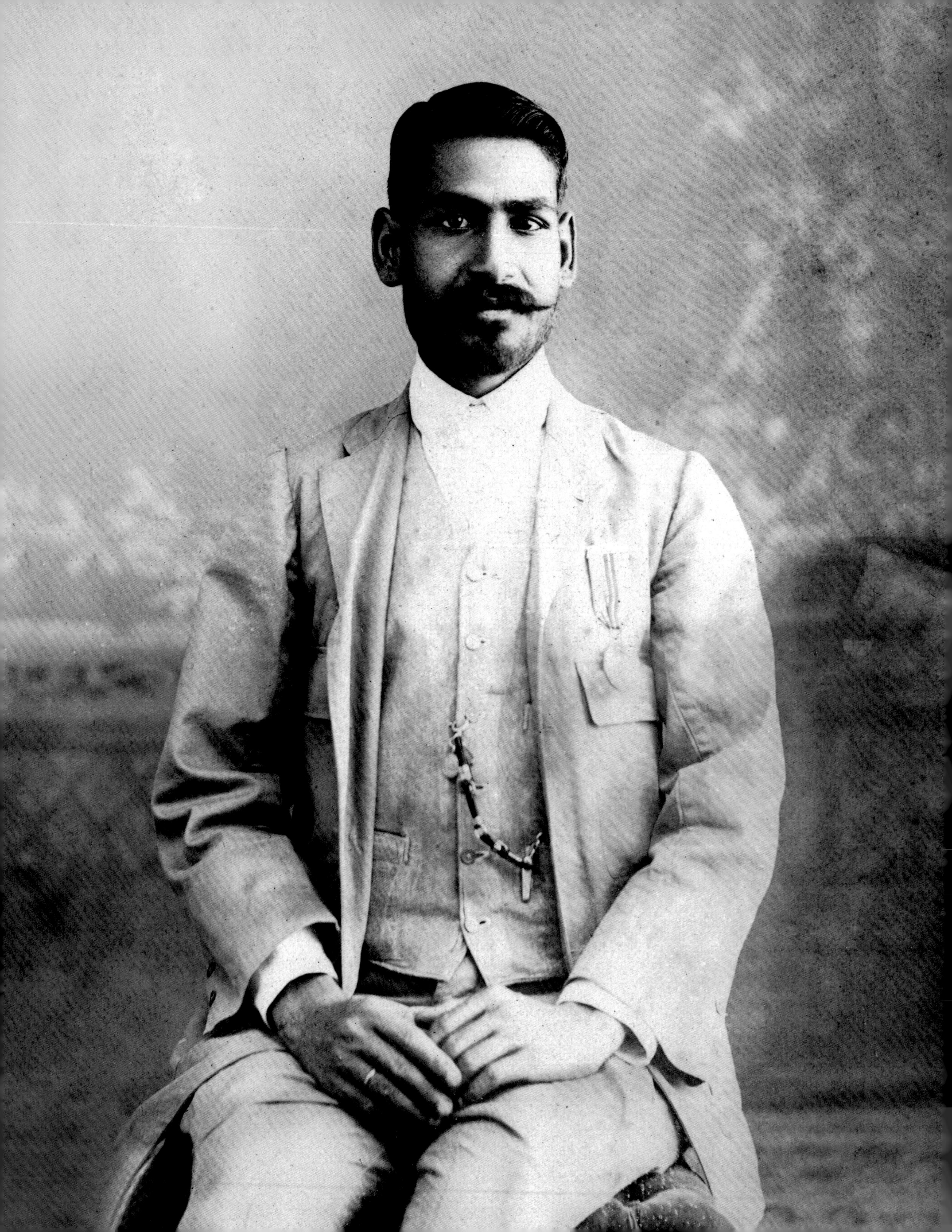

BRITISH RAJ

1856-1947

BRITISH RAJ

The early hundred-year period of the British Raj brought about many changes in Awadh. The exit of the nawabs after the exile of the last nawab, Wajid Ali Shah, heralded stronger British dominion.

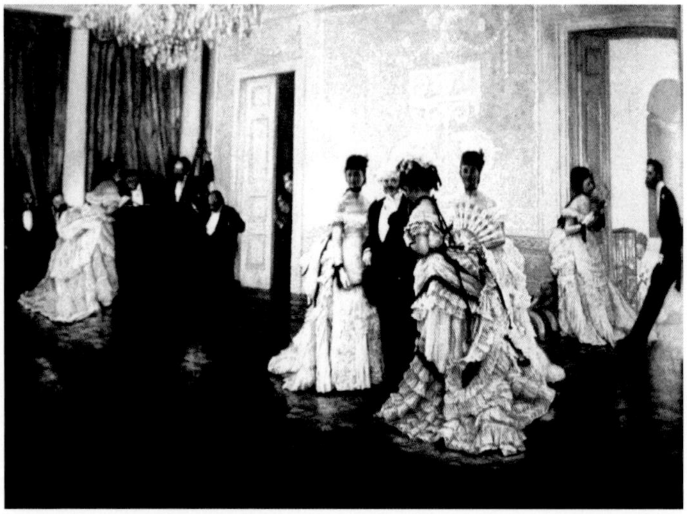

Men in black formal suits and women dressed in elaborate dancing gowns.

Previous page 96: Rai Bahadur Anand Swarup is wearing a three-piece suit over and a round-collar shirt. Pocket watch with a gold chain was an accessory of the Raj period.

Colonization led to increased interaction between the Indians and the British. Indians assumed additional roles in administration and there was increased social interaction among Indian and British women. The official language shifted from Urdu to English. These changes gave rise to a new Anglo–Indian culture that brought a mini cultural revolution in India. Elite Indians started adopting British costumes and lifestyles. They held garden parties, organized polo matches, pig-sticking and loved going for shikar. The officers of the armed forces set the trend among club members. The clothes they wore, the food they ate, the drinks they had – all became popular among civilians. By the late nineteenth century, the hukkah of the nawabs started to be replaced by cigarettes, pipes and cigars.

Western style dancing became more popular and courtesans' *kothas* (chambers) started being used as dancing halls. Men who came to dance were dressed in British attire with black suits, white shirts and bow ties, and women started to dress in long skirts and blouses. Instead of the legendary traditional *itr* of Awadh, perfumes from Paris and London began to be used.

Continental food and drinks started replacing nawabi cuisine. Whisky and champagne were introduced in bars. Bartenders and bearers who served food wore costumes that were entirely different from the Indian costumes worn by the *khansamas* (cooks) of Awadh (churidar paijamas, *patka* and pagri). Their dresses now resembled those of English butlers and attendants.

The Industrial Revolution in England in the late eighteenth and early nineteenth centuries led to the increased use of mill-made British fabrics in India. Synthetic textiles such as nylon, polyester and rayon were invented in this era. Mass-produced, chemically dyed cloths from Europe replaced the rich and hand-woven gold brocades, delicate Dacca, Tanda and *jamdani* muslins, vegetable-dyed silks and cottons, and exquisite wools of Kashmir. The traditional hand-made *jamavar* started to be industrially produced on Jacquard looms in the town of Paisley in Scotland. In this way, costumes lost the subtle sophistication and refined grandeur of the traditional hand-made textiles, which became a thing of the past. The introduction of the sewing machine in the field of stitching was a landmark change in the tailoring methods of the period as well.

With the passage of time there appeared a growing spirit of rebellion towards the British. In a span of ninety years, from the mutiny of 1857, which happened in Lucknow, to Independence in 1947, India, and particularly Awadh, witnessed a period of revolutionary change in textiles and costumes. Mohandas Karamchand Gandhi conceived the strategy of non-violence and civil disobedience for India's freedom struggle. The feeling of national pride led to the appreciation of everything native and resulted in a boycott of imported goods, which had been so popular in the earlier stages of British influence.

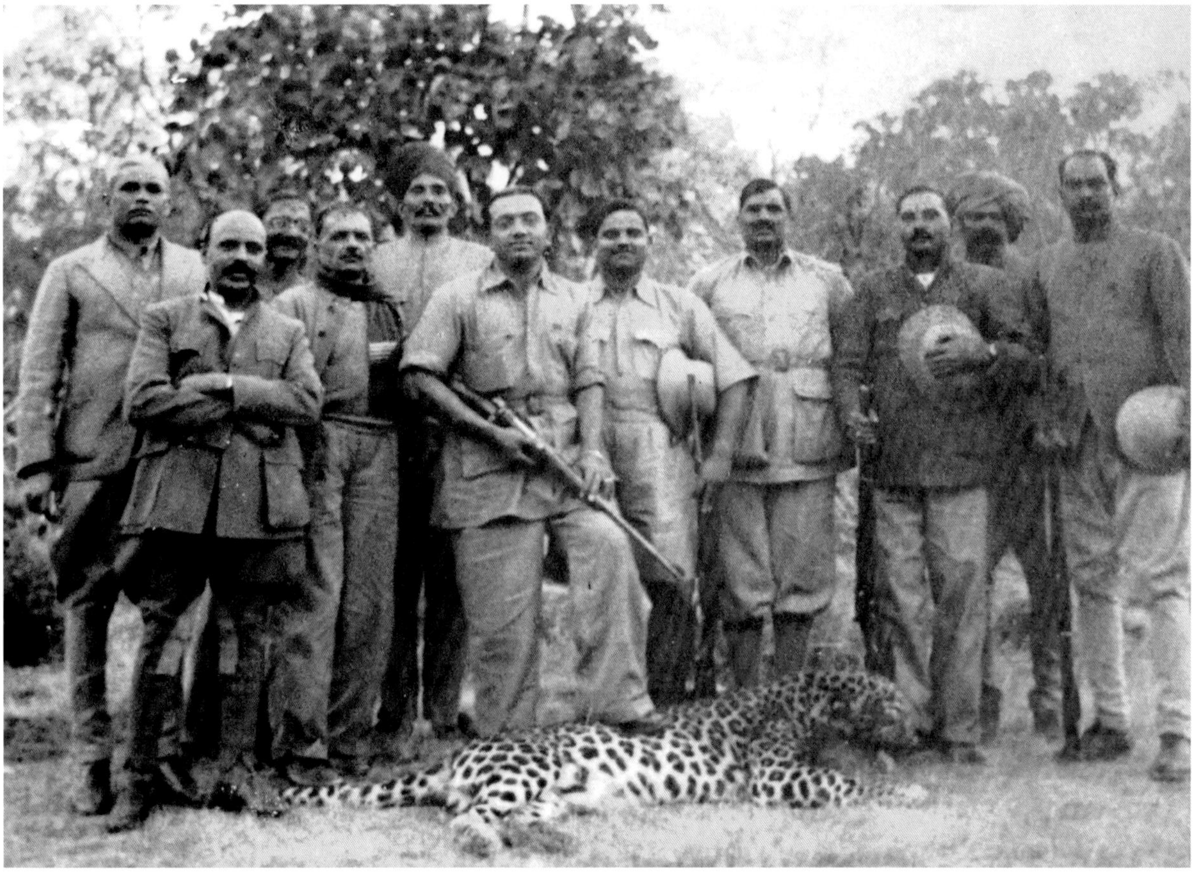

Hunting was the favourite pasttime of the Indian royalty, the British officers, bureaucracy and the Lords. Great shikar expeditions used to be planned and for months the hunting camps were set up. Safari-suits, breeches with jodhpurs, laced shoes and sula hats were commonly worn on shikars.

MEN'S COSTUMES

The full impact of British influence on the costumes of Awadh was visible only in the twentieth century. Before the British dressing style was adopted fully, the common dress code for men in Lucknow included the *chaugoshia*, *angarkha*, *arz ke paichon ka paijama* and *rumal*. The transformation in the costumes of Awadh to Indo-British styles became evident from the introduction of Western design elements and accessories such as the collar, cuffs, buttons, laces and hooks in traditional costumes.

The formal clothing of British officials, particularly their suits and shirts, were tailored in Calcutta, Madras and Bombay (now called Kolkata, Chennai and Mumbai respectively), as the tailors of Awadh lacked the appropriate skills. This benefit was extended to Indian high officials. In fact, the suits and shirts of my grandfather, who was the first Indian Chief Engineer, were stitched by the same tailors as those of the British officers. His ceremonial clothes came directly from tailors in London, namely, White Way Laidley and Rankings tailors. High-ranking Indian officials, working for the British, adopted European dresses for their uniform but dressed in their traditional wear when at home. My grandfather wore the uniform on official occasions but always dressed in his dhoti and kurta at home.

This was a vibrant period for innovations in garments for upper body. The Western influence helped transform the *jama* and *angarkha* into the *chapkan* and *achkan*. In addition, the shirt also became popular as a garment. It was worn without a collar under the *achkan* and sherwani, and later with a collar under the coat. The vests replaced *shaluka*s as an inner garment and were worn under the shirts.

The British introduced three-piece suits in addition to the classic two-piece suit in India. The waistcoat, a sleeveless garment worn beneath the suit, may have been introduced by King Charles II of England. A diary entry from 8 October 1666, written by Samuel Pepys, states, 'The King hath yesterday, in Council, declared his resolution of setting a

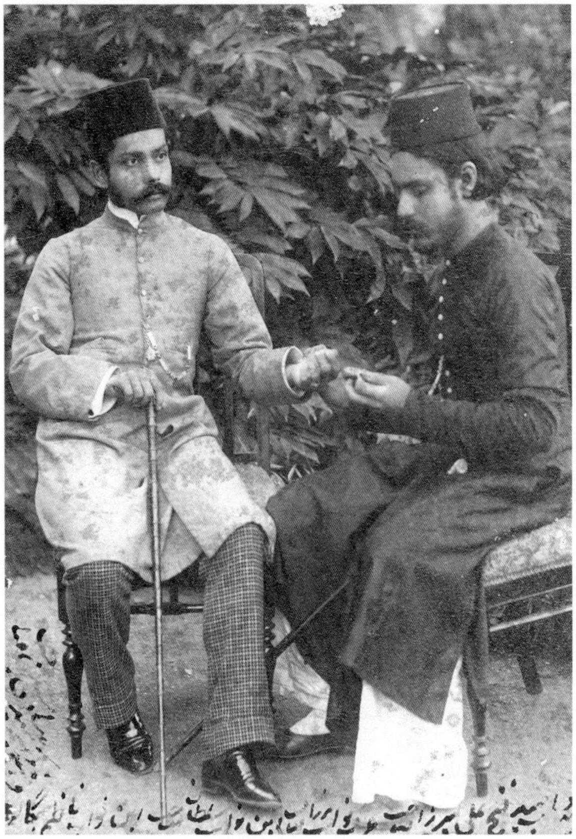

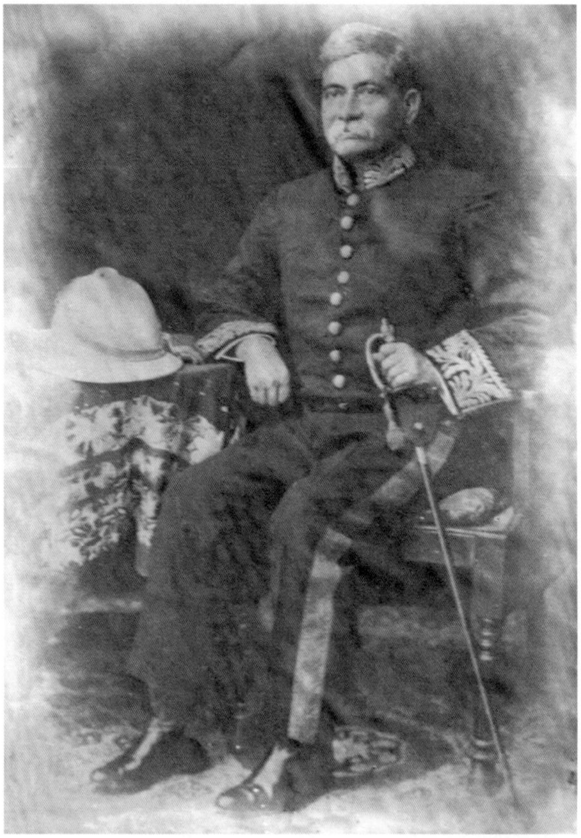

Above left: Gentlemen wearing a light-coloured brocaded *achkan* with fashionable chequered pants. The doctor is dressed in *achkan* with traditional paijamas. Both have caps and laced shoes.

Above right: Rai Bahadur Bishan Swarup wearing his uniform of a senior government official. The coat with a luxuriously embroidered high standing collar and heraldic buttons was a part of the full dress uniform that also included pants with gold stripes down the outer seam, hat and a sword.

fashion for clothes. It will be a vest, I know not well how, but it is to teach the nobility thrift.'

The paijama was still a popular lower body garment. Churidar paijamas were introduced in Lucknow and had tighter fittings at the calf than the earlier ones. They became very popular and were worn with *achkans* and sherwanis. On the other hand, the earlier *sharai* and *kalidar* paijamas became old-fashioned. Though the shape and style remained the same, men totally discarded satin and the ornately embroidered or coloured paijama and preferred white ones instead. The aligarhi paijama was a beautiful introduction that merged the existing Awadhi paijama with the British-introduced trousers. This was neither too loose nor too tight and started being worn with the *achkan* and the sherwani.

A significant change, which has carried over to modern times, was the introduction of the trousers. This had a lasting impact on the popularity of the traditional paijama.

Towards the end of the Nawabi Era and the beginning of the British Raj, the main headgears were the *dopalri* cap, *chaugoshia*, *mandel* and the *nukkadar* cap, also called babu cap by the British. The educated and the aristocratic wore the Turkish cap and *kullah* with coats and trousers. After the mutiny in 1857, the *nukkadar* cap gained popularity. When worn by nobility and taluqdars, it was embroidered with heavy gold and silver threads. The British introduced hats, which also served as protection from the tropical heat. At times, felt caps were also worn. The Lucknow elite increasingly began to wear English hats with their Indian costumes.

This period saw the introduction of British boots, laced shoes and court bow shoes. However, Hindus continued to wear their wooden *khadau* at home, as the use of leather by Brahmins and upper caste communities was prohibited. Over the course of the period, leather shoes became increasingly accepted and utilized. As the military encampments increased in Awadh, the nineteenth century came to be characterized by the predominance of boots, both for men and women.

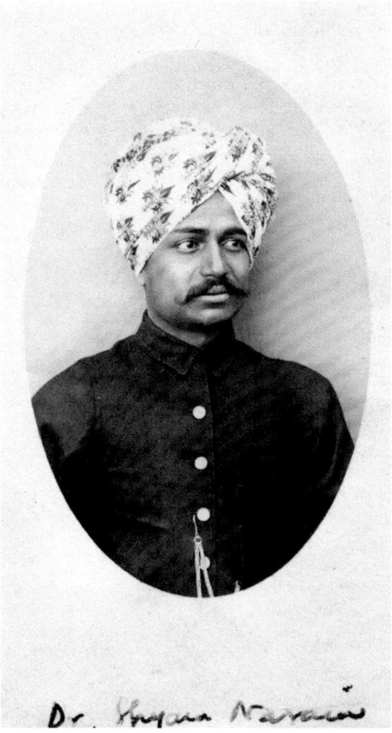

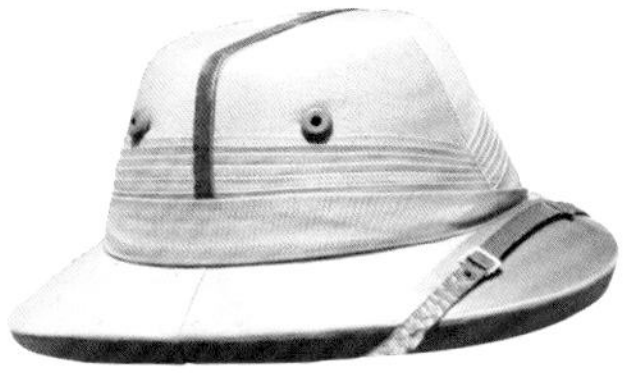

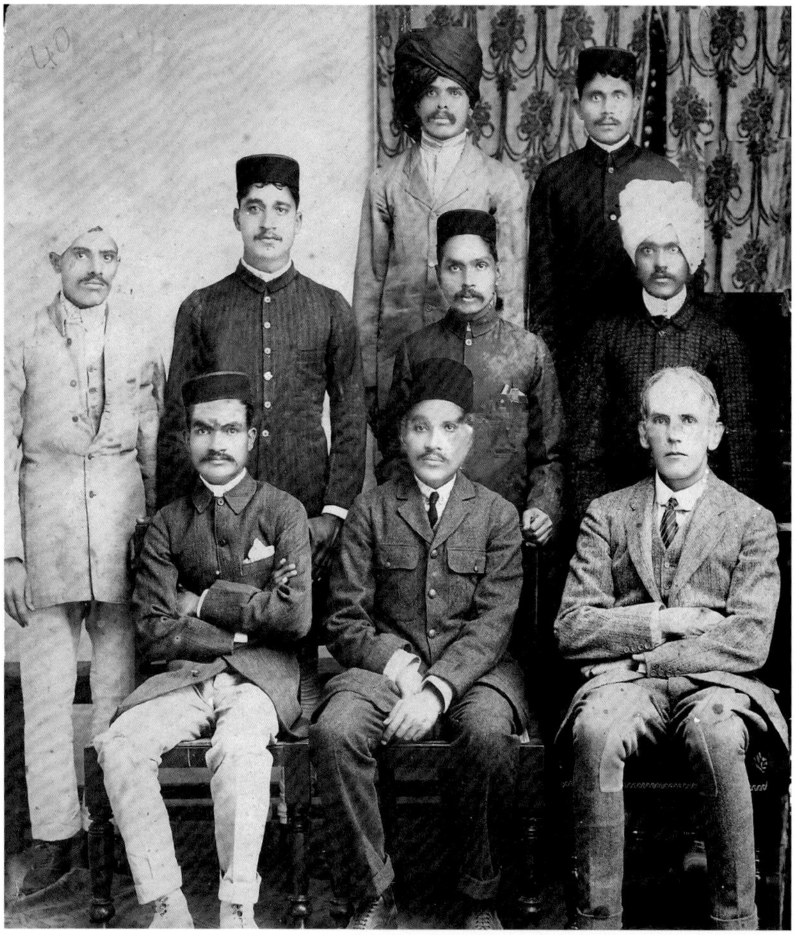

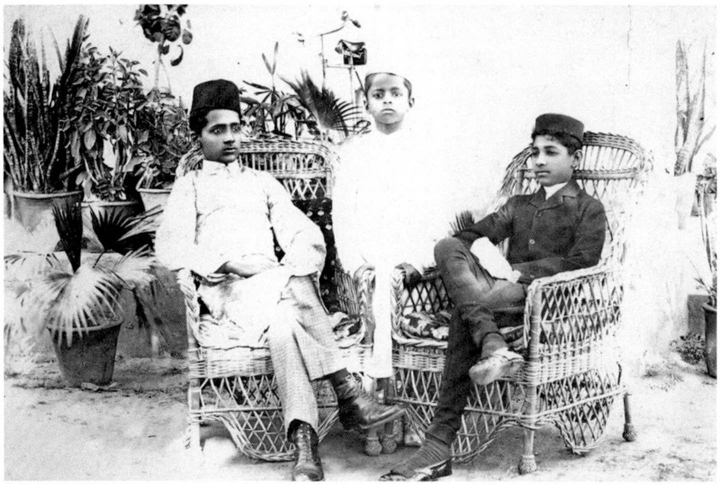

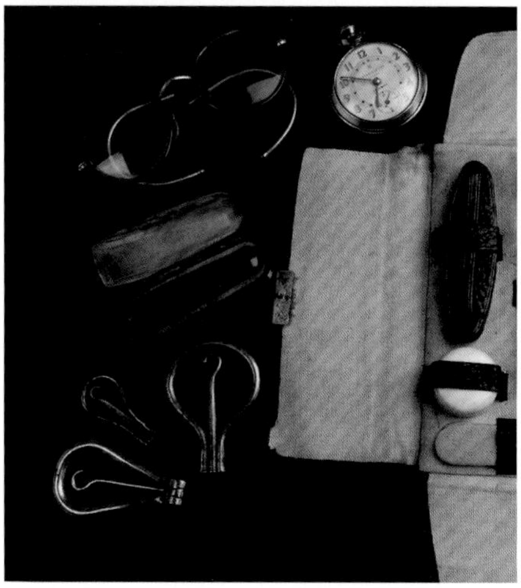

Clockwise from top:

1. Dr. Shyam Sunder, a physician, is dressed in a plain sherwani adorning a pocket watch attached to the gold chain. He is wearing a fashionable cotton printed turban with floral motifs.
2. Formally dressed gentlemen in coats and caps of various fashionable styles.
3. Accessories like pocket watch, shoe-stringers, manicure-set, spectacle and a cigarette holder. Different shoe-stringers were used to tighten the boots depending on the thickness of the shoe-laces.
4. Young boys dressed fashionably in sherwanis with chequered pants, breeches and coat, wearing stringed boots or laced shoes with socks. Caps were an essential part of formal dressing.
5. Sula hat.

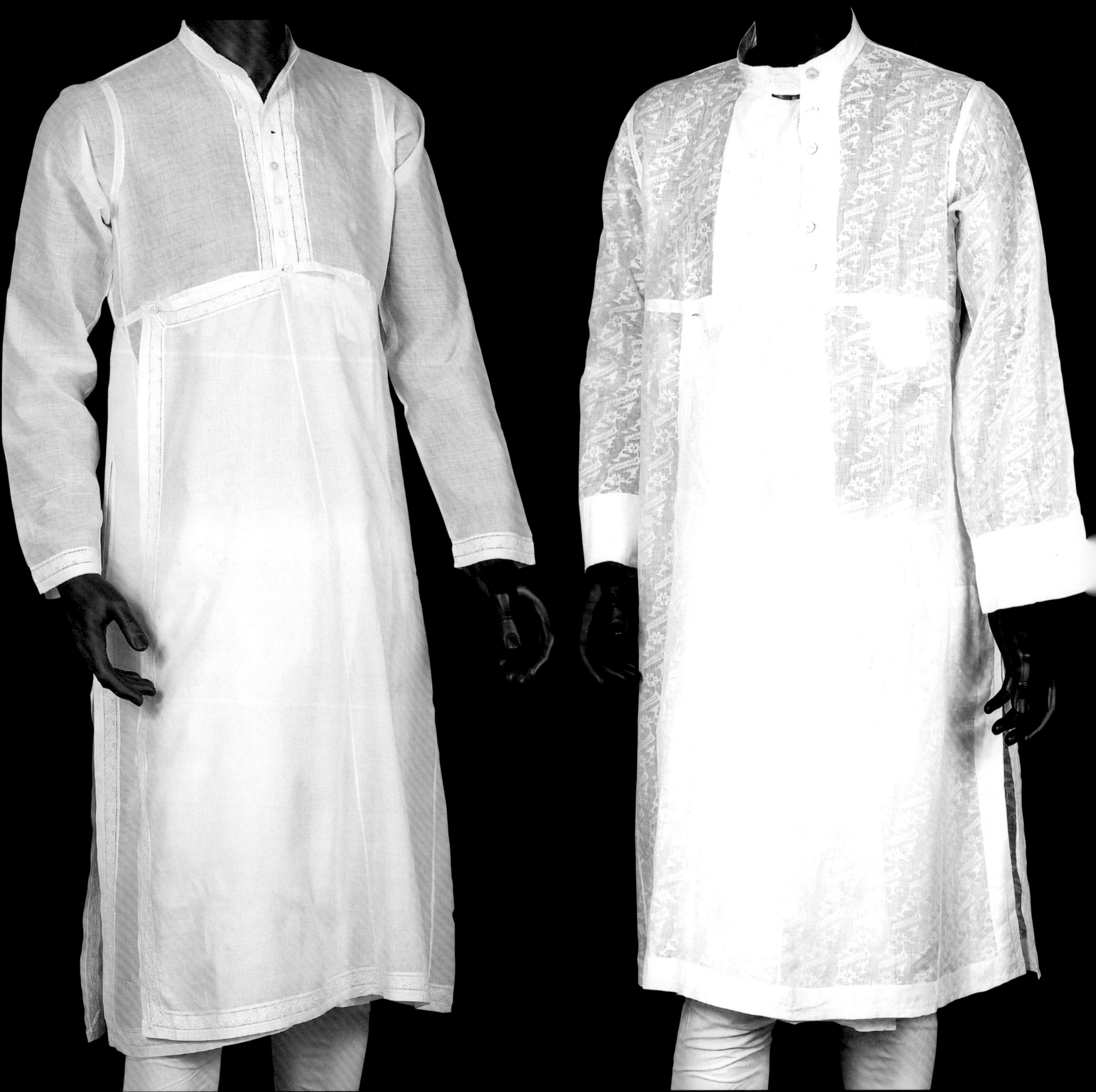

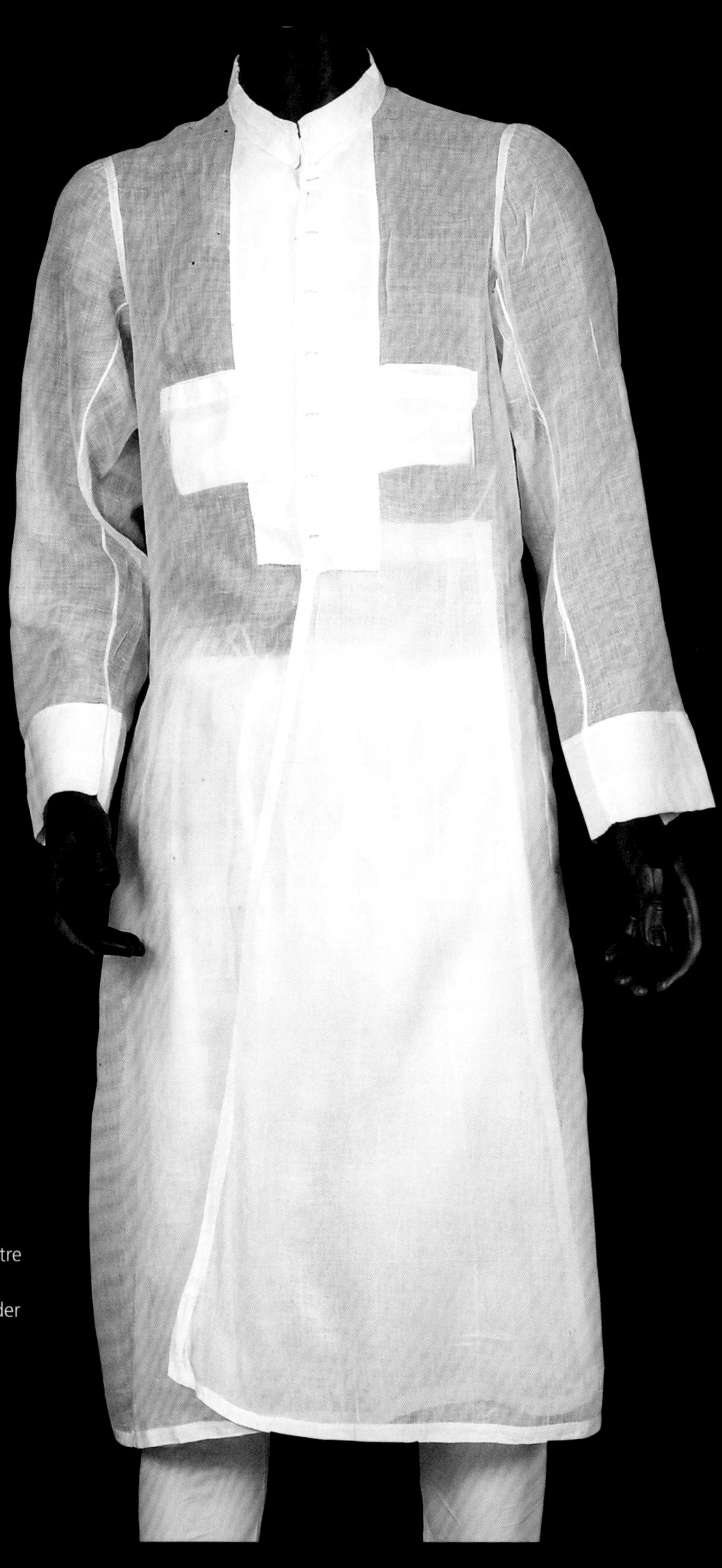

Facing page, Left: Muslin *chapkan* adopts the Western centre fastening. The left skirt panel crosses over and fastens at the side seam on the right hand side. It is edged with aureb border and embellished with chikan embroidery at the borders.
Facing page, Right: This *jamdani achkan* is fashionably tailored, with a stylised front, which is fastened with double columns of buttons.
Right: A machine-made muslin *chapkan*: Western influence is quite evident in the cut of the sleeves, similar to that of a coat. The buttons and button-holes substitute the *tukma-ghundi* fastening.

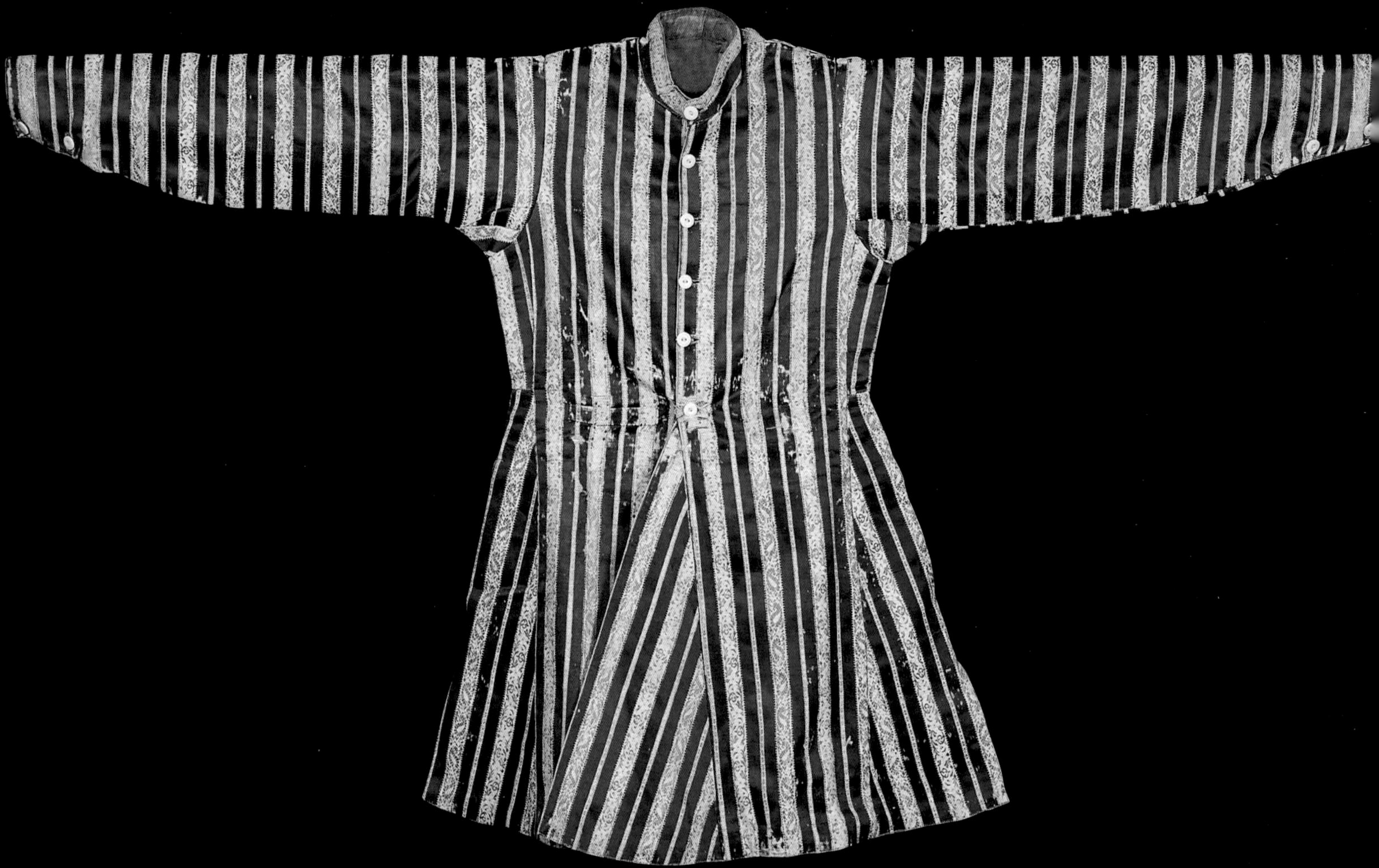

This *chapkan* is made of machine--made silk. The pattern of alternate blue and cream stripes with *turanj* motifs was woven in satin weave. The upper part is like a coat fastened with buttons while the lower part is wider and has two suspended pockets similar to an *angarkha*. No ornamentation is seen here.

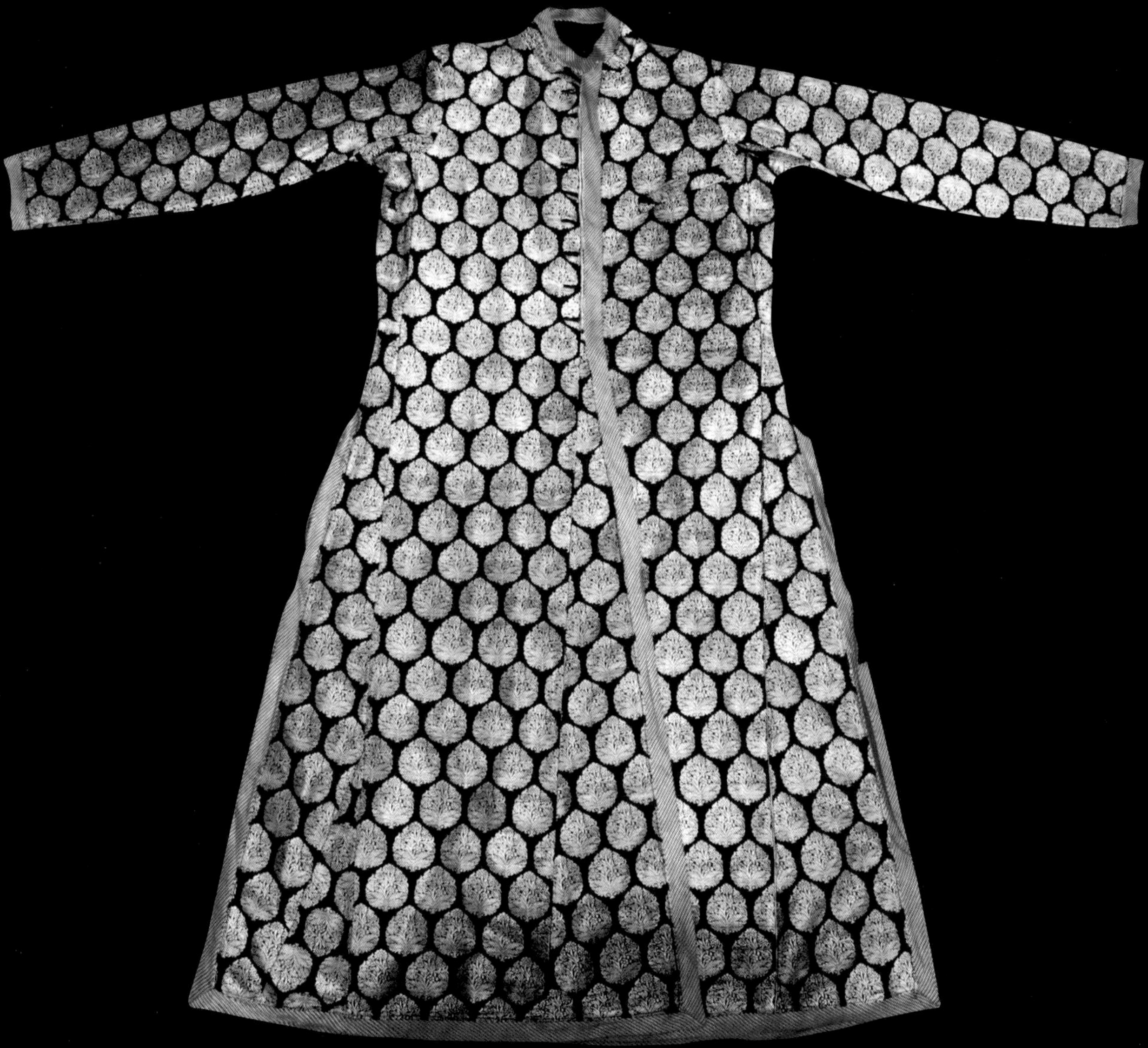

A *chapkan* made of silk brocade in gold zari with tree-of-life motif. There is no purdah to cover the chest but has a central opening with stitched button-holes (buttons missing). The sleeves are joined with *bagalia* like an *angarkha*. A red and white *laheriya* silk piping edges the raised collar, borders and sleeves

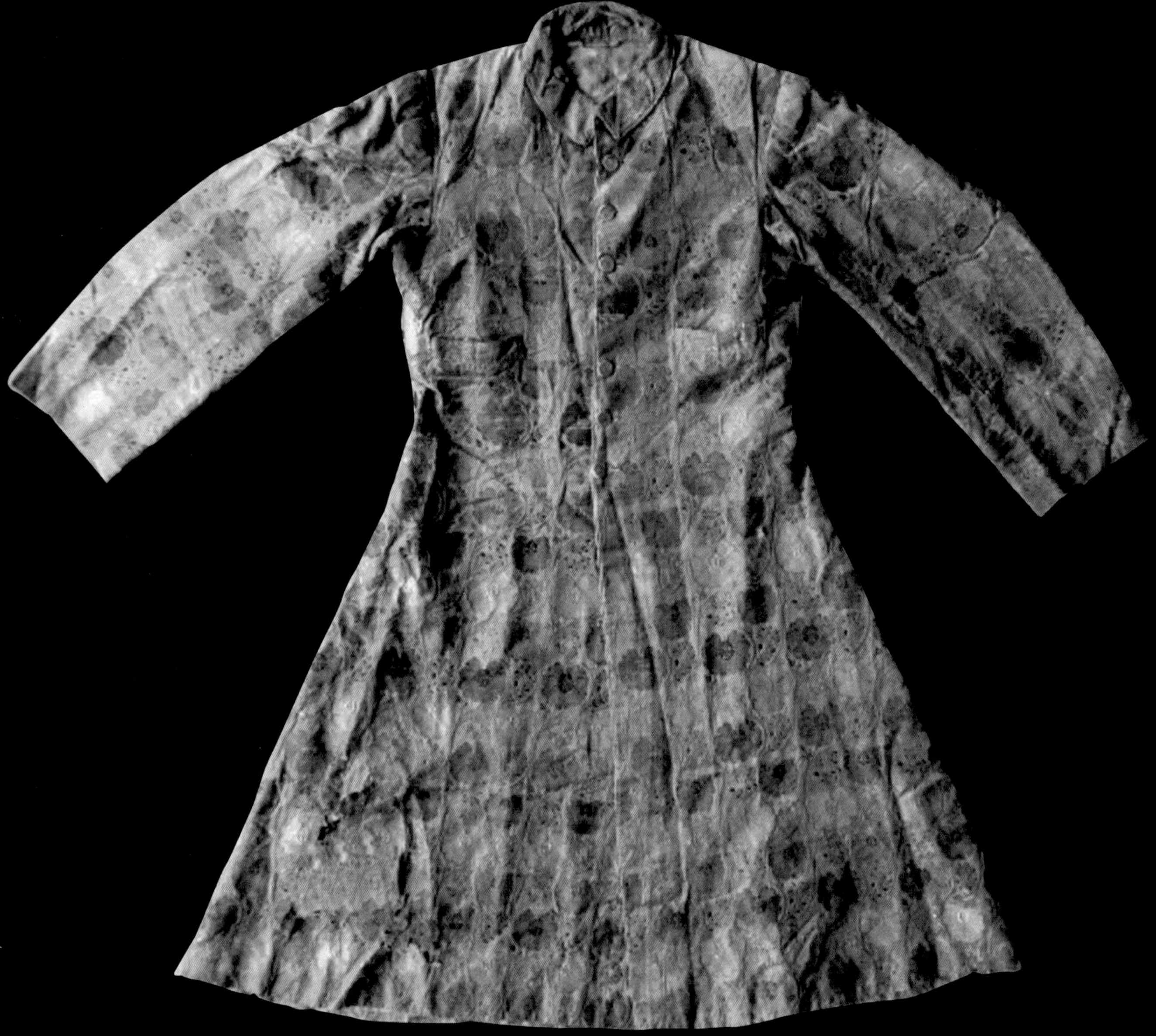

This multi-coloured *achkan* is woven in silk with *butas*. The opening is straight down the centre with eight cloth-cased round buttons and the round collar, typical of Awadh . Two small pockets are visible in slits, just above the waist.

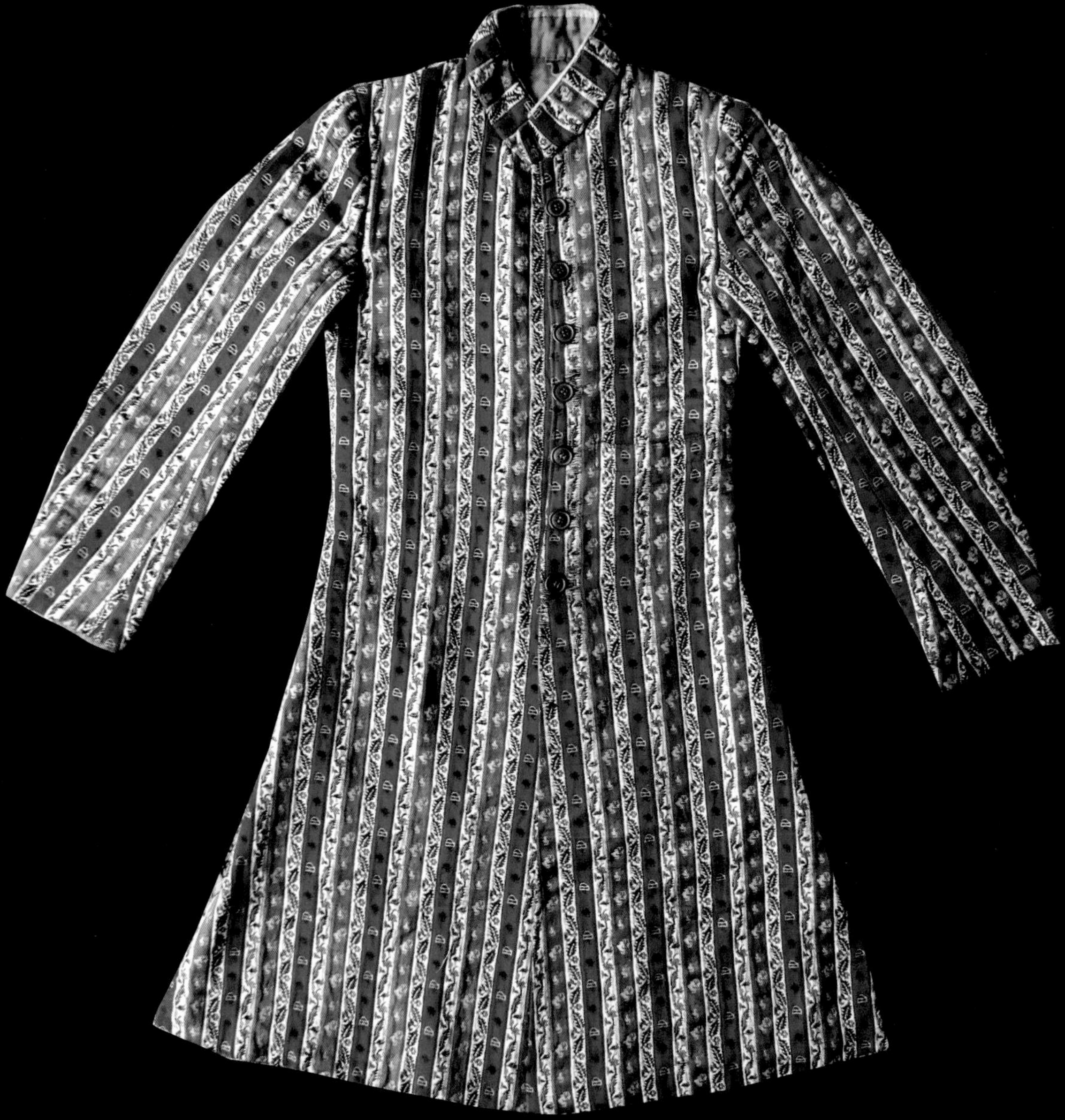

This *achkan* has tailored shoulders with sleeves shaped to fit. Around the neck there is a narrow straight stand-up collar. There are no slit pockets in the front instead they are at the sides.

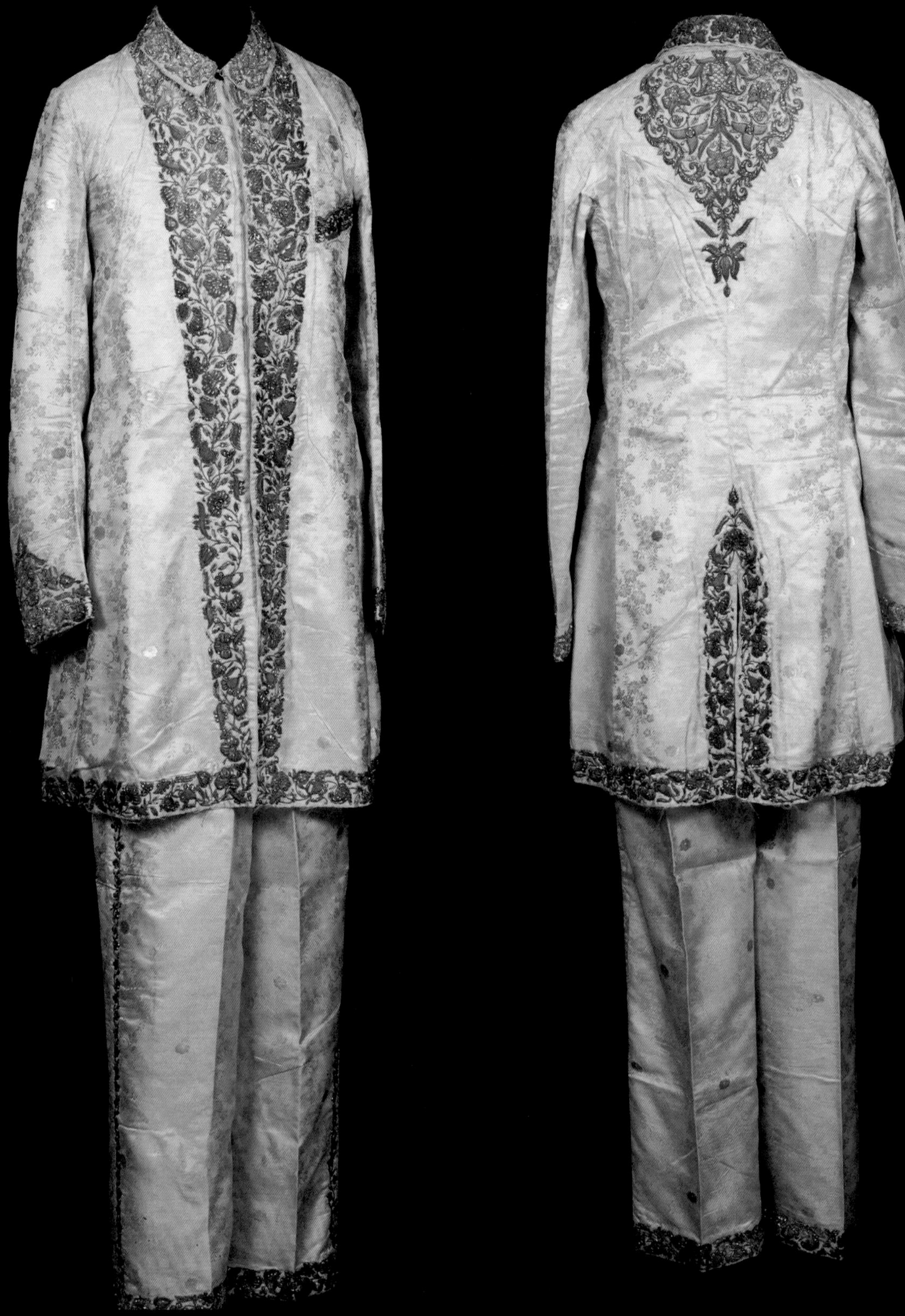

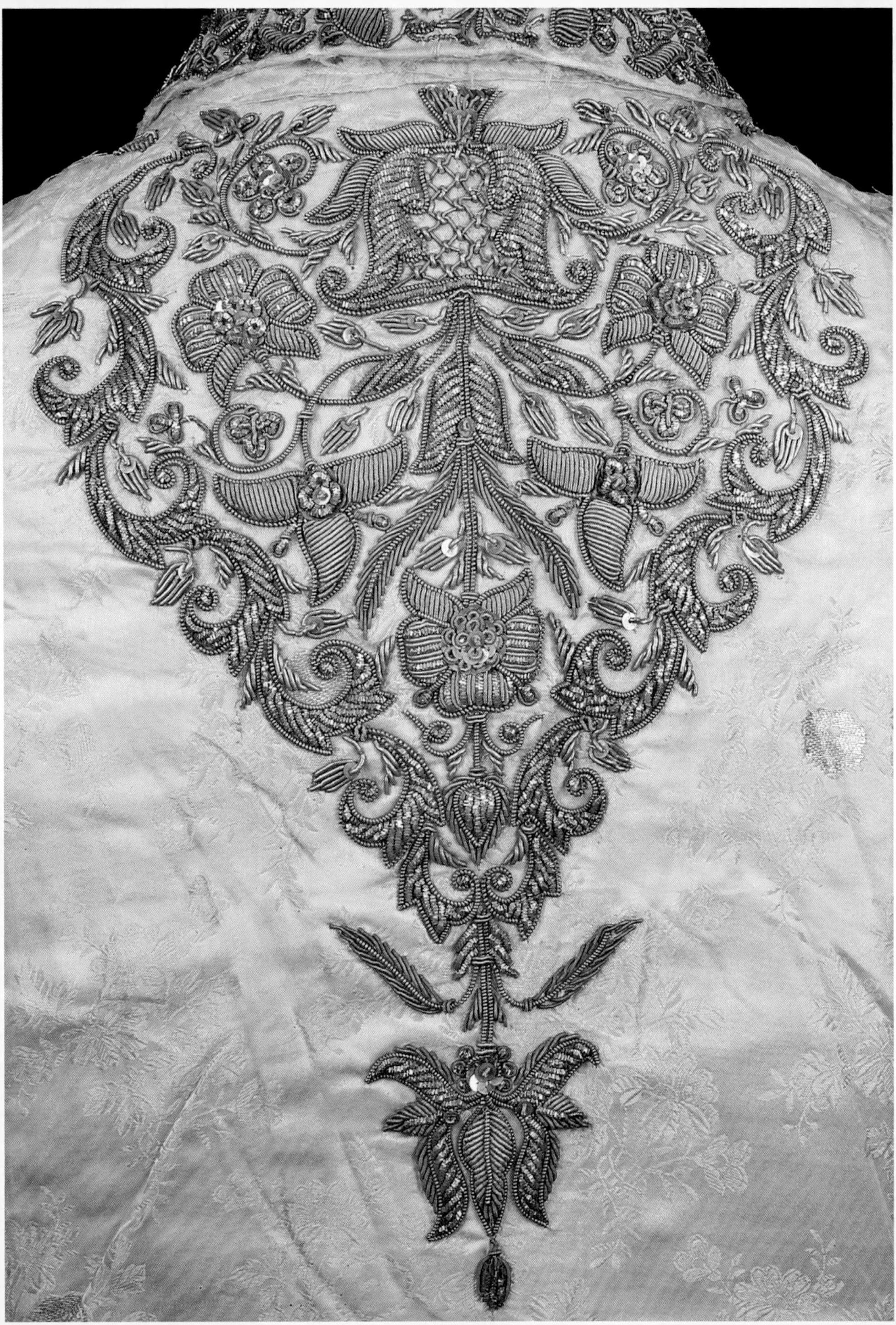

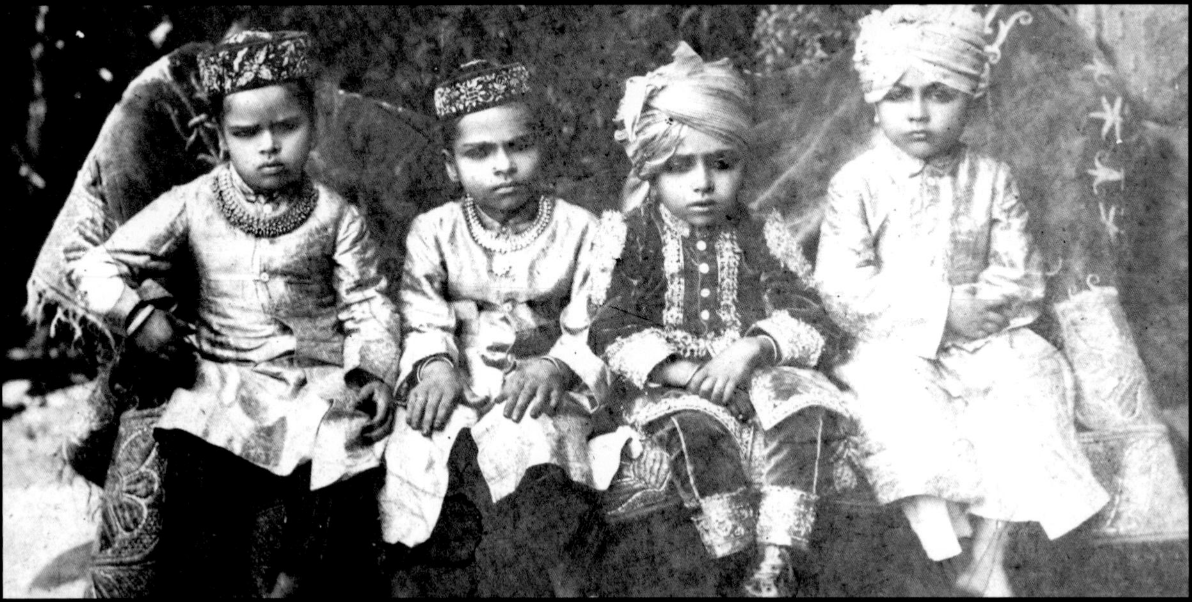

Nawab Jafar Mir Abdullah's Reminiscences About Boys' Wear

My conversations with Nawab Jafar Mir Abdullah of Lucknow revealed a more distinct fashion was introduced for children. Boys' shirts were made of *mulmul* and silk and were richly embroidered at the collar and at sleeves. Paijamas were embellished with *lachka* and *gota* work.

The shapes of the cap changed with the age of the child. The child's cap used to be round, made of soft materials like silk or *mulmul* and delicately finished with frills, sometimes embroidered with *salma* (gold or silver coil), *sitara* (round metal discs), *lachka* (broad *gota*) and *gota* work. For adolescent boys, the cap took the shape of a boat, called *kishtinuma* and frills gave way to clean cuts. The embroidery was mainly in *karchobi* work.

Birthdays were special occasions. On a boy's birthday, the child was dressed like a groom. He was dressed in rich clothes of brocade that were embroidered in *karchobi* work. *Sehra, badhi* (string of flowers worn in criss-cross manner across front and back) and *turra* (a decoration for the headgear) were important decorations for birthday celebrations. *Turra* was a bunch, usually of flowers, that was tucked under the cap. On birthdays, the *turra* was made of precious stones and pearls.

Boys used to wear plus-four knickers, which were ankle-length pants, balloon-shaped till the knee and then fitted till the ankle. Knickers were also worn, often with half-sleeved shirts or full-sleeved shirts and a jacket. Pants were held in place with the help of suspenders and the hem of the pants was turned towards the outside. Eventually, suspenders were replaced by belts, which were fastened around the waist to get a better fitting.

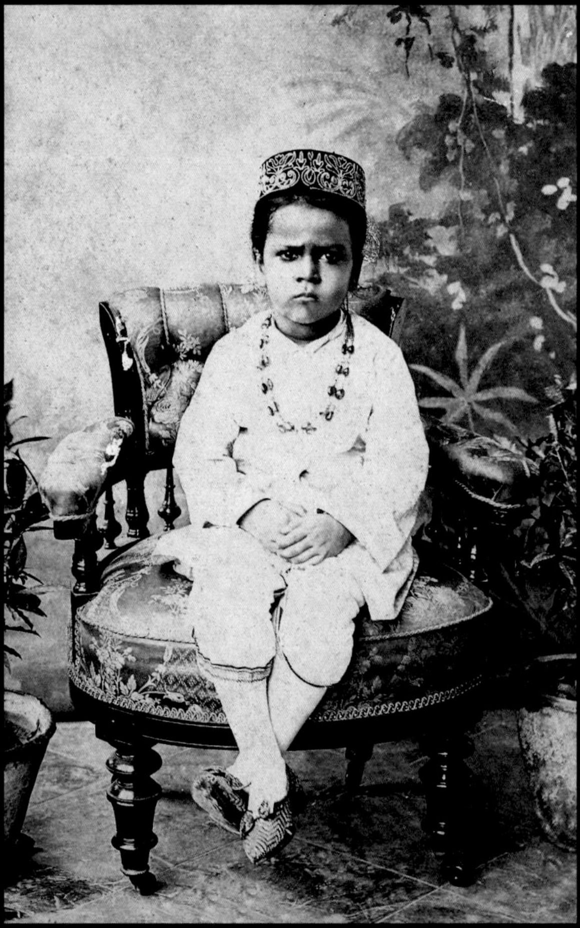

Above: The plus-four knickers are worn with a coat, round topi, designed pump shoes with knee-length socks. An important two-stringed necklace as part of a formal outfit was essential.
Above Left: Two boys are dressed in brocade *achkans*-paijamas and topis which are richly embroidered in **zardozi**. Another wears an ornate velvet coat and pant suit with laced shoes.

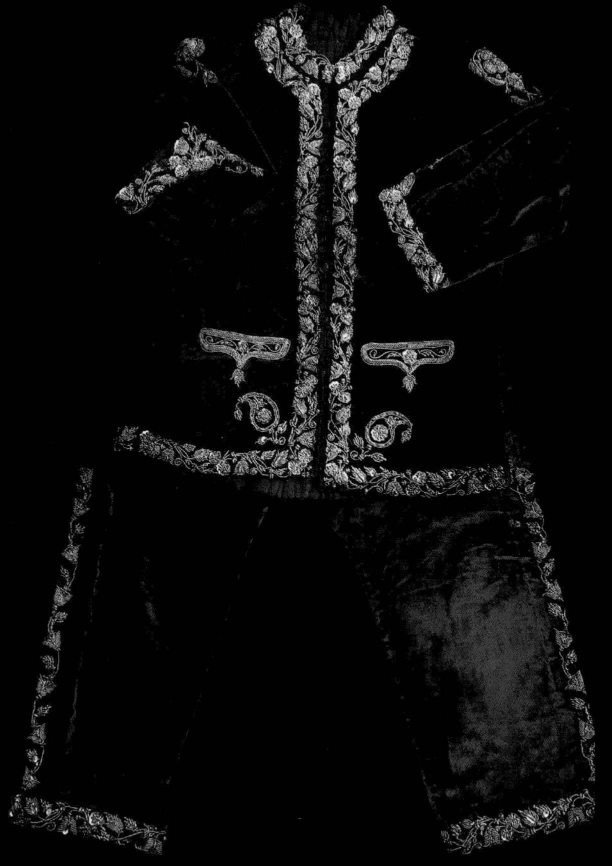

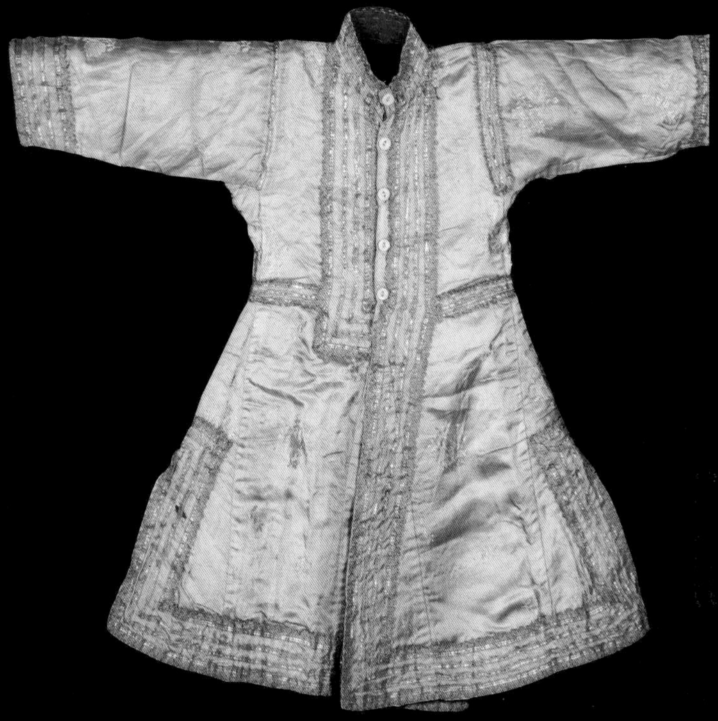

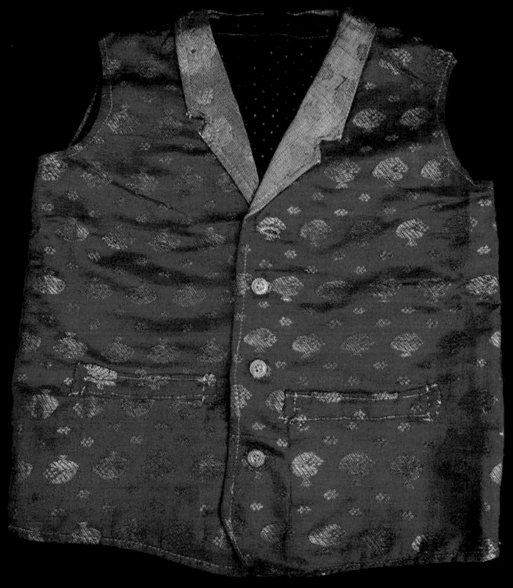

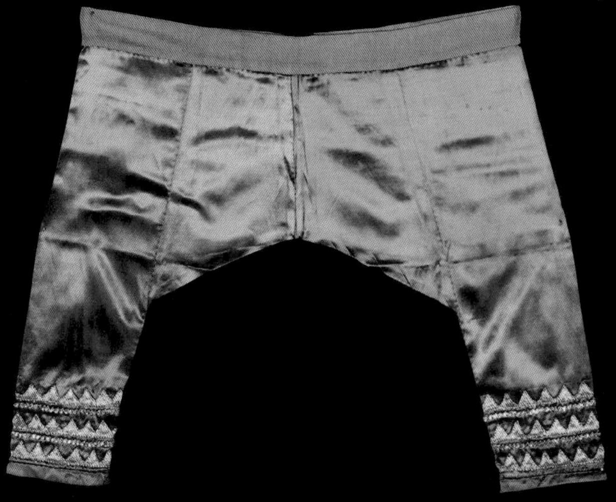

Clockwise from top: 1. A child's velvet machine-stitched coat and pant tailored with a Western cut but adorned with Awadhi ornamentations. The rich embroidery in zardozi makes this garment gorgeous enough to be worn for a celebration.
2. This ceremonial peach-coloured *chapkan* is made of Chinese silk with woven floral motifs, embellished with a gold braid and narrow *gota* ribbon.
3. *Sidha* paijama in *atlas* silk has beautifully decorated *mohris* in applique work in *gillori* (triangular shaped) design. The *nefa* for the *izarband* is in contrasting red cotton.
4. A red waistcoat made of *bafta* brocade with a black cotton lining. It has a contrasting green collar and slit pockets on both sides. While the waistcoat is machine stitched, the button-holes are hand-finished.

WOMEN'S COSTUMES

Changes to women's dress came slowly with the gradual decline of the purdah system during the British Raj. Gradually, the initial differences reflecting the Hindu and Muslim cultures receded as there was increased interaction between the two cultures. It should be remembered that the vast majority of Muslims in India had been Hindus, who loved to continue with their traditional clothes. Elder women still wore traditional clothes, even when they had to entertain or attend social functions. My grandmother always wore her lehenga, blouse and chunni even when she attended parties at the governor's house. The *chadariya* was still worn over lehengas. Young women started wearing saris during this period. The sari, seen as a neutral dress of Hindus and Muslims combined the different dressing styles, and increasingly gained popularity in Awadh and rest of India.

The influence of the West also became visible in the upper garments of women. The increasing importance of tailoring and tighter fitting led to the evolution of the modern blouse. The jacket-coat was introduced and embellished with Awadhi ornamentations. These were typically worn over the sari.

Among handbags, clutch purses and purses with handles were introduced. Some of them were embellished with beads and some were embroidered in petit point. The *batuiyas* of the nawabi period were replicated in different shapes and materials, such as leather. Gradually, they lost their appeal and declined in fashion. Interestingly, shoes began to be worn under saris.

Younger girls generally wore frocks over paijamas. A new variation of the paijama came into existence that resembled a gharara. Instead of gathers at the knee level, like in the gharara, pleats were inserted in the lower part of the garment as is done in English petticoats.

Below left: Seen here is a lady wearing a sari with machine-embroidered scalloped skirt border worn in *sidha pallav* style and a blouse with lace. The little baby is wearing a frock.
Below right: A *chadariya* made of Chinese silk-cloth decorated with a black velvet border. The flowers made of coloured ribbons, are hand-stitched making a separate motif.
Facing page, left: A British influence: to the extreme left the girl is wearing a frock with salwar, while the girl on the right is wearing a Western frock with shoes, and the young boy is wearing half pants and high-neck sweater with a coat. Knee-high socks are worn with buckled shoes.
Facing page, Right: A family portrait. Sherwani worn with churidar paijama by the man, sari in *ulta palla* style worn with tailored blouse by her and young girls wearing Western frocks and young boy wearing shirt with half-pants complete the dressing style of mid twentieth century.
Facing page, Below: Young girls are wearing '*bachkani*' sari in sidha-pallav style, adorned with embroidered border. The muslin and brocade blouses have puff sleeves.

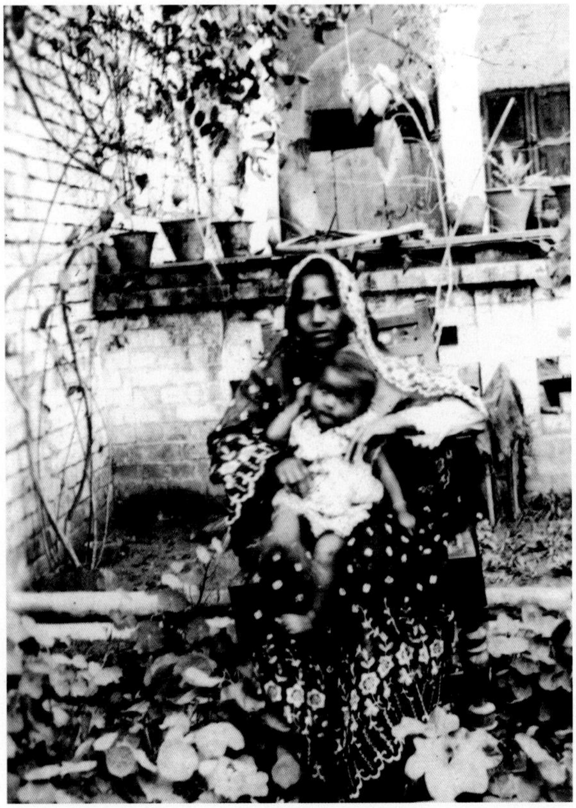

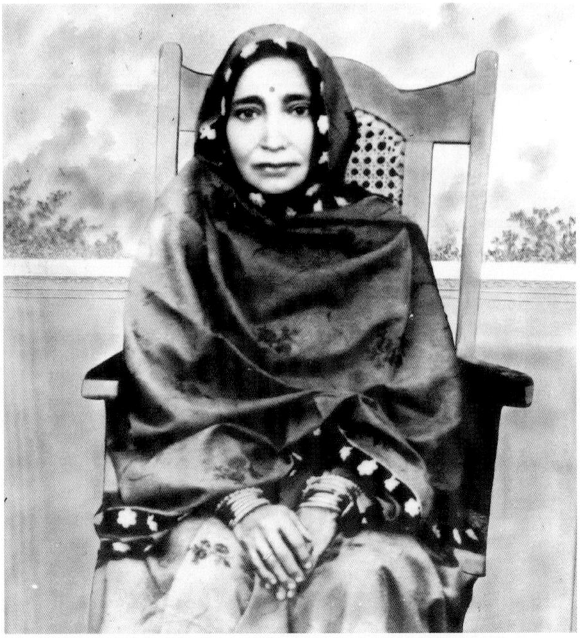

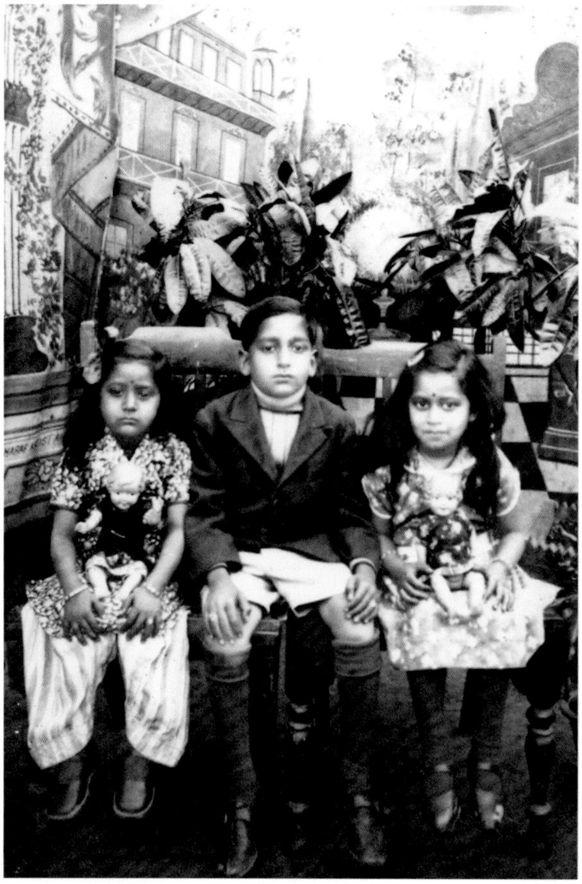

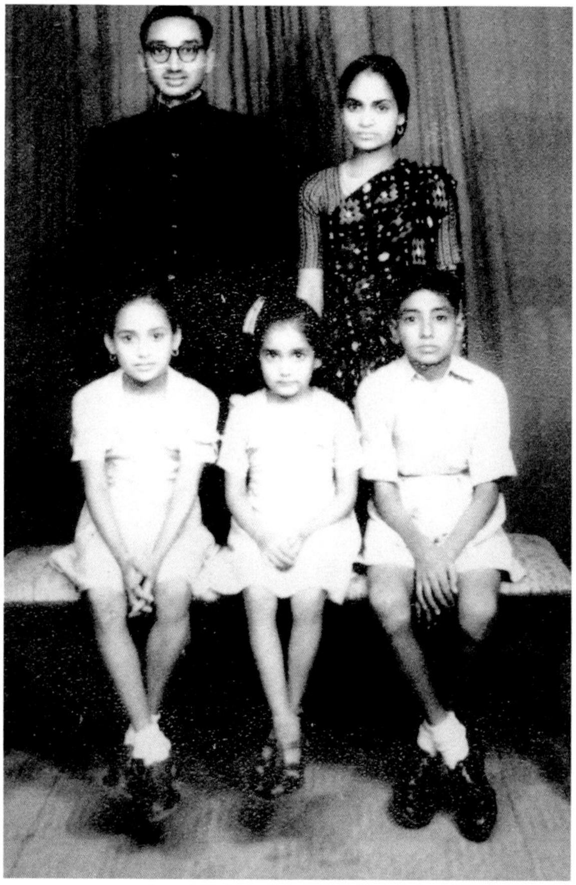

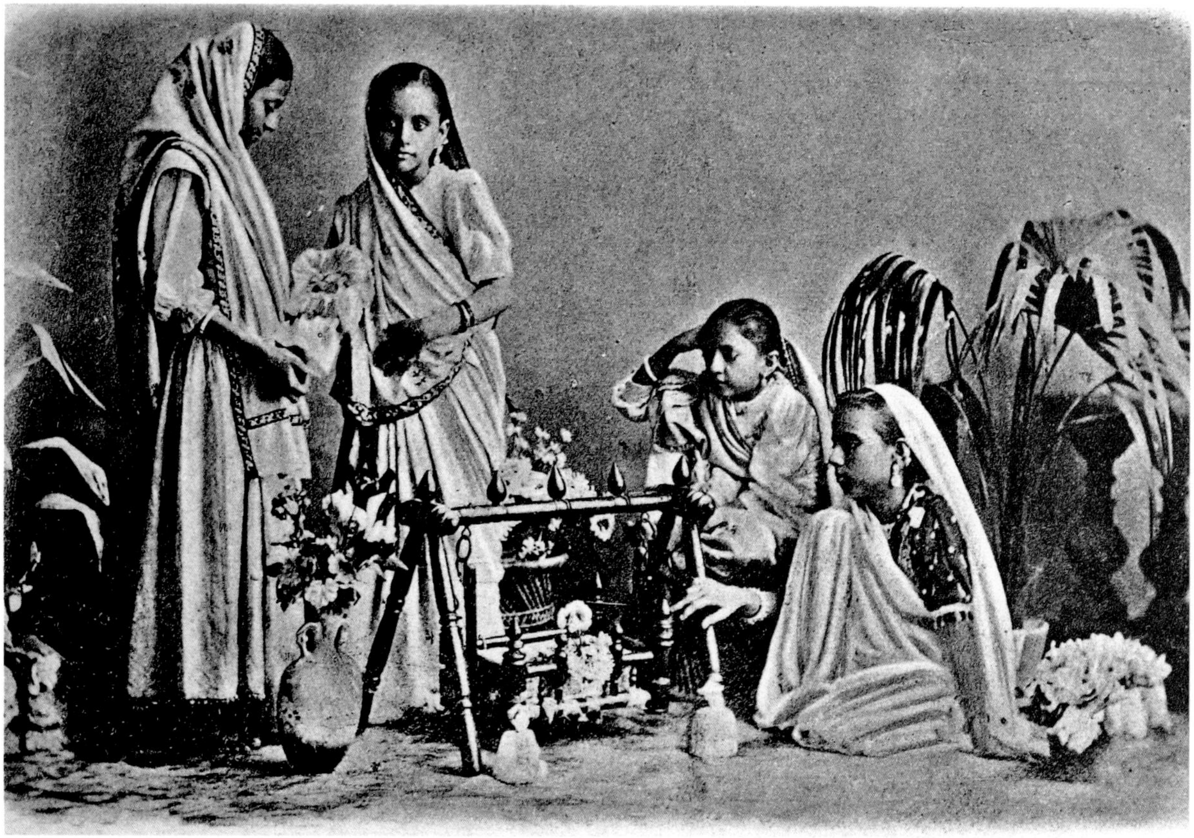

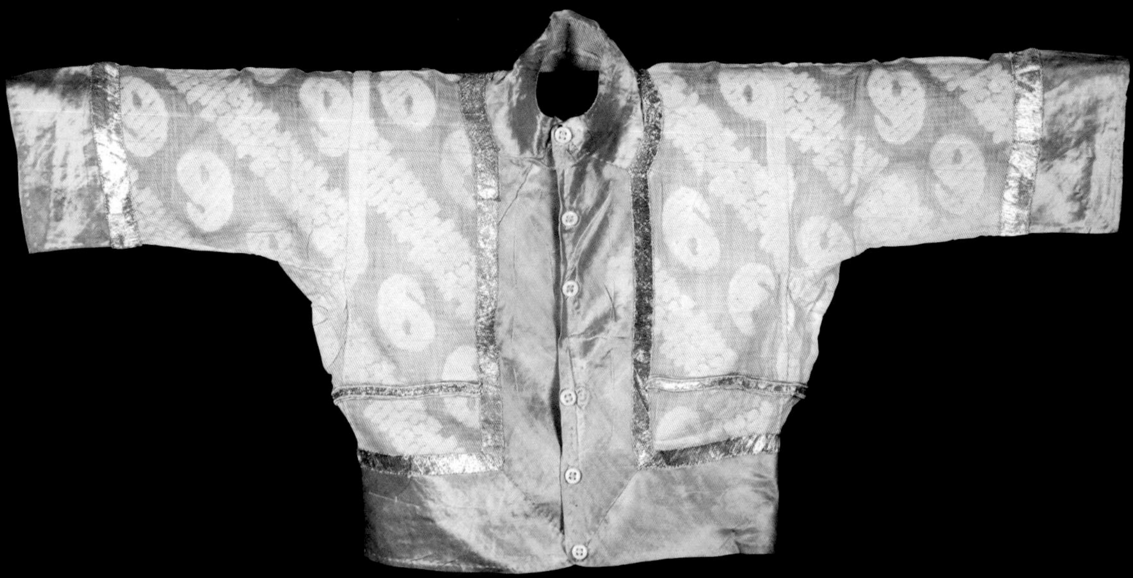

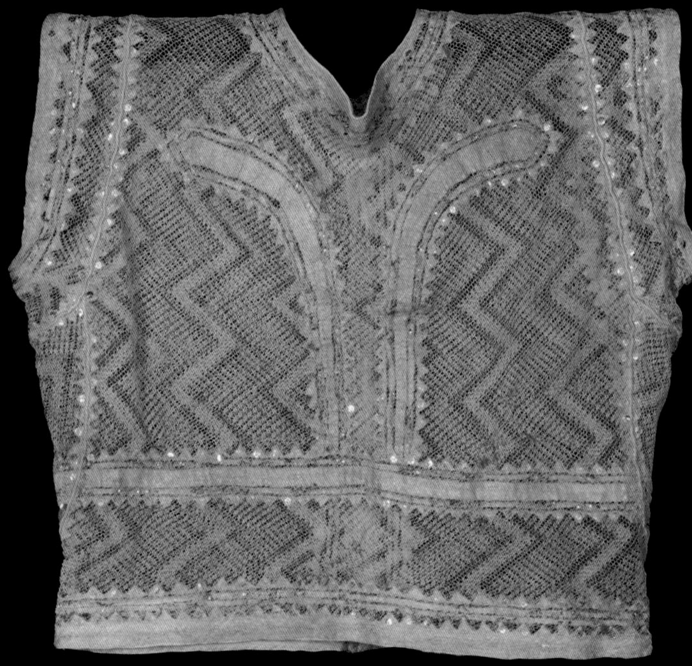

Above: This pink *jamdani* blouse incorporates some elements of Western fashion. The length is longer than the *angiya/choli* as this was worn with a sari rather than with a lehenga. The *katoris* disappeared, fastening moved to the front instead of the back and buttons replaced tie-cords. The ornamentation was more linear.
Below: A tailored net blouse with mega sleeves. The applique work is outlined in *kinari* motif and embellished in *badla* work.

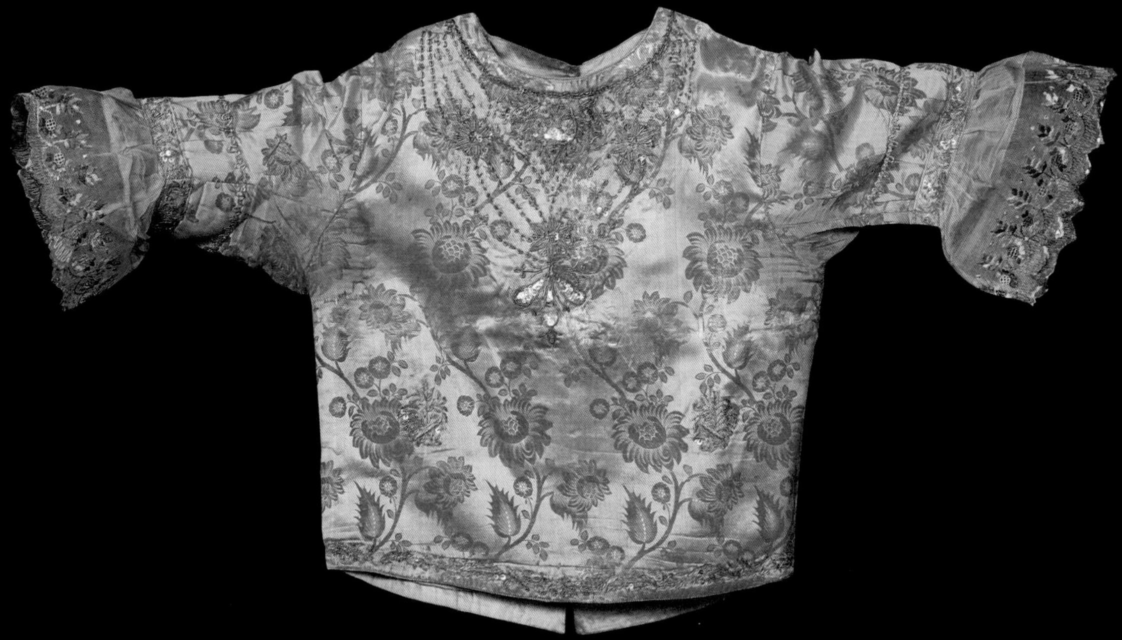

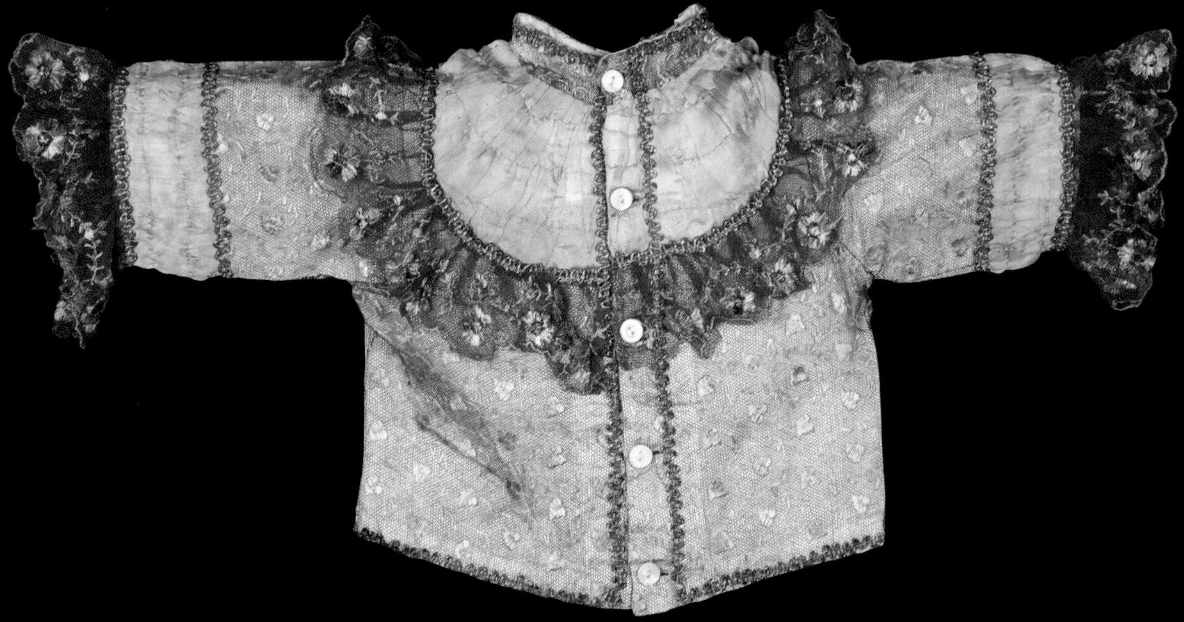

Above: A pink blouse, made of silk brocade from China, has a necklace-like motif embroidered in **zardozi** with real gold *kalabattun*, *salma* and *sitara*. The lace borders on the sleeves give it a Western touch.
Below: This blouse of red net fabric has white silk lining. A contrasting green-coloured yolk in the front and borders at the sleeves are used for the design. French machine-made matching red lace is added to the yolk and sleeves as ornamentation in addition to Awadhi element of *gota* of *bakuri* type.

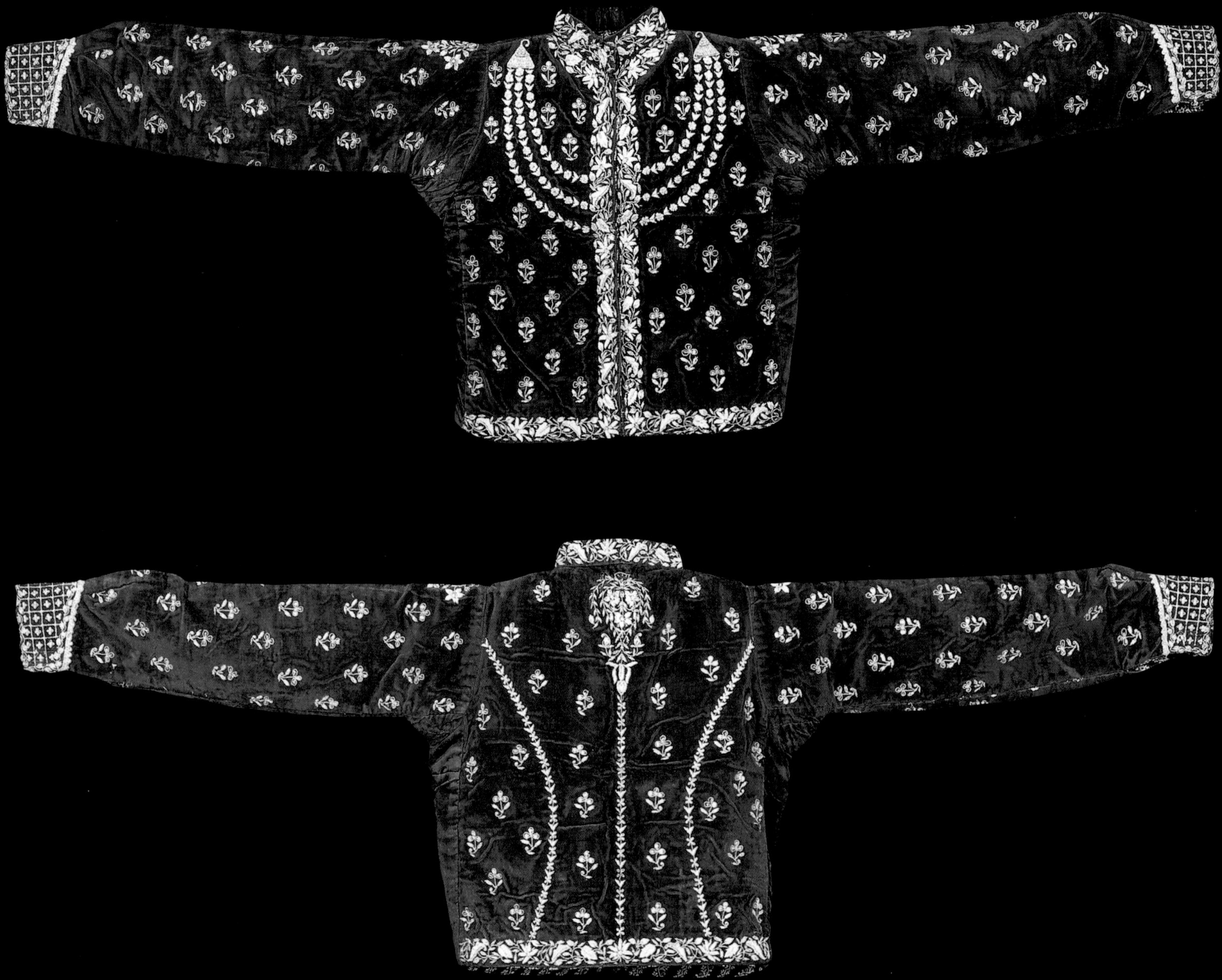

European influence can be seen in the tailoring of this jacket-blouse; the neatly cut armholes, fitted look at the back and the distinct collar and cuffs.

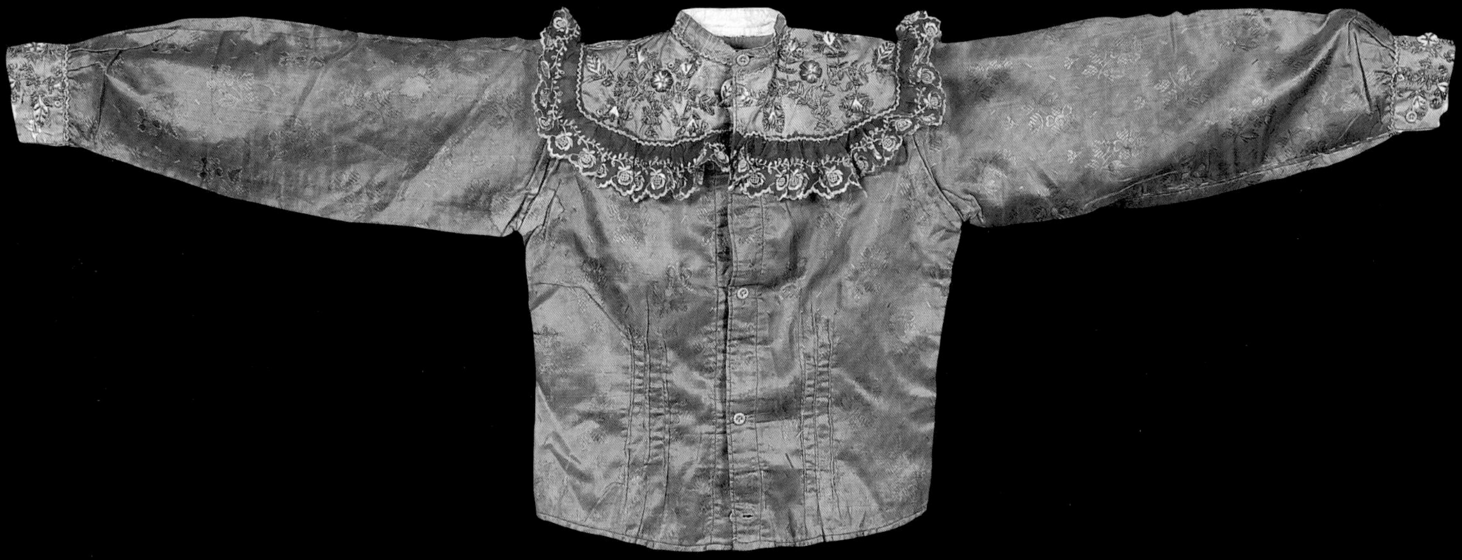

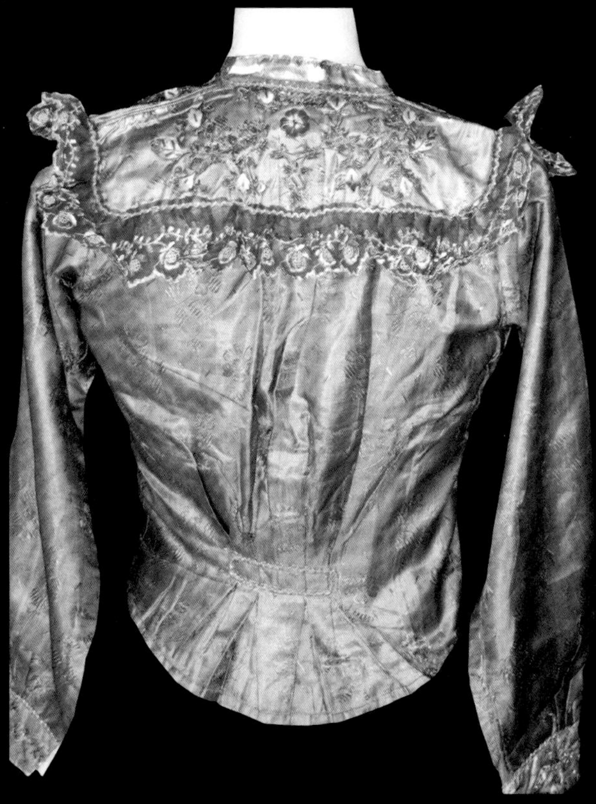

Above: This Chinese silk jacket-coat was worn with sari. The machine-stitching and embellishments on the yolk with frilled lace depict the adoption of Western elements of fashion.
Below (detail): The jacket coat has pleats at the back for silhouette fitting.

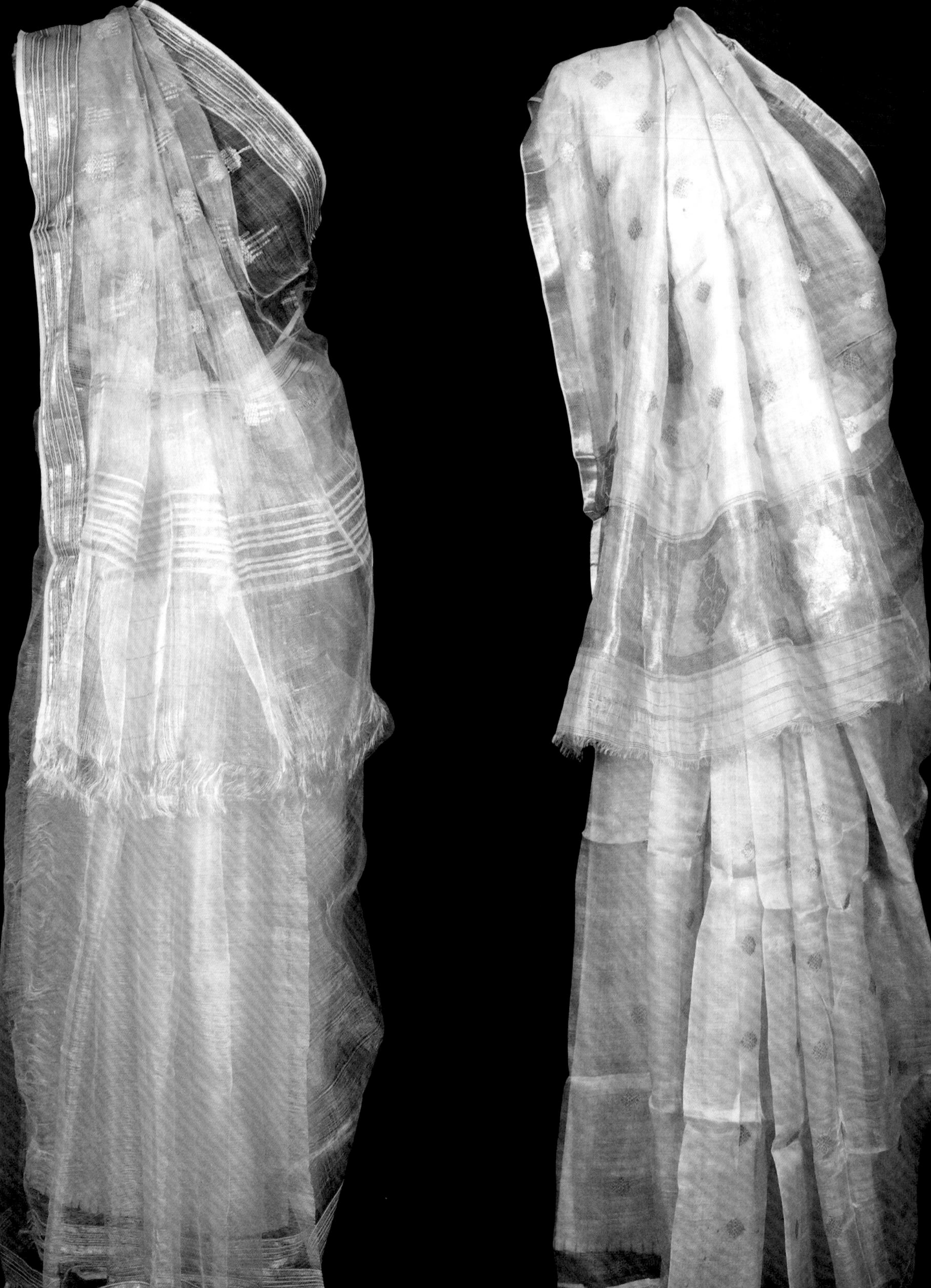

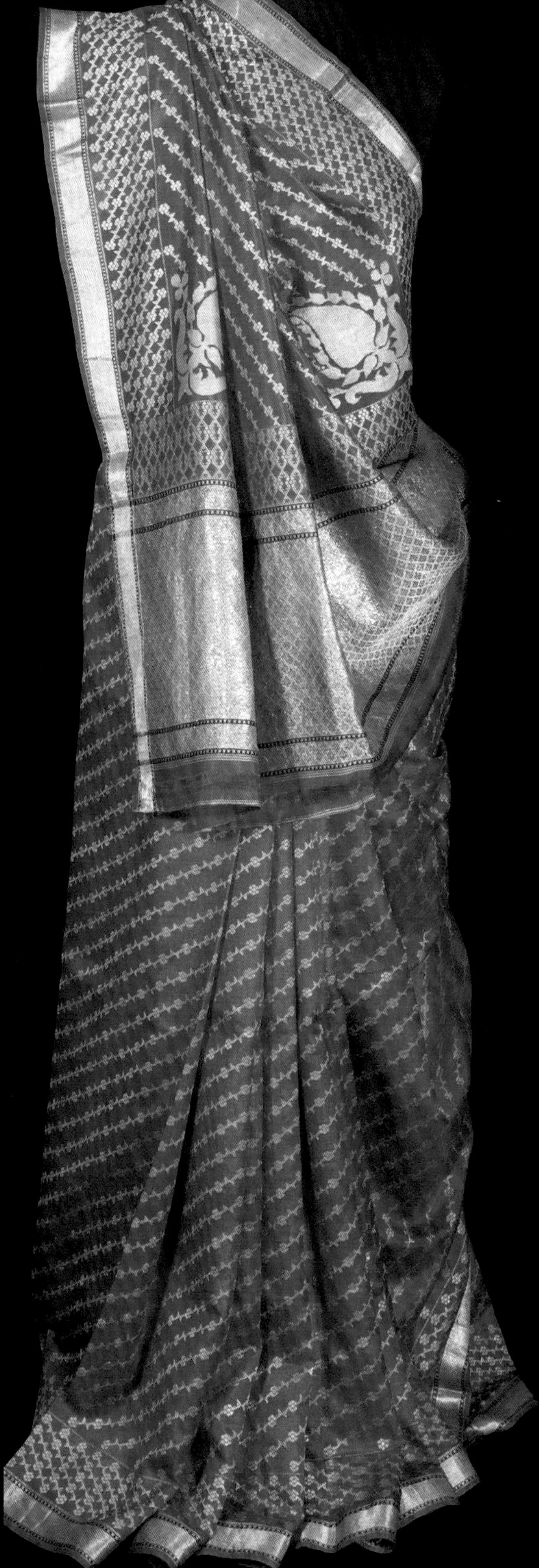

Facing page, Left: A tissue sari has a very fine silk warp and *zari* weft, giving the cloth a metallic sheen and lustre. The use of purple silk yarn in the border and lotus *butis* in gold and silver zari on pista-green base creates a Ganga-Jamuni effect.
Facing page, Right: A lightweight organza silk sari, woven at Banaras, has its ground scattered with *asharfi* (coin) motif. The *pallav* is elaborately woven with a stylized tree-of-life motif.
Right: This crimson red sari is hand woven in *bafta* brocade. The *pallav* is intricately woven in *ekpara kinkhab* with *chasm-e-bulbul* pattern. A *turanj* motif can be seen on the corners of the pallav. To Hindus, *turanj/ambi* design connotes auspiciousness.

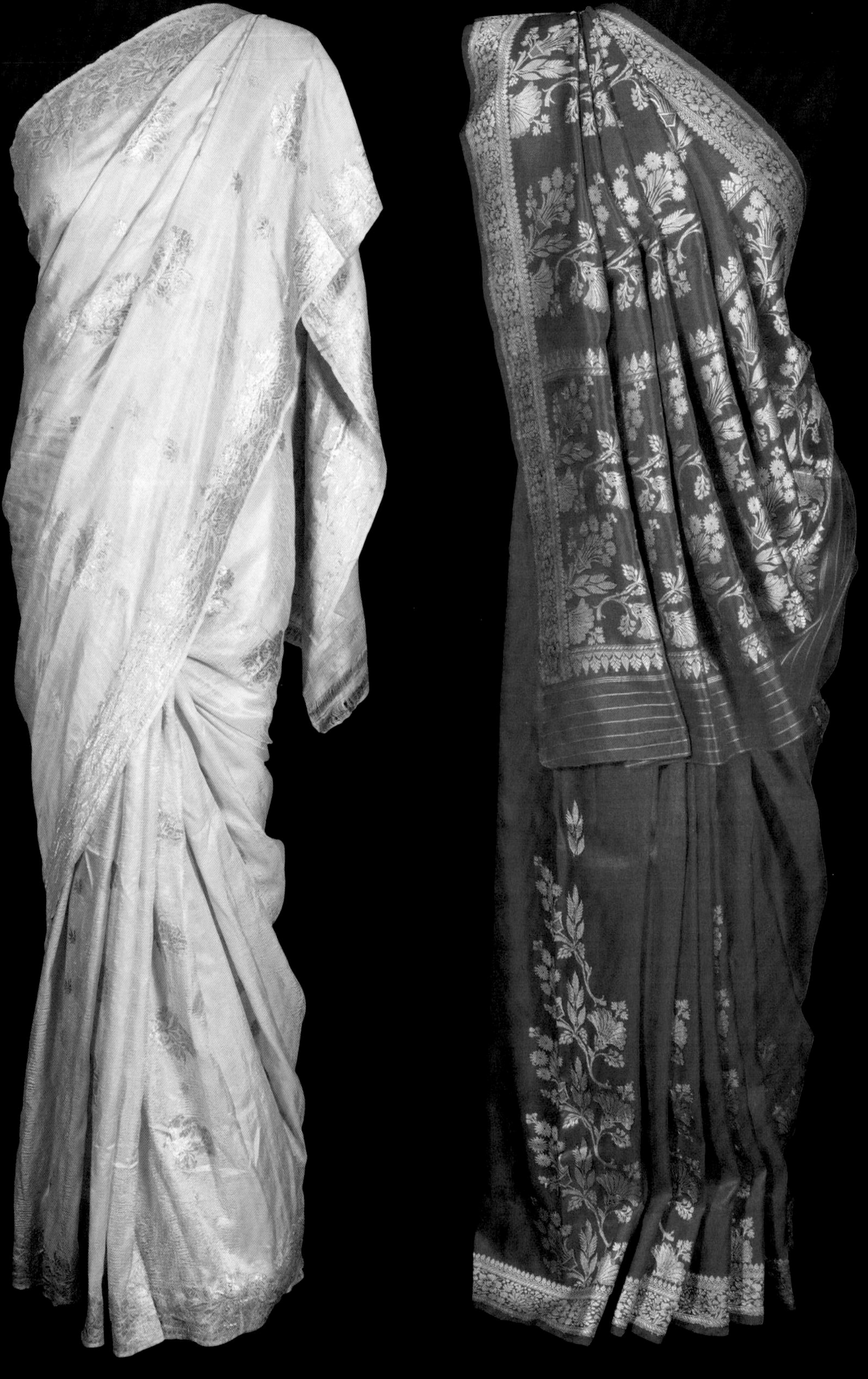

Clockwise from top:
1. An evening purse (seen from both front and back here) made of cream-coloured silk is embellished with four-petaled white flowers in the front and ornately worked with white beads, outlined with brown beads, at the back.
2. An evening purse with gold-tone sequins on a cream fabric base (seen from both front and back here). The handle is delicately decorated with beads and pearls.
3. This evening bag features intricate petit point needlepoint with rose floral motifs, a snap top closure and a metal chain.
4. This pink leather bag, inspired by the typical *batuiya* of the nawabi period has drawstrings made of twisted yarns.
5. A black cotton bag decorated with glass beads with a matching draw-string for closure, similar to the *batuiya* of the nawabi period.
6. A black Rayon evening bag with a snap lock closure.

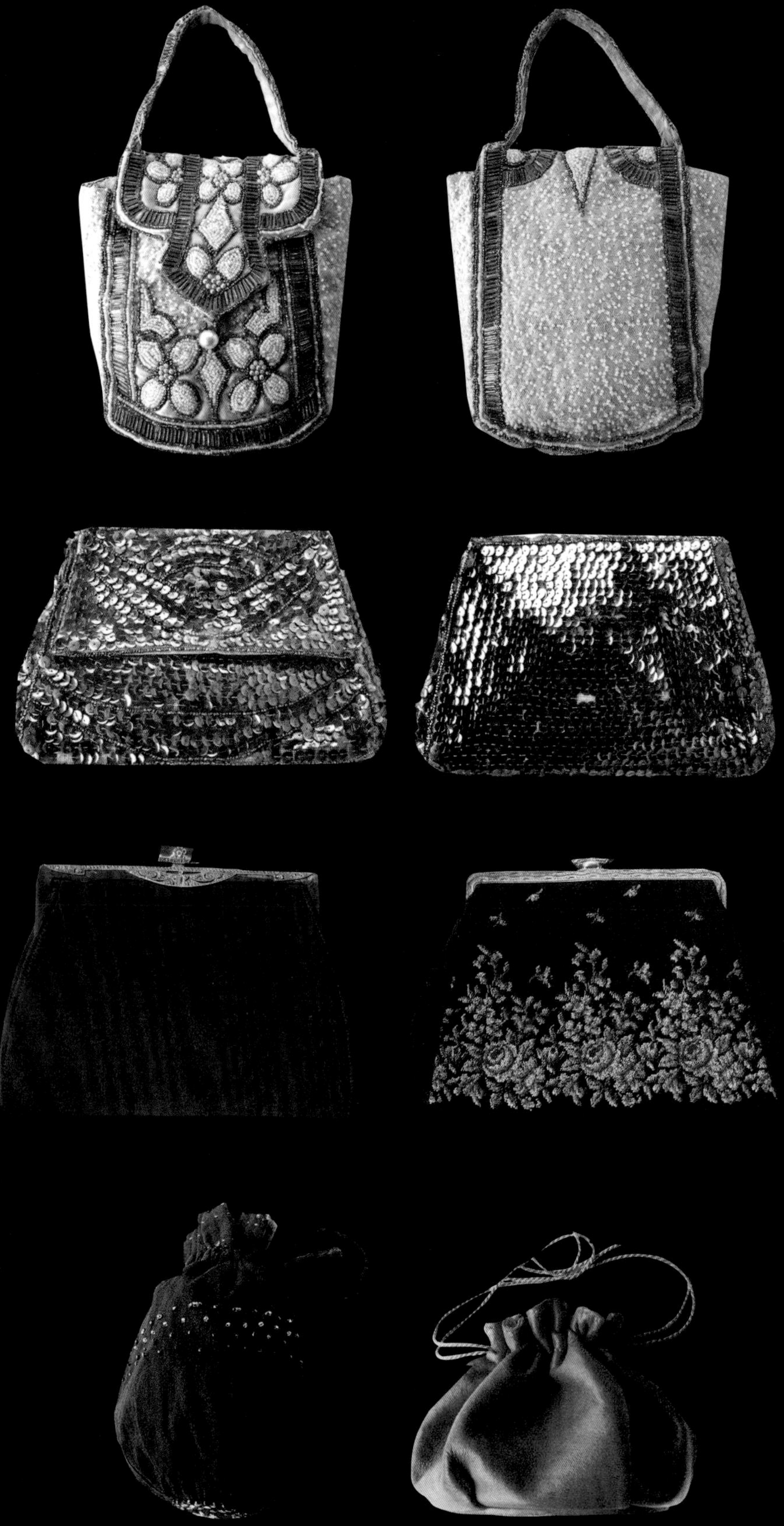

Facing page, Left: This *bafta* brocade sari, worn in *ulta-pallav* style, is hand-woven and brocaded with a gold floral border, *butas* and smaller *butis* fill the body. The powder pink colour signifies softness and tenderness, an example of British influence.
Facing page, Right: This vibrant *gul-e-anari* sari is made of *amru* silk. It has a unique design of floral *buta*s arranged vertically. It has an intricately woven *pallav*. The use of green and blue silk threads interwoven amongst the flowers gives a *minakari* effect.

Vishnu Narayan Agarwal of Lucknow, national awardee (1991) for miniature painting, narrates his personal story.

'In my ancestral haveli (palace-like house), there were separate halls for men and women and no male member, not even a boy of twelve years was allowed to enter the women's quarters, without informing in advance. His great grandmother used to wear a white gathered lehenga, chunni and 'jumper' kurti-like garment with handmade shoes of white cloth. She and the other women of the household wore *angiya* (blouse) made of fine muslin. They also wore a chadariya when going out. For festive occasions, his aunts used to wear lehengas made of a rich satin-finish atlas fabric from Banaras. One special lehenga that he still remembers was made of seven colours and was known as satrangi. The younger girls used to wear bachkani dhoti (child size) till the age of eleven to twelve years with *shaluka* and *kurti* or suthanne, a kind of paijama with a kurti.'

Hazira Begum and Taj Ara Begum of Sheeshmahal, Lucknow, reminisce about their childhood and about the time when they were seven or eight years old (c. 1940).

Taj Ara Begum remembers, 'We used to wear lehengas with full-sleeved collared shirts, accompanied by chunnis or dupattas that were embellished with *kamdani* work. Our *ghatela* shoes were made of velvet, matching our dresses, and had *ghungroos* (tiny bells) attached to them. These *gunghroos* made a merry tinkling sound when we would walk around. During *saawan* (the rainy season), all the girls would dress in green clothes, crinkled dupattas, green bangles and earrings. The crinkling of chunnis was done with the help of a small stone and the dhobis were experts at it.

Hazira Begum recalls, 'They used to wear *bar ke paijamas*, made of 16 yards of cloth with *asafkhani* (bodice with flare) blouses under the sherwanis. The *farshi paijama* was made of 18 yards and the *kalidar* paijama of 9 yards. They wrapped *dushalas* (big shawls) around themselves in winter—these were made of pashmina wool obtained from the fleece of the underbelly of the rare Tibetan wild mountain goat. The *peshwaz* was made in umbrella cut (diagonally cut) as opposed to the straight cuts of earlier times. Only on Fridays did they wear churidar paijamas. Salwars were worn only by the cooks and servants, while other attendants wore clothes of the same style but of rougher material.'

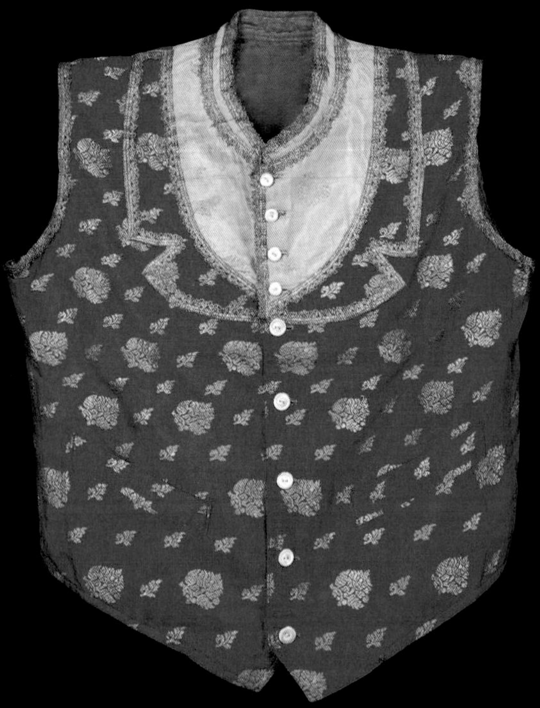

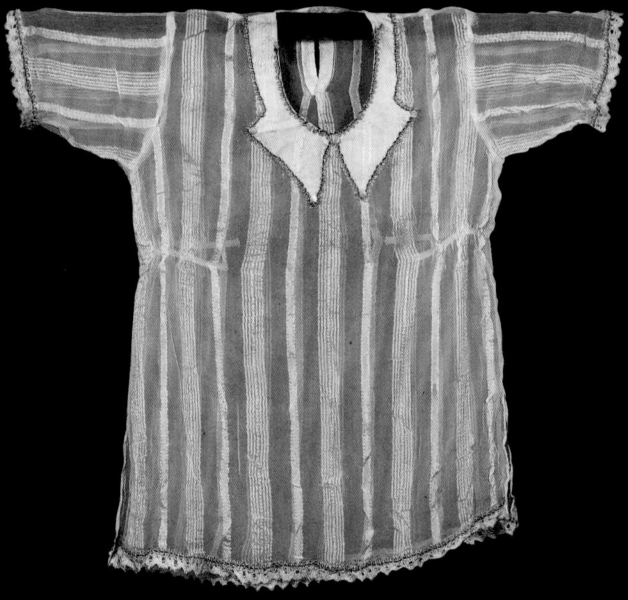

Top: An European style tailored silk brocade waistcoat with a cream-coloured front piece opens in the centre. There is a special attention to detail: uneven settings of buttons and a buckle on the back to make it a better fitting garment. The embroidery in braided gold **zari** gives the effect of a collar.
Bottom: S*haluka* (upper garment) made of machine-made silk chiffon is embellished with fine *gota*-work. A collar is designed through appliqué work and an elastic band is inserted for better fitting.

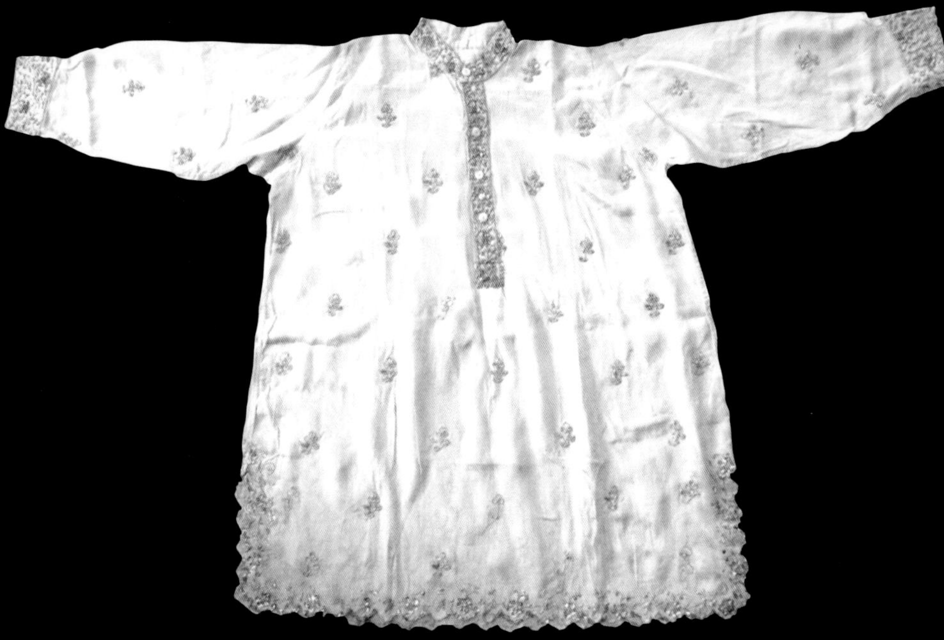

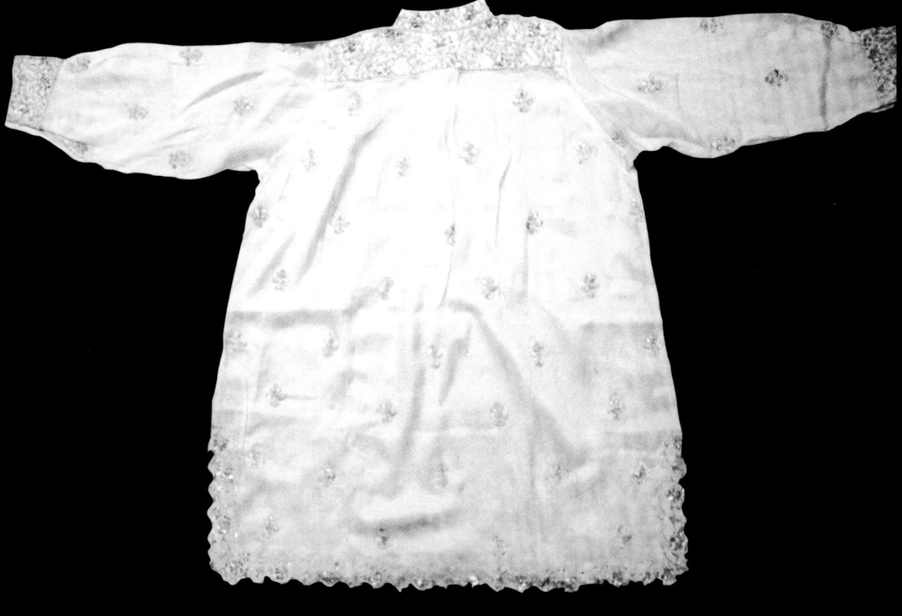

Above: The front opening and cuffs of this cream-coloured silk kurti is embroidered with *tilla* and sequins in gold. The embroidered scalloped hem and slits were typical of Awadh during British Raj.
Below: The back of the kurti has a *tira* (yoke- the part of a shirt that stretches over the back shoulders, usually made out of a doubled piece of fabric) with matching embroidery.

TEXTILES

COTTON

In the early twentieth century, hand-spun cotton, khadi, became a key symbol of the Non-cooperation Movement in the battle for independence from British rule. Mahatma Gandhi urged Indians to wear only homespun khadi and asked for the public burning of British mill-made cloth. The cotton khadi costumes came to be identified with political awareness and patriotism. Khadi replaced other textiles and led to a transformation in the costumes of Awadh, from the delicate clothing of the nawabs to the rough khadi fabric. Freedom fighters developed a distinct code of dressing. The khadi kurta and khadi paijama were worn with the Gandhi topi, and the Jawahar bandi (waistcoat). The *nukkadar* cap of the nawabi period, made of velvet, shawl cloth, embroidered with gold and silver and overall a symbol of luxury, was now simple, made of khadi cotton and became a symbol of the freedom struggle.

SILK

Many European design styles were woven in silk by Indian weavers to the taste of the British rulers. As pure gold and silver became too expensive, imitation zari began to be used for brocades around 1852-1854 and plastic *zari* around 1890. Imitation zari is made from copper wire and plastic zari is made from a chemically coloured metallic yarn. A significant evolution in this period was the addition of silk and silk-based textiles produced on power looms introduced from the West. The dresses and gowns of British women made Indian women try new diaphanous silk materials such as chiffon, georgette, tulle, organza and silk tissue. The fabric Georgette is named after a French dressmaker of the twentieth century, Madame Georgette de la Plante.

All these textiles added a new dimension to the existing costumes of the period as the diaphanous look, which was previously only used for chunnis, started appearing in kurtis, *shaluka*s and, most of all, in saris. Contextualizing this change within the decline of the purdah system makes it even more interesting.

Below: Gandhiji clad in his loin-cloth in Noakhali 1947. The freedom fighters adopted kurta- *dhoti/* kurta-paijama with Gandhi topi and Jawahar *bandi* as their costumes. Women actively participated in the movement and preferred wearing salwar-kurta-*odhni* or a sari made of khadi.

Facing page: An auspicious mill-made cloth used for religious ceremonies. It depicts auspicious symbols, an elephant, a peacock and *rangoli.* The *Purna-Kalasha* in the centre refers to a pot filled with water and topped with a coronet of mango leaves and a coconut. It is considered a symbol of abundance and 'source of life' in the Vedas.

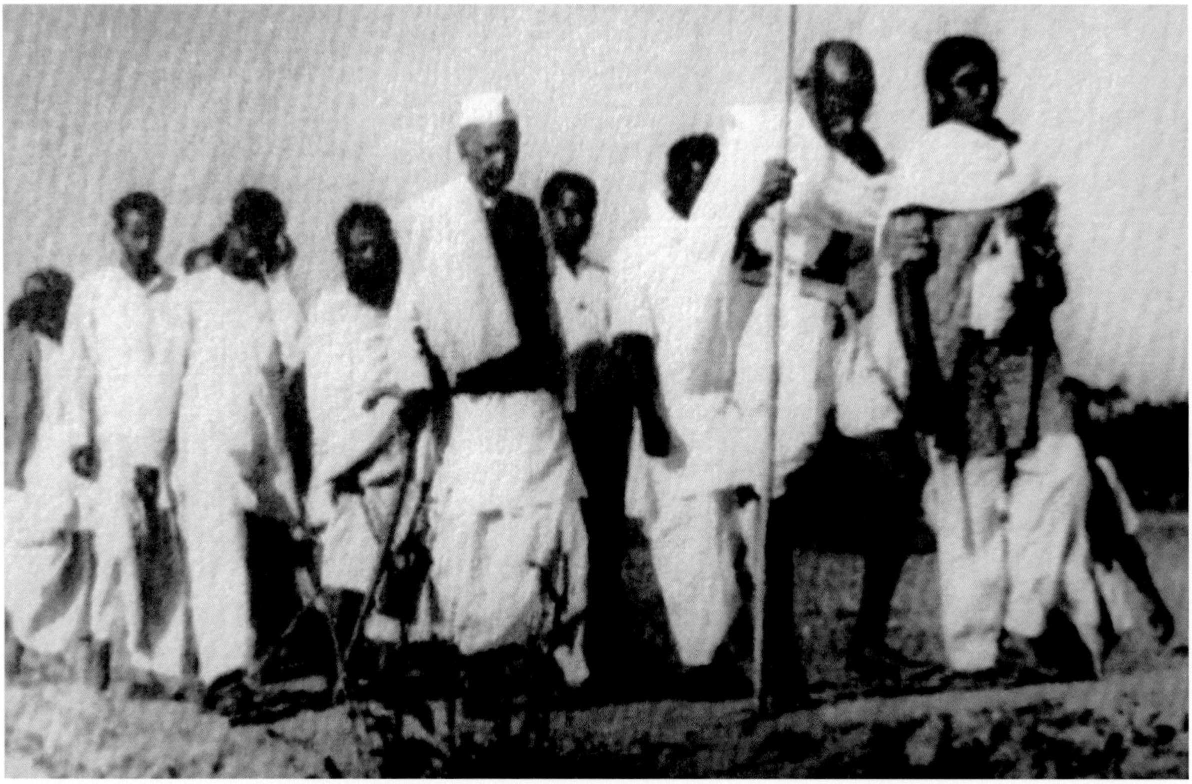

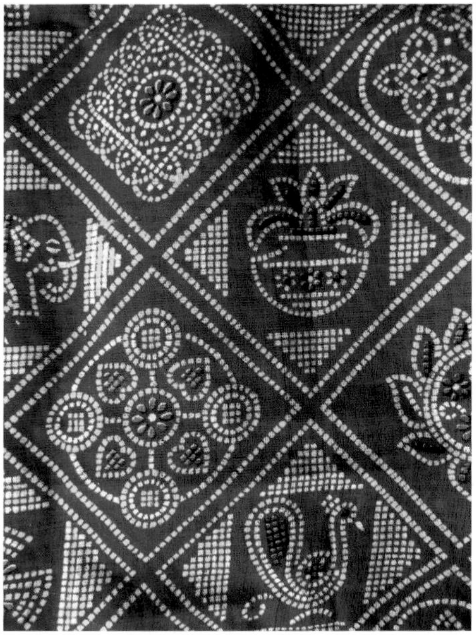

Shahjahan Ansari, a weaver from Banaras, explains, 'Chiffon and georgette are soft, lightweight fabrics of plain weave, usually made of natural yarns of silk or one of the man-made fibres. In pure chiffon, both the two-ply threads are of silk, while in artificial chiffon, one is silk thread while the second one is substituted with artificial silk called kela silk made with the bark of banana tree. Georgette has a grainy texture: first, the twisting is done on the machine with two silk threads and while twisting, one thread is kept tight and the other relatively loose to give this *danedar* (grainy) feel or texture. In one inch of two-ply silk thread there are eighty twists, which are difficult to notice with a naked eye. Georgette is slightly heavier and more opaque than chiffon.'

Although they are delicate in appearance, they are relatively strong fabrics and can be dyed or printed. In Lucknow, they were dyed and then embellished in *badla* and *kamdani* work. Organza is a thin fabric of plain weave made only with one ply, traditionally made from the continuous filament of silkworms. Tulle is a fabric created by silk threads or man-made threads that are intertwined to create a transparent but very stable network. It is technically a gauze-like fabric produced on bobbinet machine, forming hexagonal holes. Its name comes from the French city of Tulle.

WOOL

The popularity of knitted wool eventually reduced the use of Indian quilted garments. Knitted wool became extremely popular, partly due to its accessibility as a form of occupation and skill. The high quality hand-woven *jamavar* shawls became extinct by the end of the British Raj and were replaced by paisley shawls for the Awadhi elite.

The man-made or synthetic fibre industry began in 1910 with the first commercial production of rayon in France. The inventions since then have been many, such as nylon, acrylic, polyester, spandex, polyolefin, microfibers and are commonly used for clothing purposes.

The rise and fall of the cotton industry in Awadh

Cotton was grown and spun in the region of Awadh since time immemorial. The fertile land and hot and humid climate helped farmers produce the finest quality of cotton. This cotton was spun on a charkha in villages and woven on handlooms by a community known as Ansari and they were called *julaha*s or *katwas*. The farming of indigo was also developed, giving a parallel occupation of dyeing the cotton fabric, which took form of an art under the nawabs. A large population of rural Awadh was engaged in growing, spinning, dyeing and trading cotton.

The trade of cotton flourished in the area of Awadh with its centre in Cawnpore (British name the beginning of the eighteenth century. With the growing interest of the British in this region, the textile industry started growing in the late nineteenth century. Elgin Mill was the first cotton mill of the city established in 1864 and Muir Mill was established in 1876.

This growth continued even in the twentieth century in the United Provinces of Agra and Oudh (named Awadh in 1902). The period of the First World War (1914-16) witnessed phenomenal growth with increased international demand. More mills were established, such as J.K. Cotton Mills, British India Corporation (BIC) with five companies, Cawnpore Textile Mills (1922) and Atherton West Mills (1923). Post-war effects started to be felt by

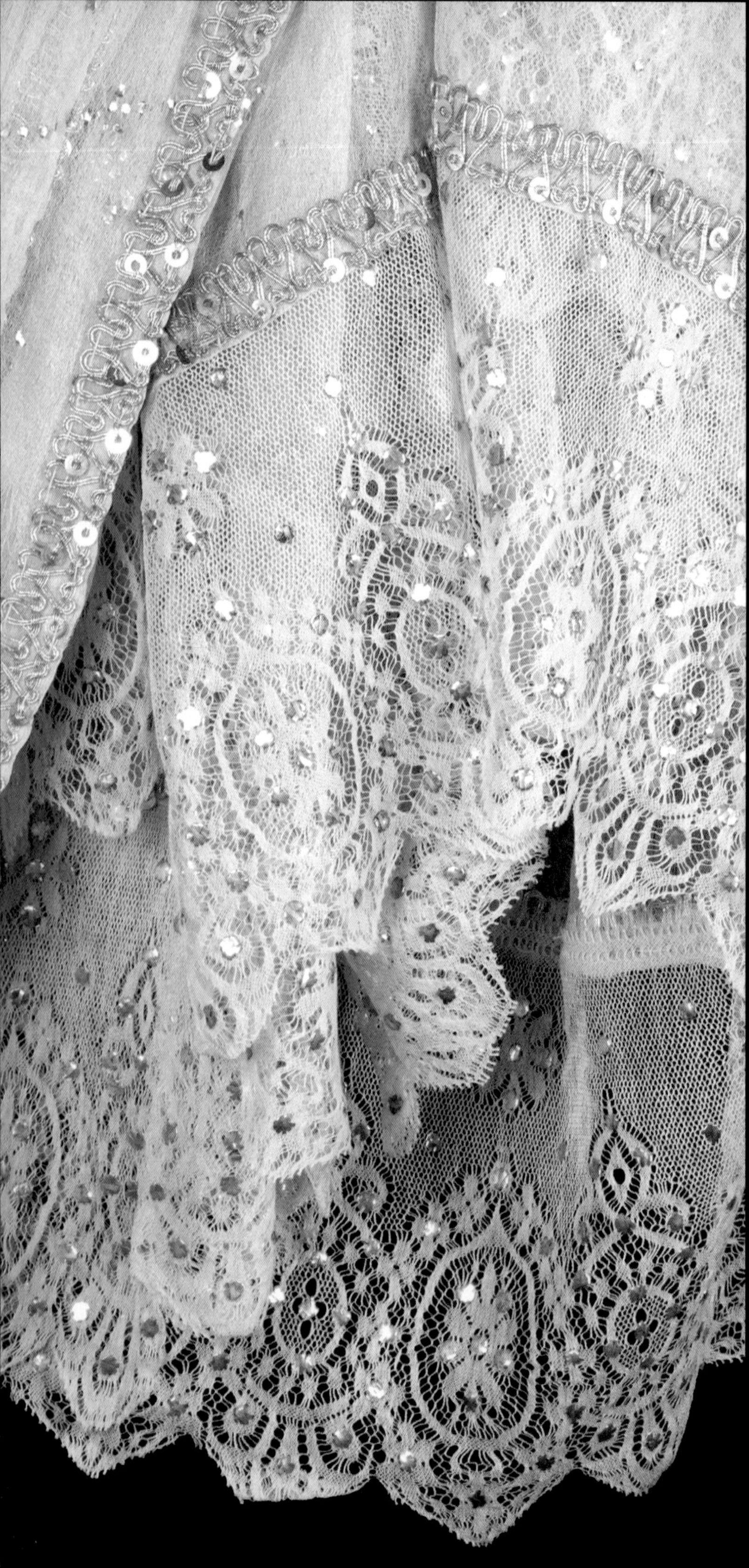

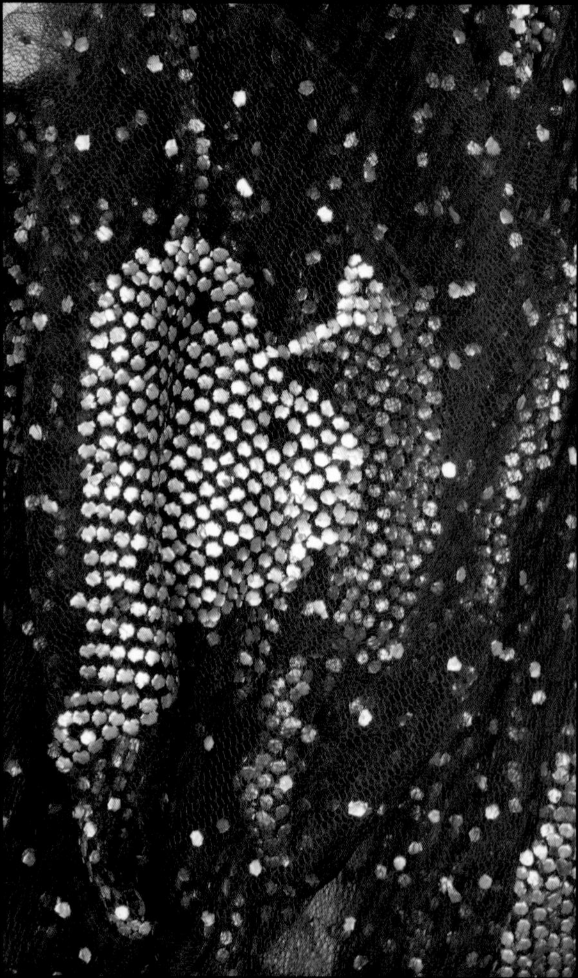

Left: This ceremonial *odhni* made of French net, tulle, is embellished in *mukaish fardi buti* and with *peepal* motif by creating a cluster of *fardi butis*. This *peepal* leaf motif of ancient origin is found on the pottery and seals of the Indus Valley Civilization.
Above: A silk georgette *odhni* of plain weave ornated with diagonal *rows of badla* work. The borders on two sides are embellished with intricately woven French lace border. A strip of braided gold *gota* at the joints of lace and chiffon cloth and silver *kamdani butis* gives it the Ganga-Jamuni effect.

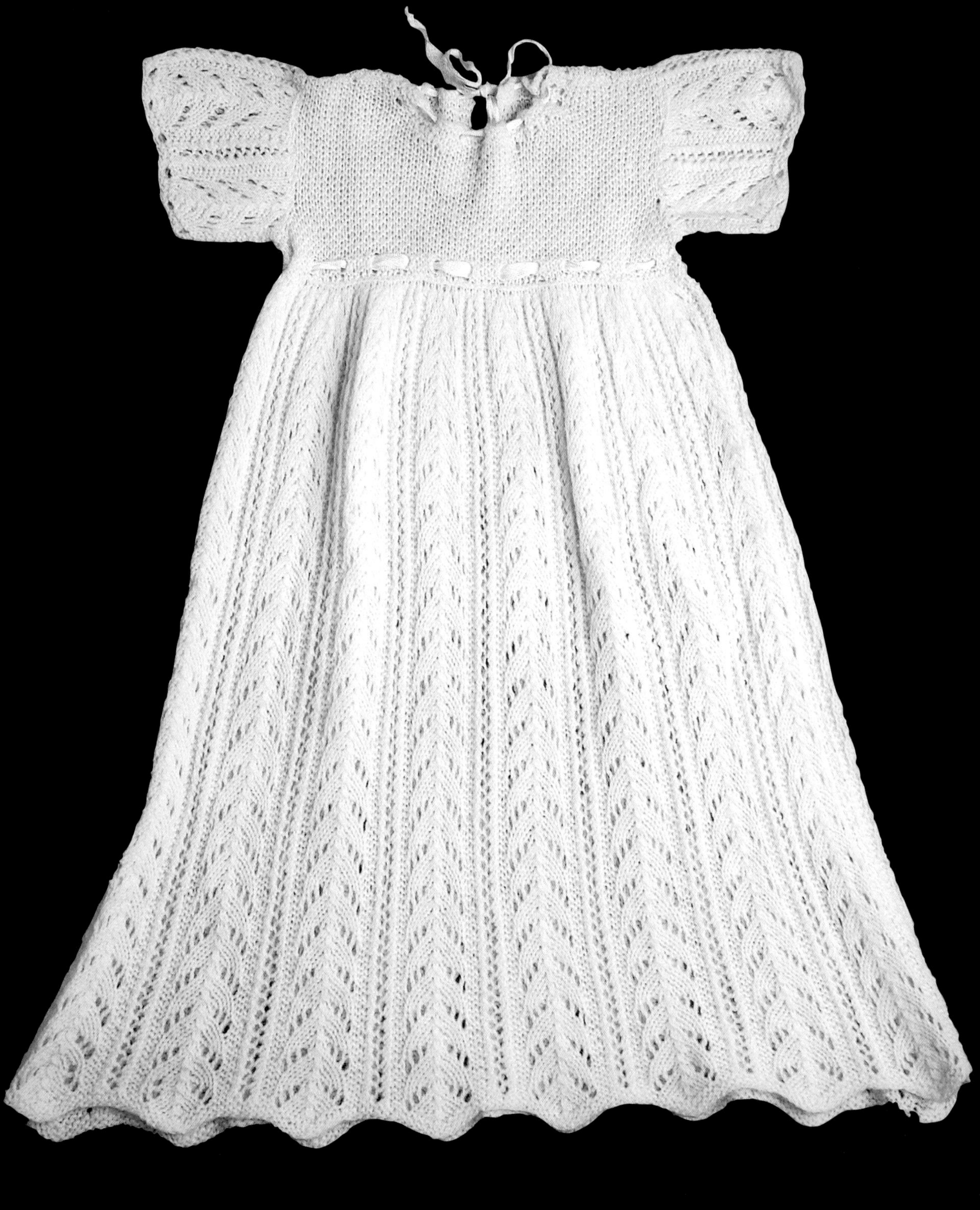

A white coloured infant's winter dress is hand-knitted in 'jours en angle' and 'jour vertical' patterns. The bodice is in 'point de riz' stitch. The silk ribbon around the neck and the waist can be adjusted according to the flair needed.

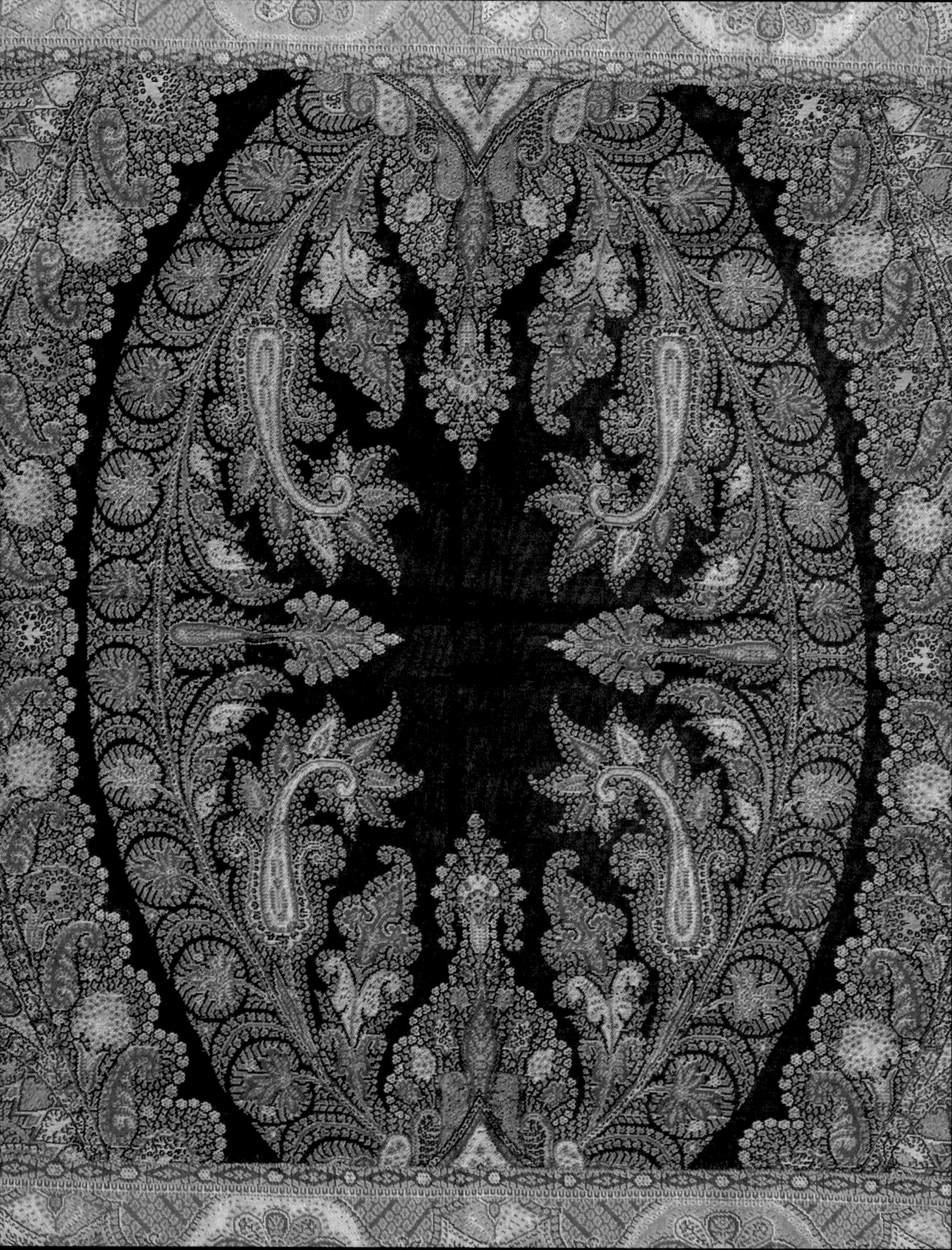

Paisley shawls were imitated from the jamawar shawls of Kashmir but instead of being woven with *tojli*, they were made on jacquard loom. They became a popular fashion item in the

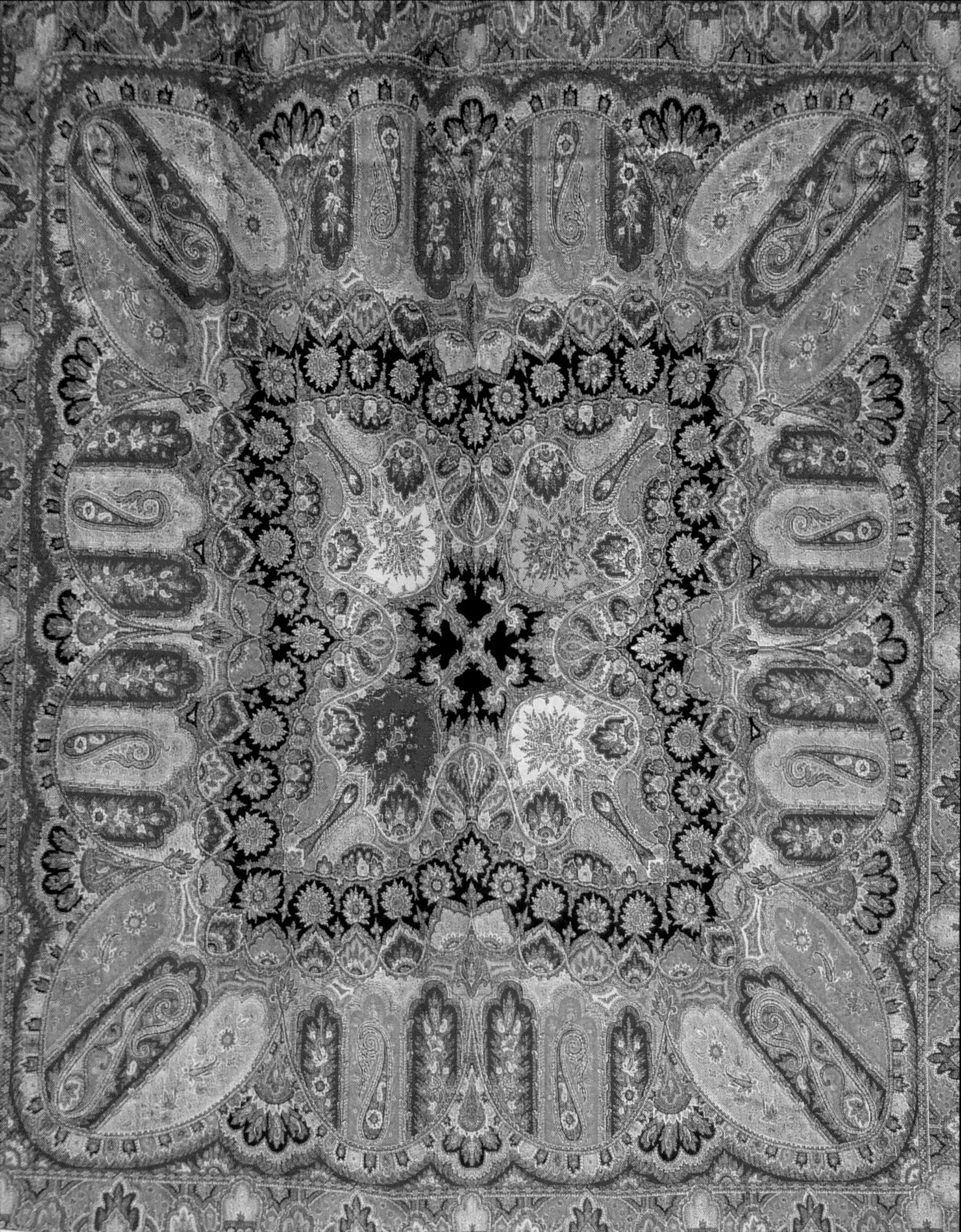

This square tablecloth in paisley is in typical Kashmir design woven on a jacquard loom. It has rich colours of burnt red, turquoise, yellow and greens. The centre of the piece displays an ornate shape in red, ochre yellow, pista green, turquoise and black. The fringes on each edge are multi-coloured. A mix of motif is intricately woven.

ORNAMENTATIONS

The British Raj did not see any significant ornamentation in costumes but new designs were incorporated in the repertoire of Indian designs for trade purposes and some new techniques were brought from England and France such as lace work, smocking and machine embroidery. The traditional forms of hand-embroidery such as *chatta-patti* and *kamdani* witnessed an overall decline. *Chikankari* and zardozi continued to be one of the most important industries of Lucknow. It found its use in cuffs, collars, caps and night dresses.

Crochet is the French word for 'hook' and involves the use of a hook made of metal, wood or plastic. The basic pattern is a chain, formed in length with as many loops as needed to finish a work. This craft was used mainly to decorate collars, cuffs and simple decorative edges. Cotton threads of all thickness are suitable for crochet work. This craft was brought to India by Portuguese missionaries. Crochet work partially substituted the traditional *daraz ka kaam*, which was popular in the Nawabi Era.

Lace was novel to Awadh. It was a European invention, possibly from Italy, or Dalmatia in former Yugoslavia. It became popular in England only in the fifteenth century and was brought to India by Christian missionaries. In 1818, machine-made lace was produced in France for the first time. In Awadh, lace work was used mainly for women's and children's garments and was popular for blouses and kurtis.

Smocking was mostly used for decorating children's clothes. It is a technique in which the fabric is firstly gathered then embroidered with decorative stitches to hold the gathers in place. The gathers must be uniform and are made in the ratio of 2.5:1 to allow 2.5 inches of fabric for every 1 inch of finished work.

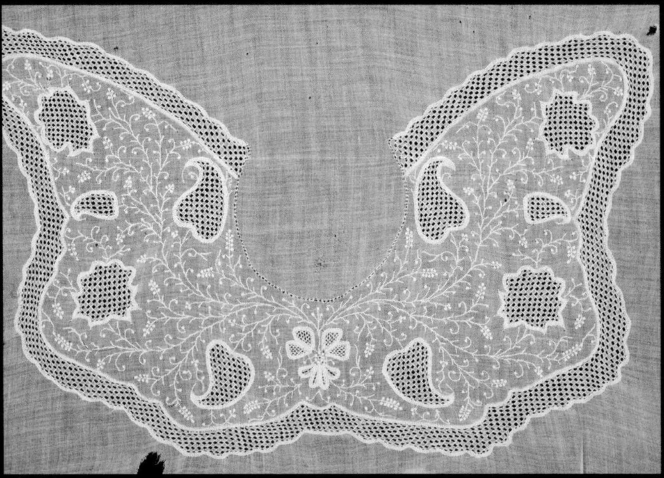

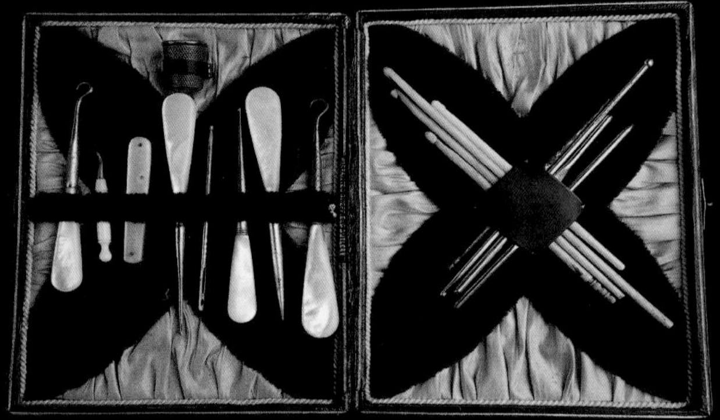

Above: *Chikankari* was also used for decorating the collars. Different *jaali* stitches have been used in this pattern: *siddhaur jali* (oval holes), *bangla jali* (square holes) and *hatkati* (single row). *Bakhiya* stitch has been used for trailing stems and leaves, while *mundi murri* has been used for buds.
Below: Crochet needles.
Facing page, clockwise from top:
1.Especially carved wooden block for collars in *chikankari*.
2. Yolk of a frock embellished with machine made laces as well as hand embroidery.
3. A floral motif in machine embroidery.
4. The gored panels are inserted below the knee-level to give flare to this petticoat. The crochet work replaced *daraz ka kaam* for joining *kalis*. A shell-designed crochet lace runs along the hem.
5. A Western frock, gathered in the front, is embroidered with contrasting pink thread in running stitch and pleats in the hem.
6. The porpora cuff is embroidered with gold zari threads in chequered design outlined with *gota-kinari*.
7. Pink silk sleeves having gathered cuff on the ladies blouses started boasting applique work with ribbons and embroidery in zardozi. It incorporates ornamentations of the Nawabi Era and the British Raj.
8. Cuff of another blouse with French machine-made laces together with *gota* braid.

Following page 132: Nine yard embroidered border with a variety of interwoven motifs from all realms: people, carriages, guns, ships, flora and fauna like horses, elephant, deer, parrots and peacock. The peacock motif often represents courtship and love. It is also the mount of Kartikeya, the god of war, thus it is associated also with death and immortality. It is the national bird of India for its unparalleled beauty.

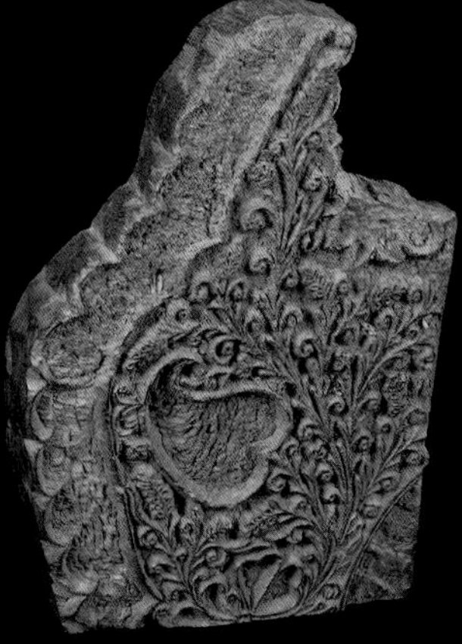

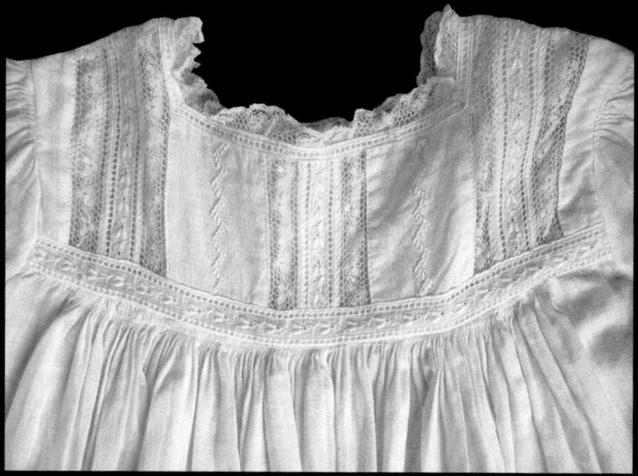

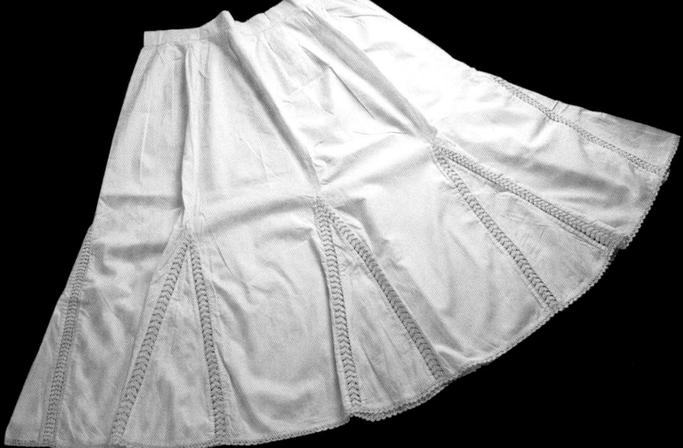

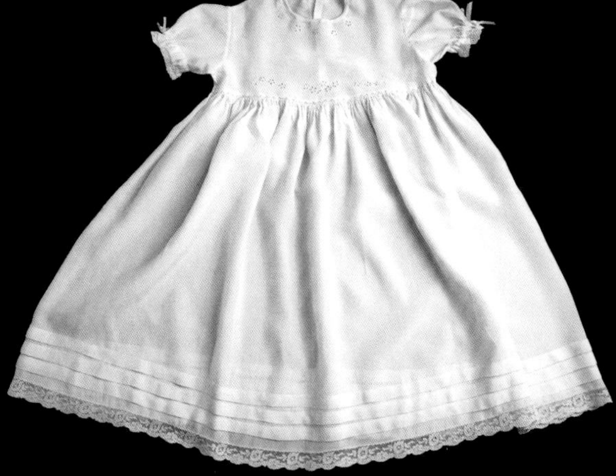

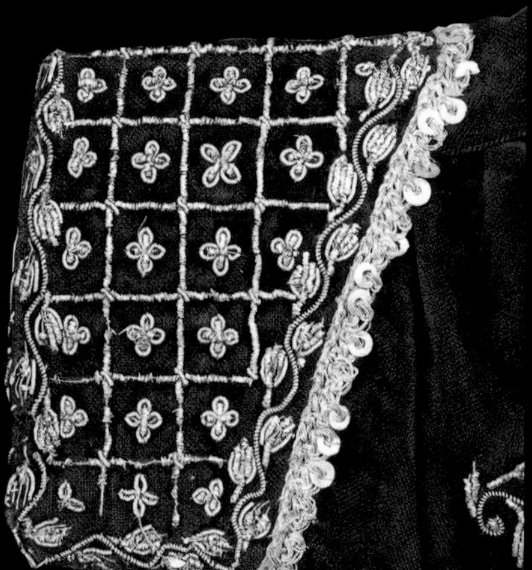

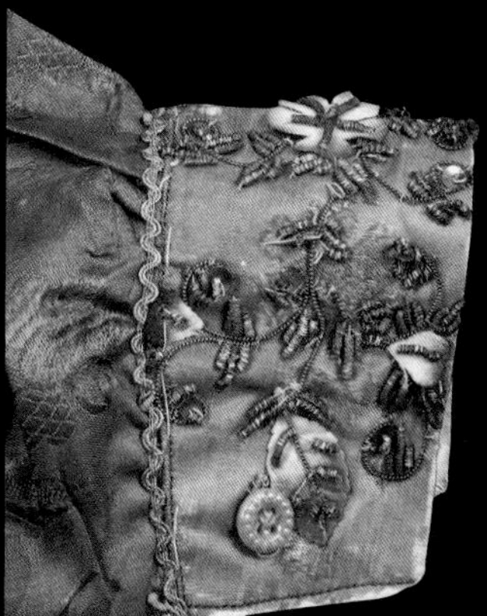

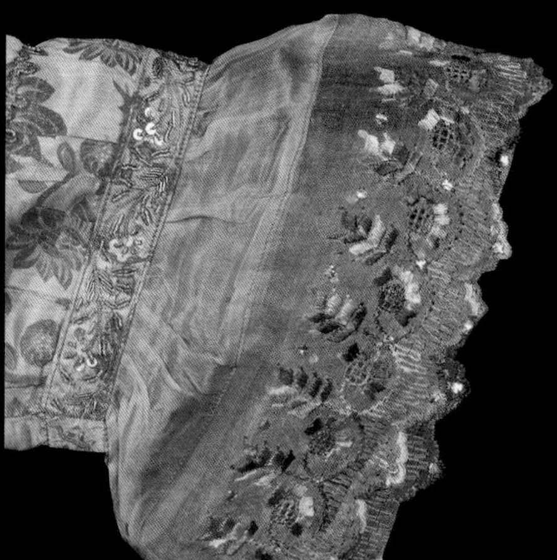

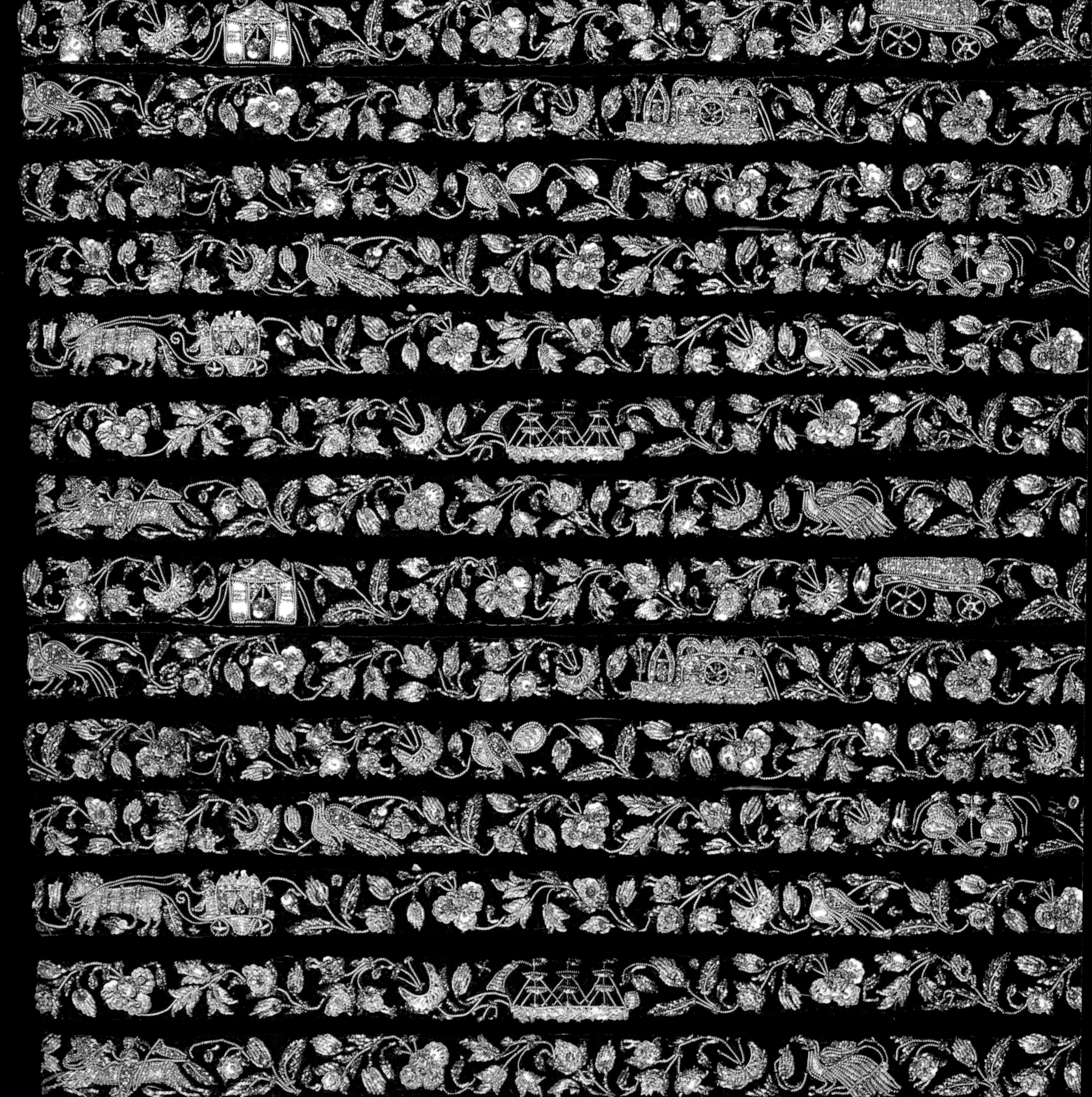

EVOLUTION OF MOTIFS AND COLOURS

1722-PRESENT

EVOLUTION OF MOTIFS AND COLOURS

Motifs and colours are not only embellishments, but form an integral part of costume. Not only do they add to the beauty of the garment, but they vividly reflect the times and tastes of the different eras. It is also through the evolution in motifs and colours that one can appreciate the changes in contemporary tastes of society, the preferences, the trends and the styles. Motifs and colours are intricately intertwined with the textiles and ornamentations, and add an extraordinary dimension to the appreciation of textiles and costumes of Awadh.

EVOLUTION OF MOTIFS

Motifs are greatly influenced by the customs of society and are symbolic of the everyday life of people, and have evolved through history. Changes in their use are evident in the weaving styles and embellishments of the different eras. The technique and purpose of the craft also determined the choice.

Motifs are used in weaving cotton and silk material. They would be printed or embroidered and were applied either over the entire garment, called *jaal*, or only at the corners, called *konia*; they could either be small (*butis*) or large (*butas*) and applied singularly or in groups. Sometimes, a particular motif was used on a single garment, while at other times a combination of various motifs was used.

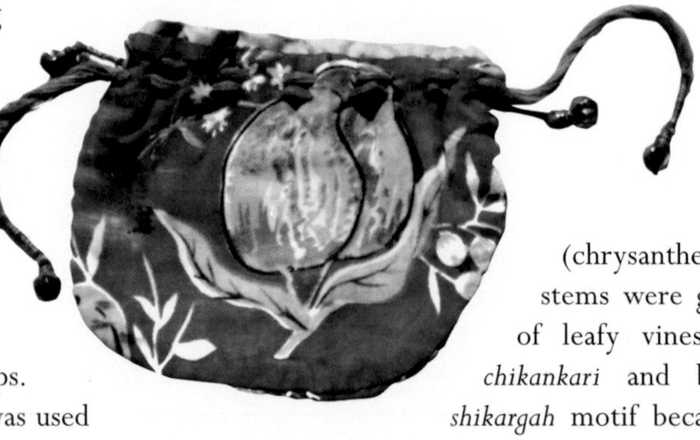

Cotton *batuiya* with *amiya* motif

NAWABI ERA

Even before the Nawabi Era, Awadh was endowed with a vast repertoire of motifs, as this region was the hub of various cultures and faiths. In fact, traditionally, most of the motifs had an auspicious or inauspicious value. Religion plays an important role in the choice and use of motifs. Under Islam, the motifs were mainly inspired by nature in addition to geometric and arabesque shapes. A flower in blossom, trees and large leaves symbolizing the Garden of Paradise were popular themes. Hindus made extensive use of stylized flowers, birds like peacocks and parrots, rooster, swan and animals like elephants (traditionally associated with water, fertility and with royalty and regal power), fish (first incarnation of Lord Vishnu) and tortoises (second incarnation of Lord Vishnu) as decorative motifs. Over the course of time, a different set of motifs started being applied to both Hindu and Muslim costumes, reducing their diversity and increasing their harmony. Motifs were also chosen with respect to the nature and climate of the place. The most popular motif known by different names in Awadh is the *amiya/ambi/turanj/kairi*. The *amiya* (raw mango) motif was borrowed from the abundant mango groves of Awadh, while the *jalpariya* or fish was also used profusely as Awadh falls in the Doab region.

During the Nawabi Era, certain motifs became more popular and new motifs were also introduced. Motifs of flower patterns like *champa* (magnolia), *motia* (jasmine), neem (margosa tree), *genda* (marigold), *guldaudi* (chrysanthemum) and flowering stems were greatly used. The motif of leafy vines was predominant in *chikankari* and brocade weaving. The *shikargah* motif became very popular with the nawabs of Awadh. This particular design was developed by Muslim weavers of brocades from Banaras who were inspired by the Mughal emperor's love of hunting. As the *kathavachaks* (storytellers) gained the patronage of the nawabs, textile artisans started depicting the stories and everyday life of people. The concept of everyday stories depicted as motifs was the characteristic of the Nawabi Era. For contrast, the baluchari saris of Bengal depicted mythological stories inspired by the Ramayana and Mahabharata. With the increasing

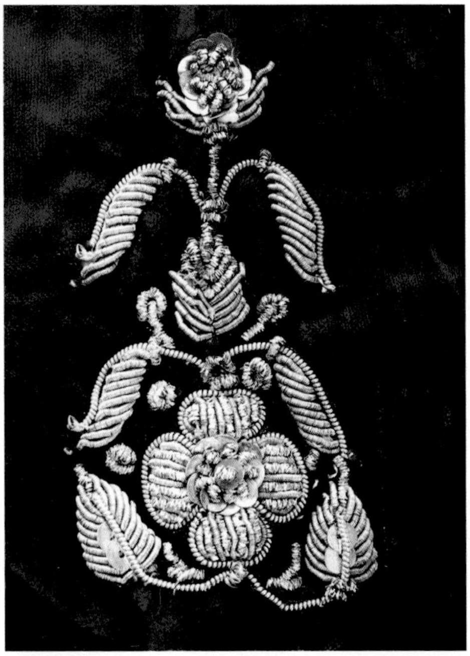

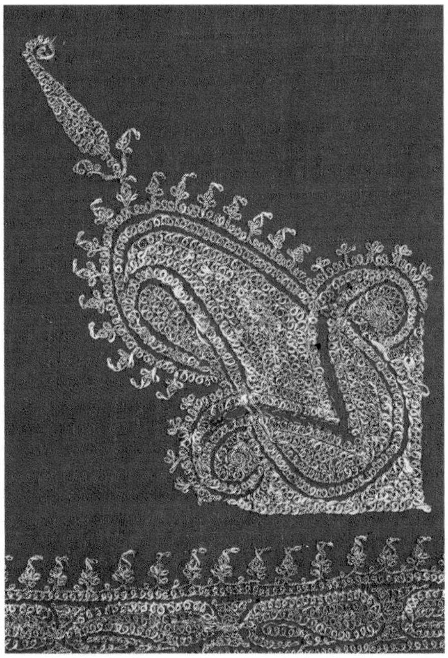

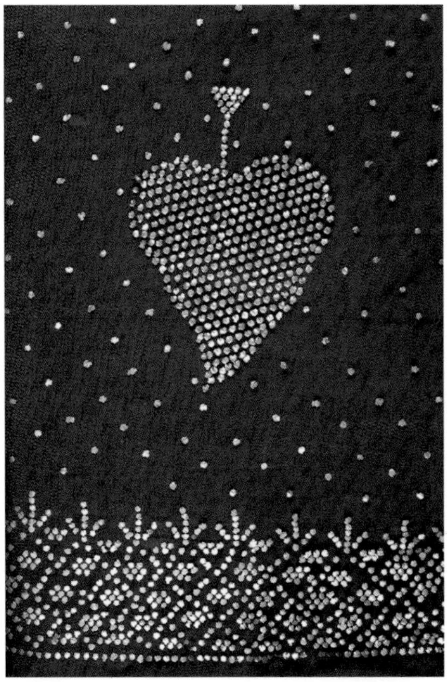

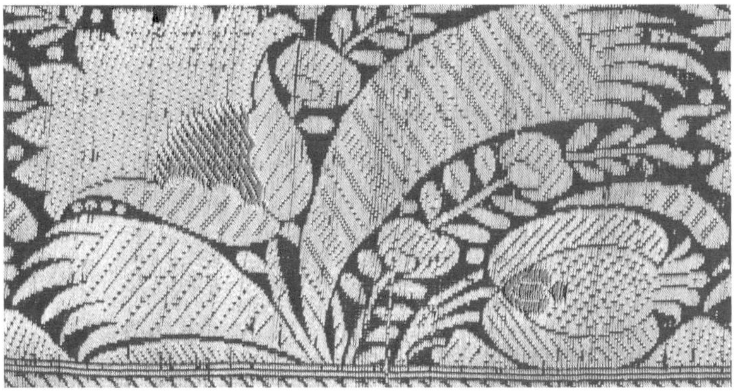

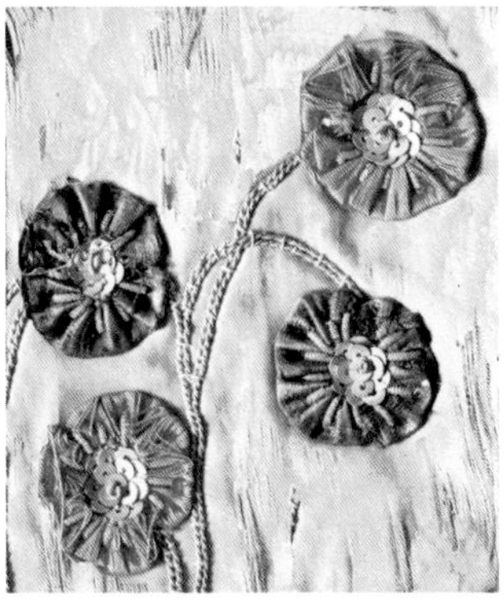

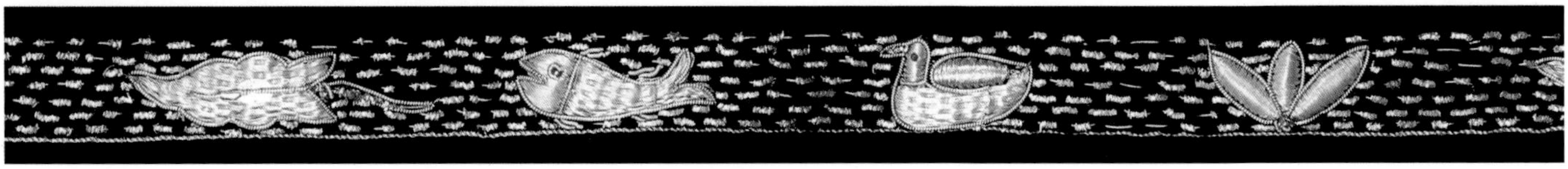

influence of British in contemporary life, new motifs such as the carriages, guns and warriors were also illustrated in embroideries. As the nawabs gained the title of kings by the British, new motifs such as the crown motif became very popular with royalty. This is found particularly woven into saris and in the *jamdani* fabric from which kurtas and *chapkans* were made (knee-length coat-like garment for men, the upper half of which is similar to a Western-style coat and lower part resembles an *angarkha*). This motif was also used in chikan embroidery.

Left to right (first row): Left: A *buta*. **Centre:** A *turanj* motif embroidered at corners called *konia*. **Right:** Peepal leaf is considered sacred in India, as people believe that Lord Vishnu and many other gods would rest under its shade.
Left to right (second row): Left: In Hinduism, the pomegranate symbolizes prosperity and fertility, while flowers are symbolic of good luck, health and prosperity.
Centre: The crown motif became popular after the nawabs were conferred with the title of 'King'. **Right:** Vibrant pink and blue applique flowers on a bright yellow base.
Final row: This black velvet border is embroidered with auspicious motifs like fish, geese, buds and leaves. Hindus consider the fish as an avatar of Vishnu, the preserver of the trilogy. It also represents food, wealth as well as the generative powers of the Nature.

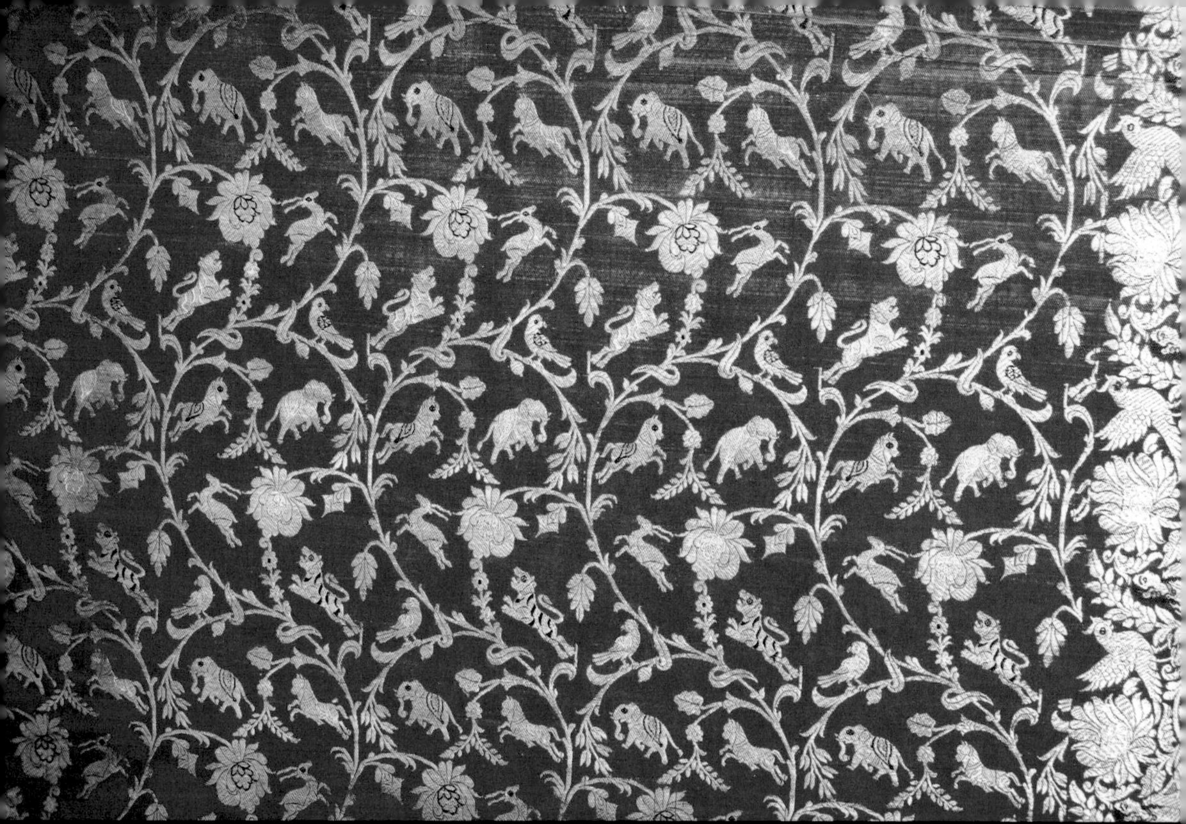

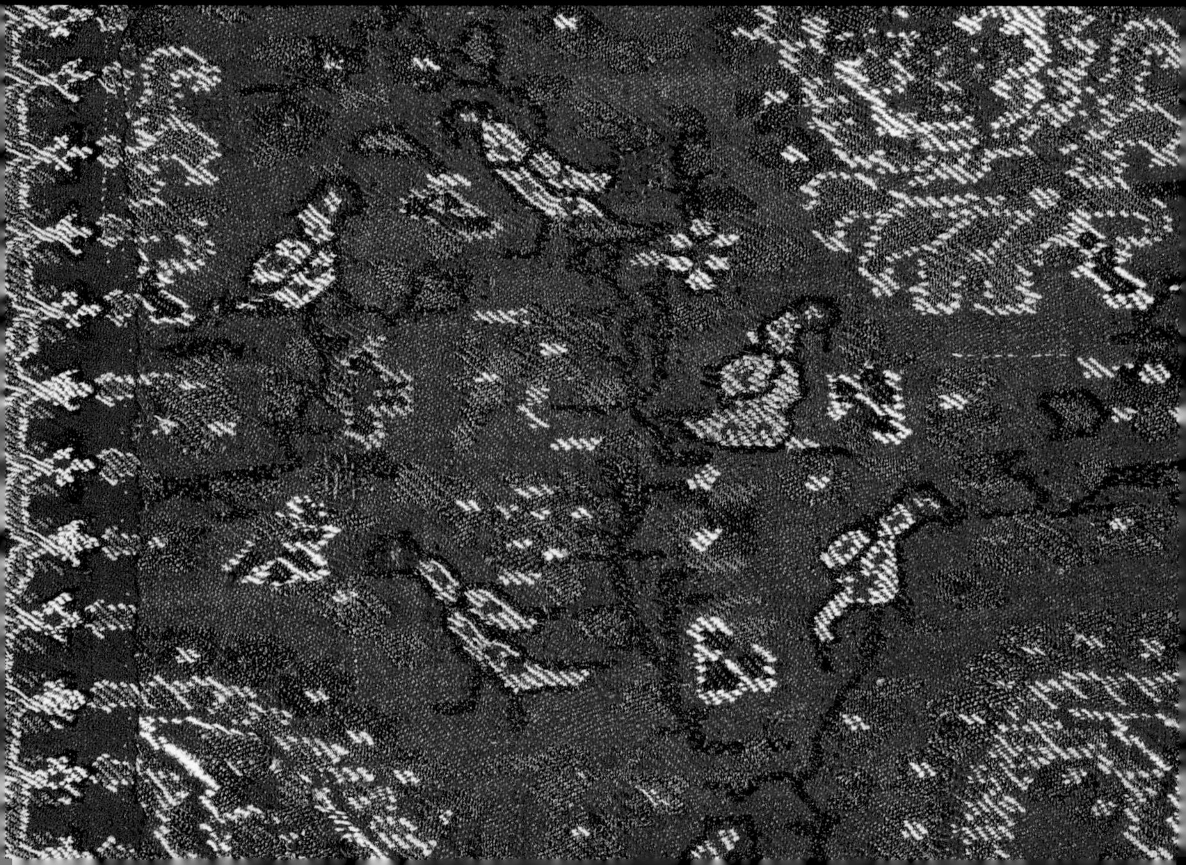

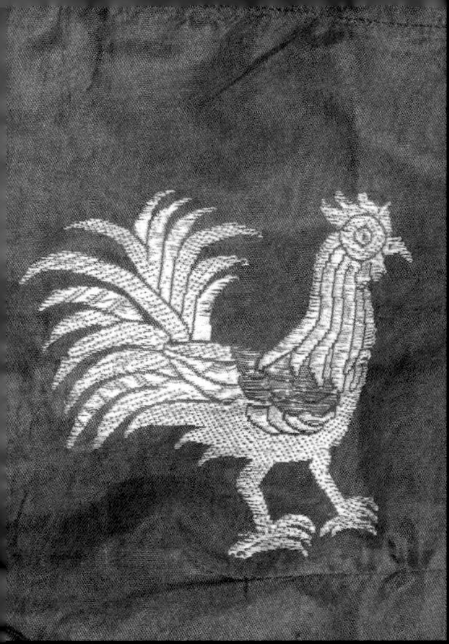

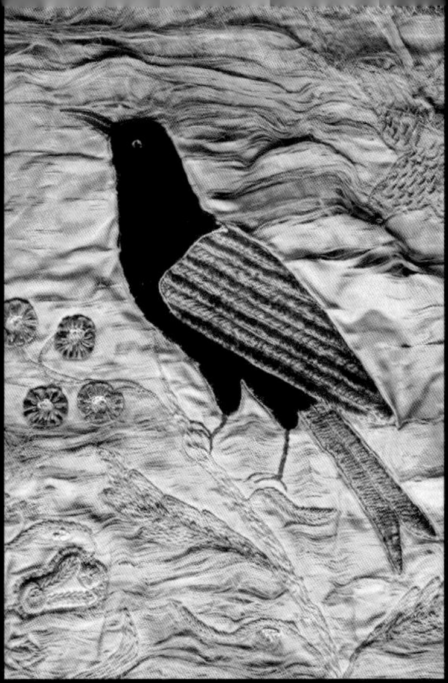

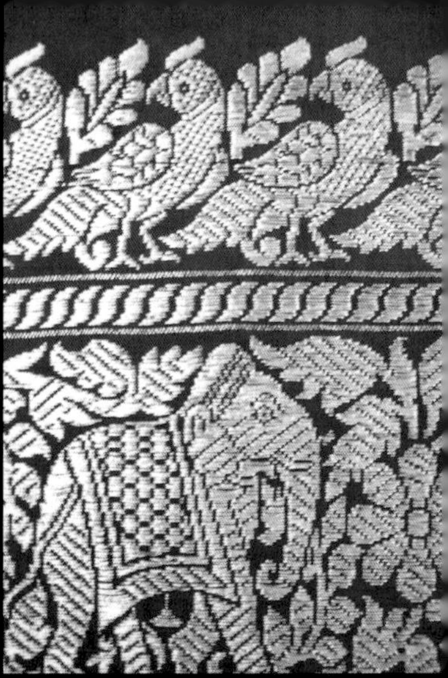

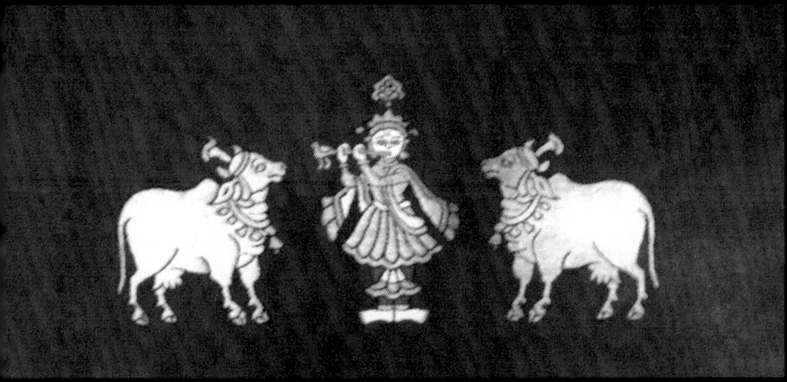

Facing page above: *Shikargah* — the abode of hunting, The moving figures of animals like elephants, horses, deer, tigers, lions and birds are intricately woven together with flowers and leaves. The lion symbolizes power, might and royal dignity.
Facing page below: Colourful parrots woven in jamawar. Parrots are generally associated with Kama, the God of physical desire and love.
Clockwise from top:
1. The cock motif symbolizes humility. Here, it is embroidered against the colour purple symbolizing aristocracy and extravagance. The Egyptian queen Cleopatra explains this extravagance perfectly. To obtain one ounce of Tyrian purple dye she had her servants soak 20,000 Purpura snails for 10 days.
2. The koel (cuckoo) is associated with the flowering of the mango tree, a fruit motif, typical of Awadh.
3. An elephant is an auspicious symbol traditionally associated with royalty, regal power, fertility and water. This association of elephants with water and rain is emphasized in the Hindu mythology where Indra, the god of rain, rode an elephant called Airavata who sucked the water from the underworld after defeating Vrta and sprayed its water into the clouds.
4. The sacred cows with Lord Krishna, the protector of cows

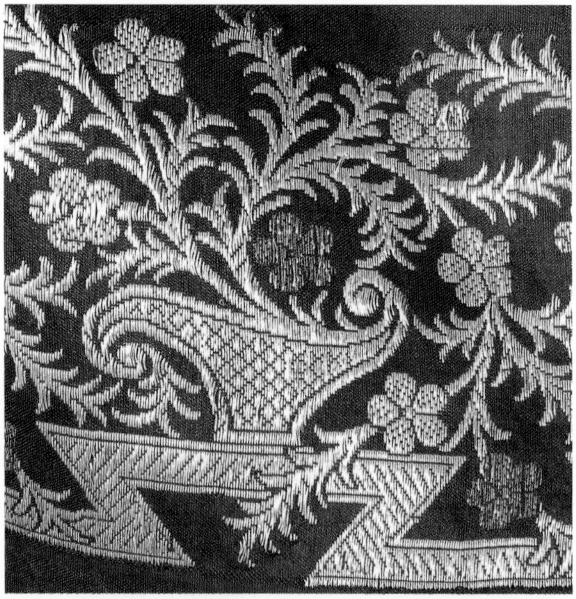

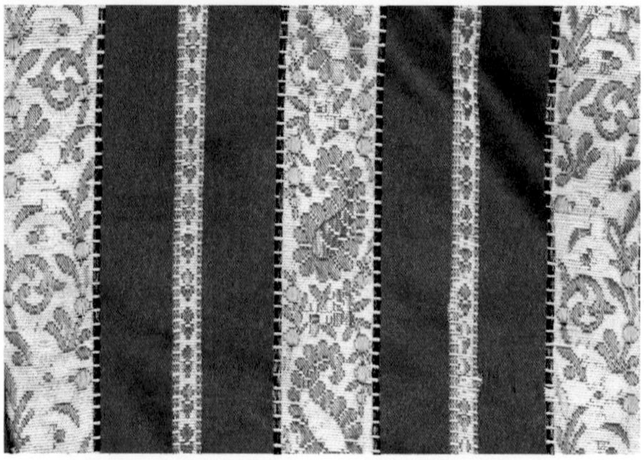

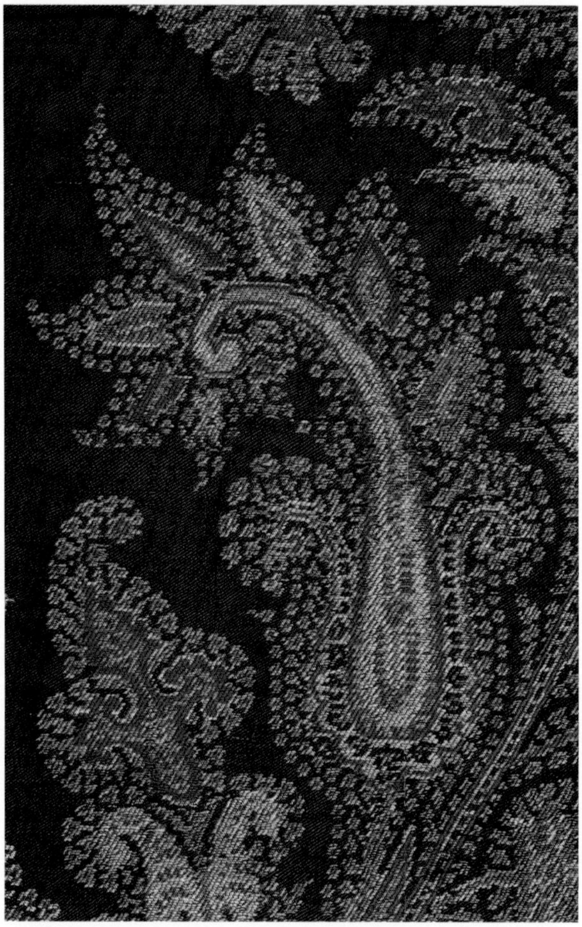

Clockwise from top:
1. A plant with blooming flowers in a flower pot. 2. Wallpaper motif, an influence of Western taste, used in eighteenth century. 3. A stylized *turanj* of a paisley shawl.

BRITISH RAJ

During the British Raj, most motifs from the Nawabi Era remained popular. New additions mainly included the wallpaper design, button roses, flower baskets, bouquets and the *gamla* (vase) *buti*. The wallpaper designs became popular in *chapkans* and *achkans* and were woven in both silk and wool for the nobility. Floral motifs were more commonly used in the saris, but instead of only being woven on borders and corners, they also started to be woven in vertically during this period.

During the British Raj, the emphasis was less on traditional embroidery and the focus was more on different stitches of crochet work, smocking and knitting. The multi-cultural influence was seen in floral representations. Delicate stems and finely drawn mixture of flowers characterized the design. As a result of the Industrial Revolution, the *amiya* motif of *jamawar* shawls was adopted for paisley shawls woven on power looms in England. This motif was used also for home furnishings.

MODERN TIMES

Modern times are witnessing both the revival of old motifs and the introduction of new ones. The more popular old motifs include floral designs, including a revival of the stylized lily or iris, the fleur-de-lis, which is an age-old stylized figure. The paisley design, also called *turanj*, has always remained popular. However, some motifs such as the *shikargah* and *gamla buti* do not have the same importance they did in the Nawabi and British eras. Reflecting globalization, designers are experimenting with geometrical and abstract designs, animal prints, religious deities and historical personalities.

EVOLUTION OF COLOURS

'[The]...yellows of northern wheat and mustard harvests, the whites and ivories of southern summers, the old rose pinks and musk blues of Islam, the shades of green that denote the rice fields or the seasons of desire, the differing shades of red which reflect the varying constancies of lovers, the indigo that records the fury of the eastern monsoon, the silvers and enamelled golds of royalty....these are the raw material of India's weaver.'

(Mehta, 2006)

Colours have always been especially important in Awadh and its costumes. Evolution in colours was affected, in addition to the preferences of society, by the availability of raw materials and the production technologies.

NAWABI ERA

Colours in the earlier period of the Nawabi Era were influenced by the Mughals and were predominantly based on combination of natural dyes. The delicate-hued palette of the Mughals included the following colours: *badami* (almond), *firozi* (turquoise), *gul-e-anar* (red of pomegranate or scarlet), *tarbuji* (watermelon red), *zafrani* or *kesariya* (saffron), *narangi* (orange), *pistai* (pistachio green), *sausani* (plum), *dilbahar* (purple), *kishmishi* or *sultanina*, *unnavi* (purple) replaced the indigenous reds, madders, indigos and ochre.

As the nawabs built their centres in Faizabad and Lucknow, they began laying more emphasis on colours inspired by the vegetation, fruits and birds of the Awadh region (versus Delhi). This led to the introduction of colours such as *amrasi*, a shade of saffron yellow resembling the colour of a ripe mango; *jamuni* borrowed from a violet-coloured fruit called *jamun* (Eugenia jambolana); *baigani* from the vegetable aubergine; *phalsai*, a shade of purple from fruit *phalsa* (Grewia asiatica); *gopi chandani* (pale yellow); *asmani* (a shade of sky blue); *totai* or *suapankhi* (parrot green) and *dhani* (a shade of green colour representing the rice paddies). Other popular colours in Awadh were the *dhoop-chhaiyyan* (sun and shade) and *mor-pankhi* (the blue/green colour of peacock's feather). In order to achieve the *dhoop-chhaiyyan* colour, the warp used to be of black colour and weft would be maroon, green or red depending on the shade, while for *mor-pankhi*, the warp was blue and weft was green. As Lord Krishna, always depicted adorning a peacock feather, was a popular divinity from the region of Awadh, the colour *mor-pankhi* also remained popular.

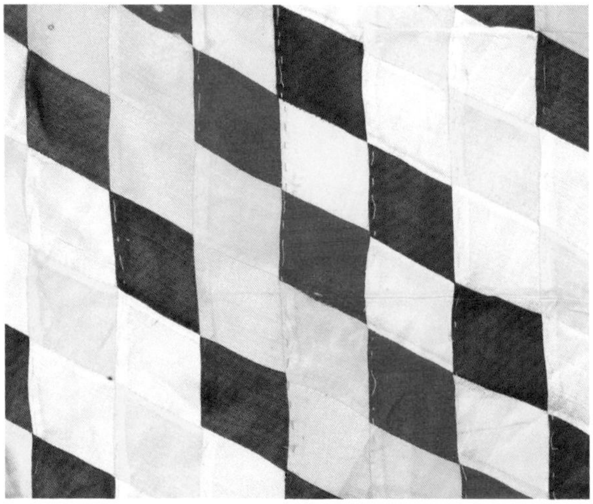

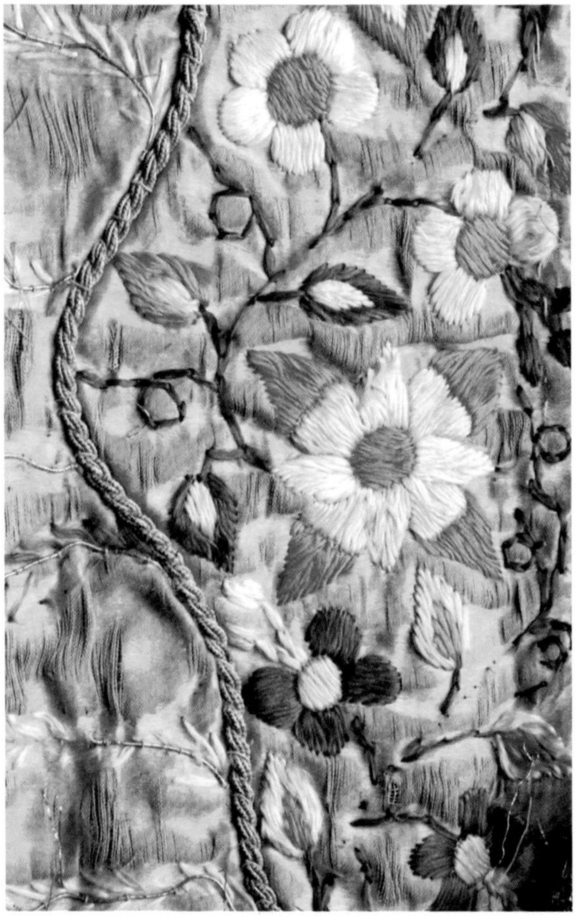

Above: Typical colours of Awadh.
Below: Yellow border embroidered in floral *bel* pattern with pink, purple blue and peach *resham*.

During the Nawabi Era, the predominant colours included combinations of primary colours, produced

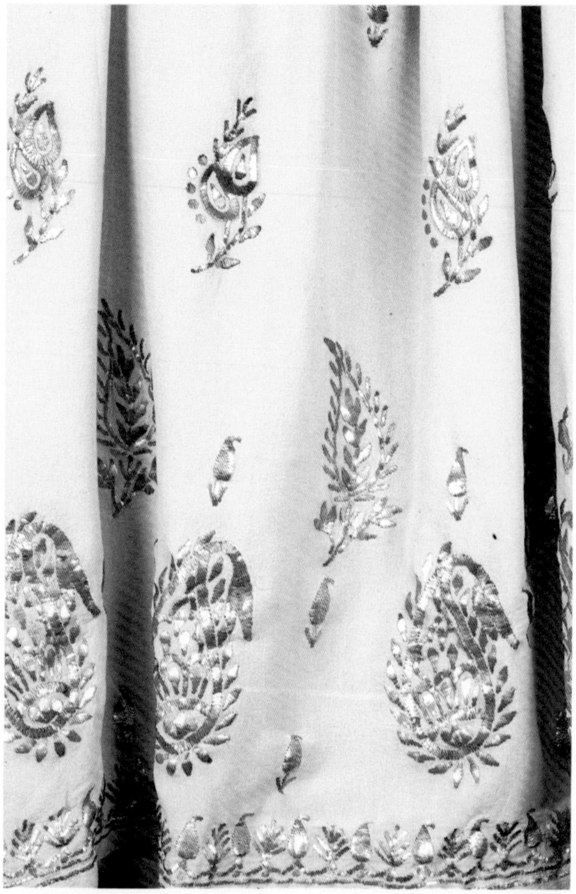

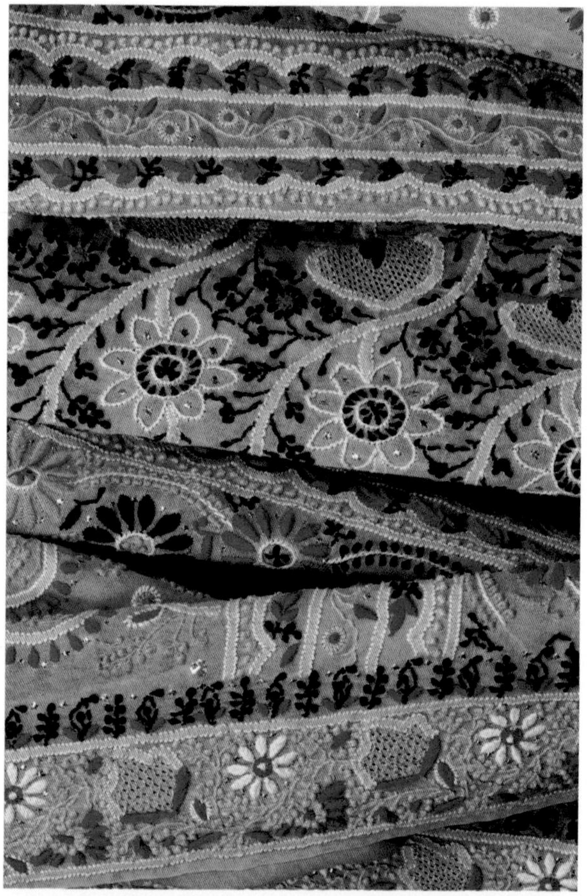

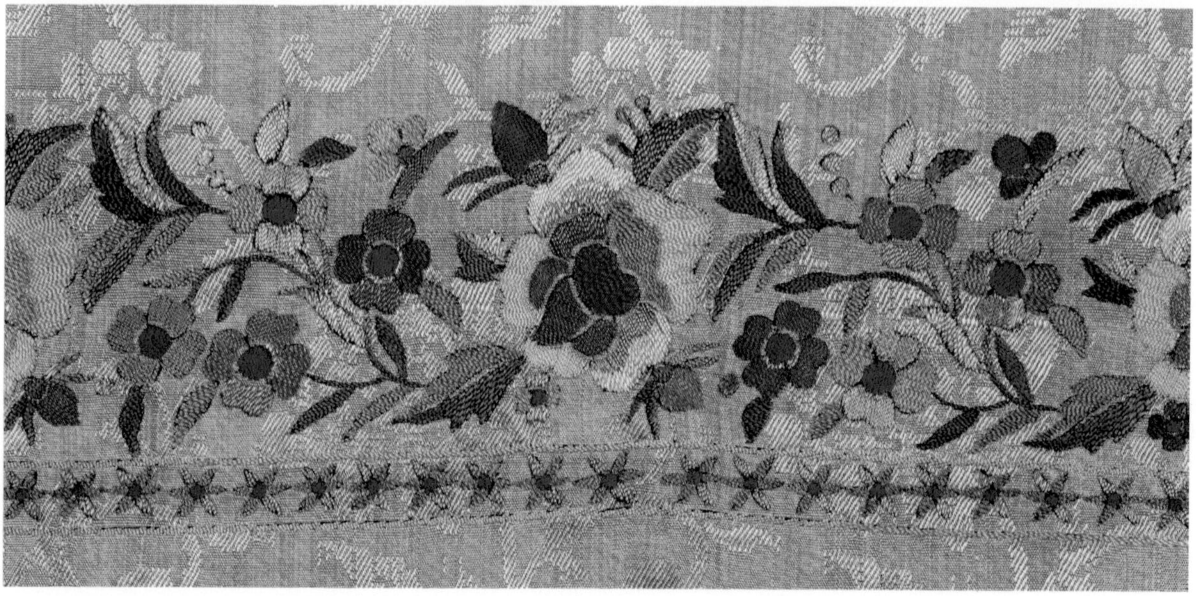

Clockwise from top:

1. A Ganga-Jamuni effect created on a georgette fabric with *kamdani work* celebrates the revival of old workmanships of the Nawabi Era.
2. Ochre sari embroidered in *chikankari* in bright pink and blue using traditional motifs.
3. Typical colours of British Raj; violet, lilac, mauve, purple, red and sea-green.

from natural organic and vegetable matter and were made from the bark, fruit rind, flowers and leaves of different plants. Some natural dyes give lasting colour without any chemical process and are known as substantive dyes like walnut (used for black) and indigo (blue obtained from the plant Indigofera tinctoria). Cochineal (purple colour), shellac and madder root (red), safflower (yellow) and pomegranate rinds for green, are not fast colours and are called adjective dyes.

Although the colour black was present in the vast repertoire of colours in India, its use was limited. The Hindus considered black an inauspicious colour as it required fermentation and was thus impure. It was, however, relied upon to ward off evil. It was used in the brocades of Banaras by Muslim weavers, in Kashmir for *jamavar* shawls and in the material for jamas and *chogas* of the nawabs. Muslims also wear black clothes on the first day of the full moon during Muharram signifying mourning.

The social structure, religious rituals, ceremonies and festivals of Awadh also helped in making its textile heritage richer as clothes were designed for specific occasions. For example, a Hindu bride would wear a *kaccha joda*, an ensemble of a *gulabi* (rose pink) lehenga and an auspicious yellow colour chunni. The word *kaccha* literally means unripe, referring to a cloth dyed in non-fast colours, symbolizing the bride's virtues of virginity and purity. Another example is the ceremony of *goad-bharai*. This ceremony is performed for the expectant mother in her mother's house, usually during the seventh month of her pregnancy. The expectant mother wears a green sari and glass bangles coloured red and green, signifying auspiciousness. The colour green was quite popular in Awadh. It is suggested that green is revered as it was worn by Prophet Mohammad and also symbolizes life and nature.

BRITISH RAJ

With the advent of the British, the process of industrialization led to the development of synthetic dyes. The first of the modern synthetic dyes were invented in London in 1856 by the chemist William Henry Perkin. Artificial dyes are synthetic dyes that give lasting colour and do not lose their lustre and brightness when exposed to light and water, unlike some of the natural dyes. By mid-nineteenth century synthetic dyes gained popularity due to their ease

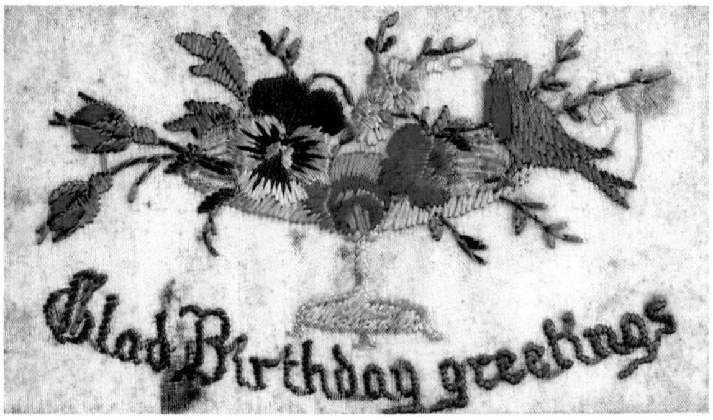

Above: Flower vase with colourfully embroidered flowers and a bird motif on a birthday greeting card.
Below: *Phool-patti* motif in bright red and green combination with a bunch of blue flowers.

and lower cost of production, leading to the decline in the usage of naturally-dyed cloth. Beige was the main colour of 1920s fashion in the West. The term originates from beige cloth, a woollen fabric left in its natural colour. It has come to be used since then for a range of light shades chosen for their neutral or cool appearance. The cream colour also became popular for formal suits, as it helped to reflect off the tropical heat.

In modern times, colours continue to evolve, reflecting the technologies, preferences and beliefs of our times. Now, contrasts of shades ranging from salmon, wine, plum, pale pinks and bright fuchsia to gold and burnt copper are used for formal wear as well as for informal, casual wear. Perceptions have also changed regarding both white and black. Earlier white was used almost exclusively by widows but now it is used by everyone. At the same time, widows now include more colours in their costumes, albeit of a lighter tone. Black is now an accepted colour in social events, although still not preferred for religious functions such as weddings.

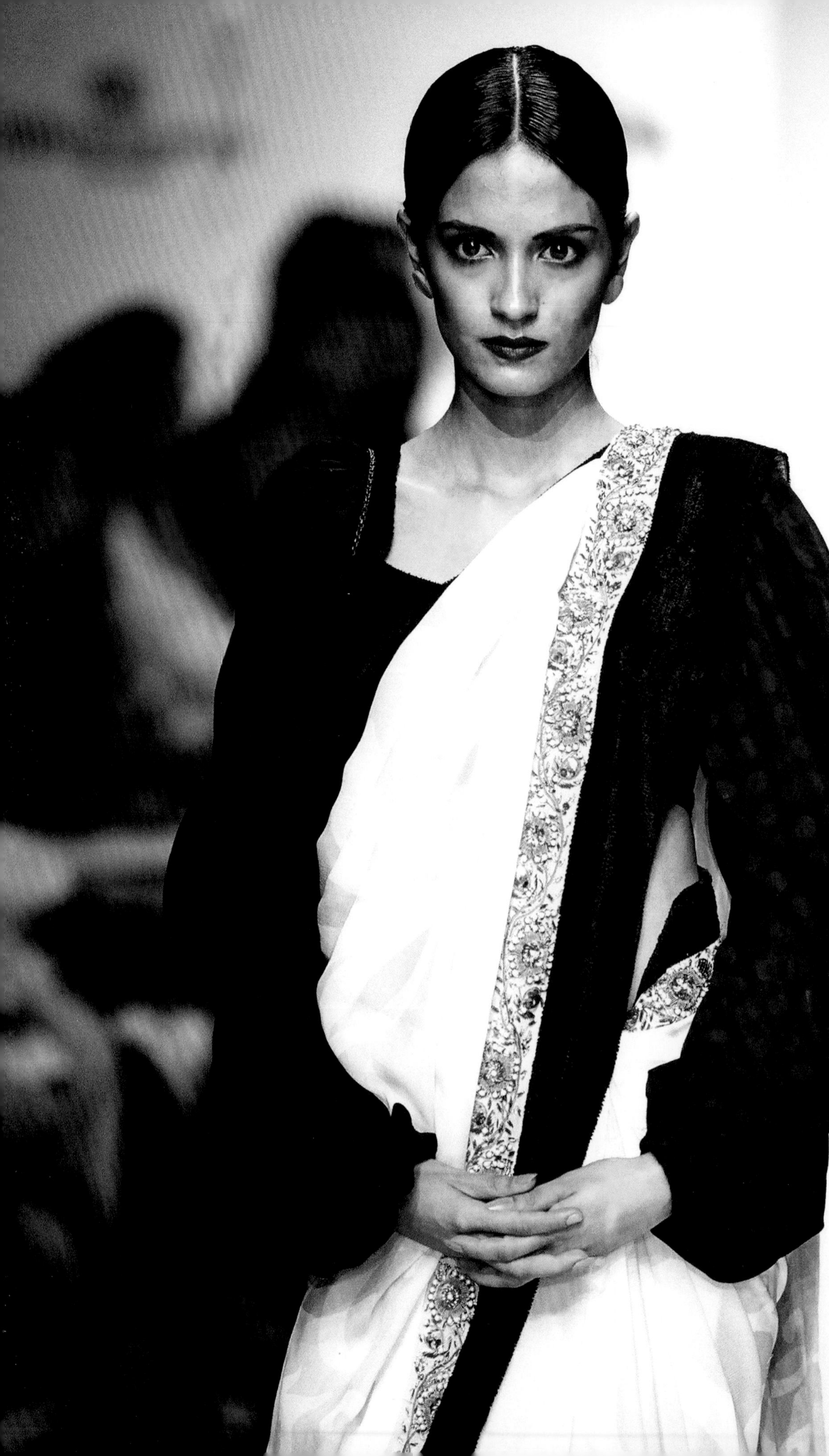

Black velvet bordered white sari embellished with zari embroidery is worm with an ornate puffed long-sleeved black blouse, called *phugga*-sleeves in 1980s.

EVOLUTION OF COSTUMES

From Jama to Sherwani

In the previous sections the changes were reviewed that took place during the Nawabi Era and the British Raj in costumes, textiles, ornamentations, motifs and colours. Combining the elements we can focus on the evolution of costumes. The modern sherwani is not just a costume, but embodies the evolution of the textiles, ornamentation, motifs and colours of Awadh and of India, and is illustrative of the contribution of the nawabs and the British to the history of fashion. The significance of these modern-day costumes can only be fully appreciated through an understanding of the historical moments that have shaped its evolution: The interactions and mutual influence of the Hindus and Muslims, the nawabi patronage leading to sophisticated textiles and ornamentations; and the increasing conformity to the British, reflected in coat-like structures such as collars and buttons, are all captured in the modern-day sherwani.
The timeline is only illustrative.

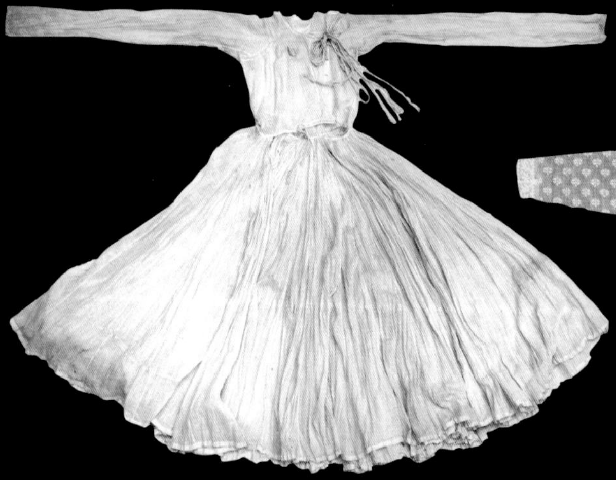

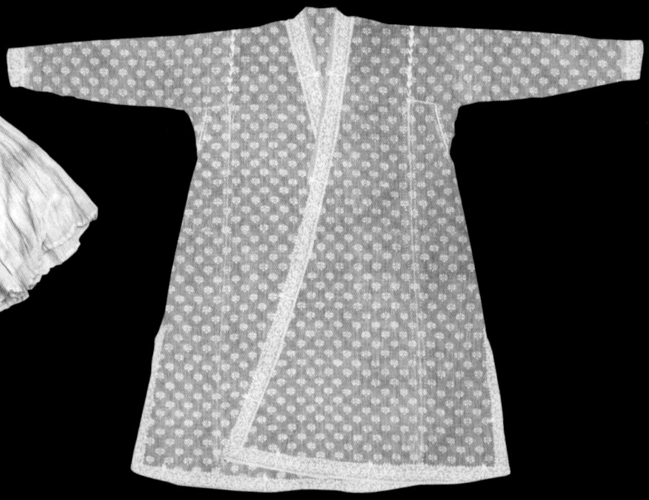

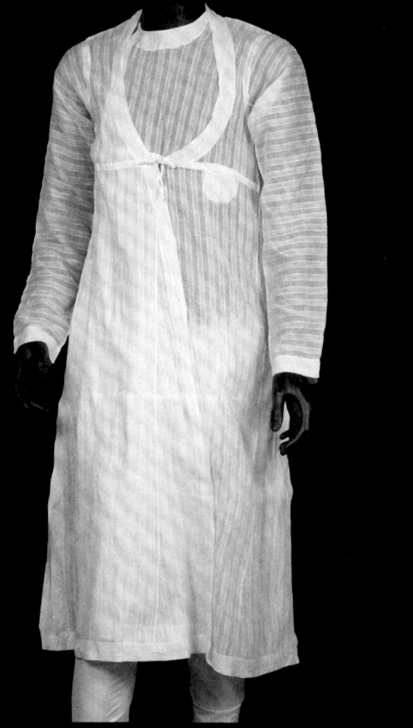

JAMA
(pre Nawabi Era – mid Nawabi Era)
The *jama* was the prevalent costume in Awadh at the dawn of the nawabi period. It became longer, the adjoining seam went up higher than the waist and the girth increased. Of particular interest is the chest fastening, where a Hindu would tie the *jama* on his left, and a Muslim would tie it on his right. This practice has been introduced by Mughal Emperor Akbar to promote a peaceful religious coexistence and was also followed by the open-minded nawabs of Awadh. This muslin *jama* is composed of a bodice and a gathered skirt with a crossed-over chest fastening at the armpits.

CHOGA
(Nawabi Era – mid British Era)
The *choga*, is a long-sleeved front-open outer garment. It replaced the *jama* as the formal dress in courts, thanks to its lavish embroidery, use of expensive materials and ornamental details. This hand-stitched *choga* is made of cotton *jamdani* material with *butis* woven all-over. It is edged with a broad border in the front, around the hemline, neck and sleeves. The seam at the shoulder is delicately worked with *daraz ka kaam*. The sleeves are tapered at the end. The sleeves are joined at a right angle and a *bagalia* (gusset) was attached to allow easier arm movement.

ANGARKHA
(mid Nawabi Era – mid British Era)
The *angarkha* is a full-sleeved knee-length hand-stitched garment. Differences from the *jama* include the lower chest-fastening, fitted bodice, reduced flared skirt and a purdah (inner panel) which was inserted into the cut out portion of the neck. The fastening was done with *tukma-ghundi* (a loop and cloth-cased button) and with a cotton tie-cord, poetically called *aashik-mashuq* (lover and the beloved). The difference vis-a-vis the *choga* lies in the cut of the armholes, which became more rounded, and the insertion of slit pockets cut on both sides. A small pouch is attached inside the waist to carry valuables and coins.

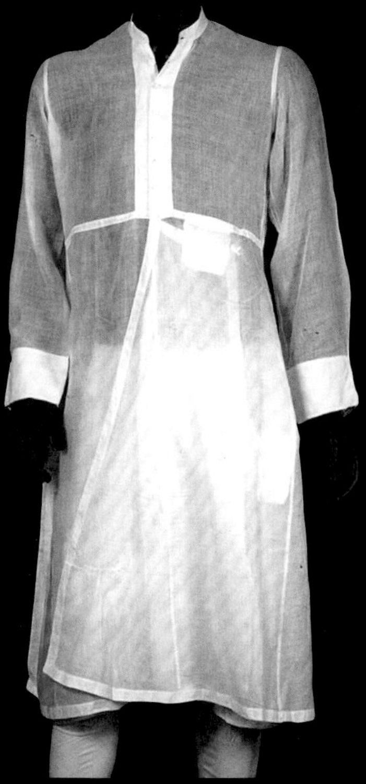

CHAPKAN
(early British Raj – late British Raj)
In the *chapkan*, the influence of the British starts to appear as increasing importance was given to tailoring and to close fitting of garments, and new elements such as band collars, buttons and machine sewing became prevalent. The upper part became like a coat while the lower part remained flared like an *angarkha*. The chest-fastening has now moved from the lateral sides to the centre, where buttons replaced the cords but the inner waist fastening was still done through the tie-cords and cotton buttons. The tapered sleeves were gradually replaced by coat-like sleeves with broad cuffs.

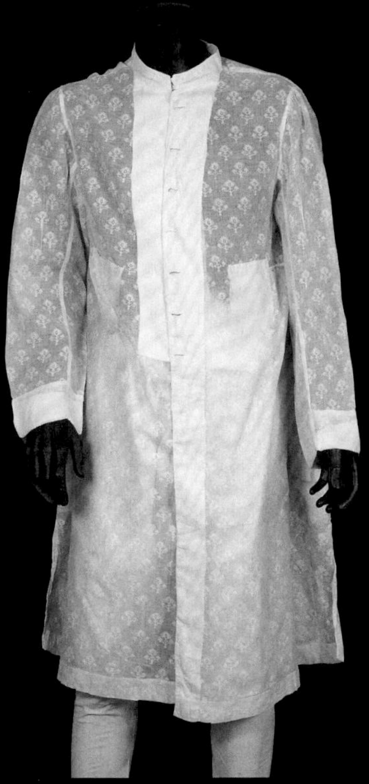

ACHKAN
(mid British Raj – late British Raj)
As the lower part of the *chapkan* became straight, it came to be known as *achkan*, which was like a long coat. The removal of the seam at the waist level in the front and back was another significant development. The tapered *achkan* reached above the knees, the fastening goes lower than in the *chapkan*, and pockets are on both sides at the waist level. The band collars were also used along with the traditional Awadhi ones. Metallic hooks and loops, products of industrialization, were introduced for the fastening of the inner flap.

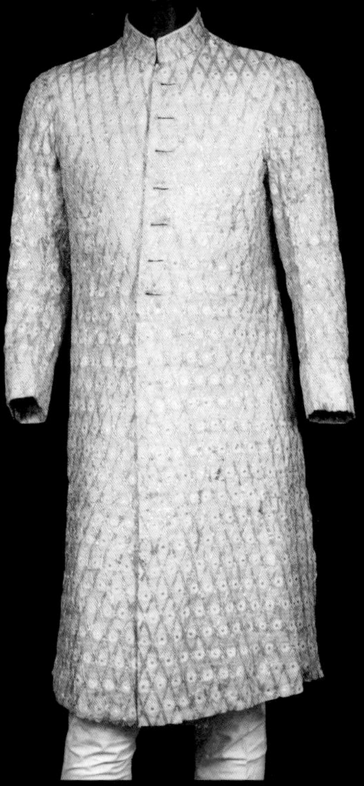

SHERWANI
(late British Raj – modern day)
The sherwani brings together the influence of the nawabs and the British. It was adopted in Awadh from Hyderabad Court of Nizams. The stark tailored, tight-fitting long coat with band collar, central fastening with buttons, created the modern-day sherwani. A breast pocket was introduced which was located on the outer left-hand side of the sherwani in contrast to pockets at the waist at the front of its predecessors. The sherwani was longer than *achkan* and reached below the knees. The sherwani has endured for many years and is still popular as a choice ceremonial dress.

From choli/angiya to blouse

Evidences from the murals of Ajanta caves, during the Gupta period which flourished during the fourth and fifth centuries AD, show women using *antariya* (dhoti) as lower garment, *stanapatta* (a wide band of cloth used for covering the breast, tied in various ways) and lots of ornaments to adorn themselves. Later certain foreign influence started to be seen on Indian clothing. An interesting change took place in the women's upper garment. Women started covering the upper part of the body with a close-fitting garment called *kanchuka* instead of *stanapatta* . This new addition in the upper garment is mentioned in Sanskrit literature as *cholka*, choli or cholika. It is appealing to realize how, for women, choli has evolved in modern day blouse. The variations in material, cuts, designs and styles, embellishments, motifs, colours and transition from hand-stitching of Nawabi Era to the machine-stitching of British period, tell us of the evolution in an exciting way.

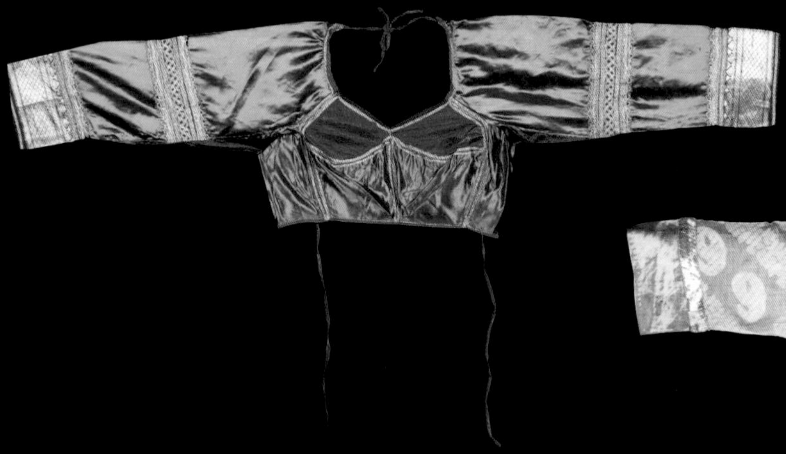

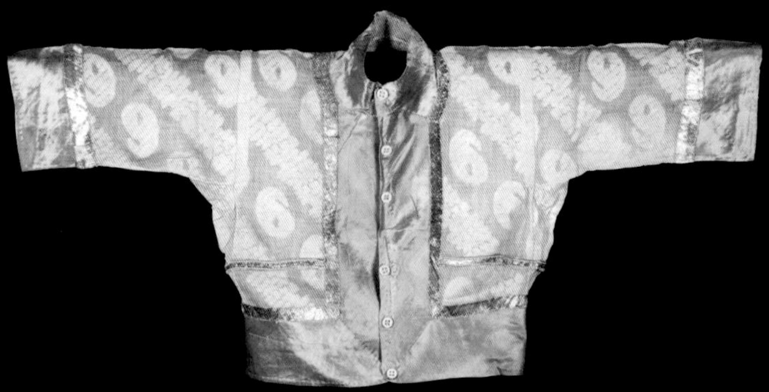

CHOLI/ANGIYA (NAWABI ERA)
(early British Raj - late British Raj)
Even before the nawabi period, women had started wearing close-fitting cholis with their lehengas in Awadh. This satin *angiya*/choli is made of two parts; the lower part at the base called *divar* (wall), providing support to the bosom, and the upper part was called paan or *katori*. The stitching on the joints of these two parts was called *chiriya* (sparrow). The cotton *bagalia* (gusset) in contrasting magenta were inserted for better movement of the arm. The back fastening is with cotton tie cords. The sleeves are decorated with *gota*.

BLOUSE
(early British Raj - late British Raj)
The earlier half of the British Raj saw the transition of the *angiya*/choli into a tailored blouse. The textile and embellishments were still from the Nawabi Era, whereas the cut was now Western-influenced and more structured. Stitching was still predominantly done by hand. The *katoris* disappeared, the length increased to cover the midriff, buttons replaced tie-cords, and the length increased and fastening to the front was adopted also for women's clothing. This hand-stitched blouse is made of *doria mulmul*. A collar has been introduced. The green border in silk and *gota* ornamentations has been used as decorations at the waist and sleeves.

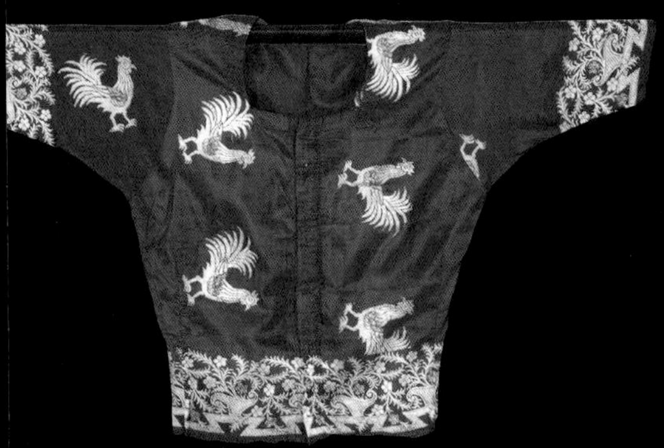

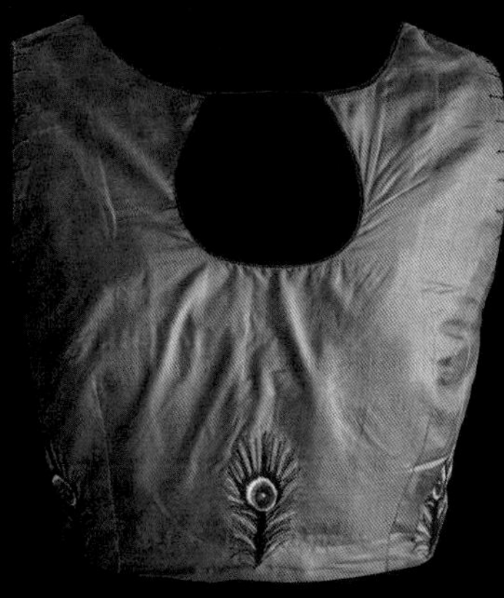

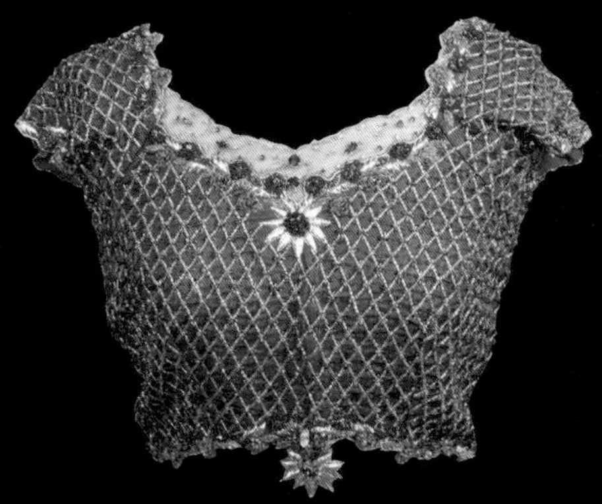

BLOUSE
(late British Raj)

With increasing industrialization, machines replaced hand-stitching. Cuts became even more structured, now with the introduction of the armhole and the removal of the gusset under the arms. The fitting was tighter and darts were introduced at the waist. It became slightly longer as the blouse was now predominantly worn with the sari instead of with the lehenga. Safety buttons replaced mother of pearl buttons/ buttonholes. New materials, new neck-lines and ornamentations were added, such as georgette, net, French laces, cuffs and collars, without replacing traditional ones like brocade. Ornamentations became part of the richly woven brocade material or cloth rather than additional elements.

BLOUSE
(modern day)

Over time, blouses increasingly became part of mainstream fashion and women started giving equal importance to blouse designs. These custom-made designer blouses can be made in an array of colours and fabrics, including cotton, silk, satin, georgette, and crepe. Originating from the choli, designer blouses are now well-fitted, have sleeves of varying lengths with differently designed necklines and are generally embellished with stones, sequins, beads and embroideries of different kinds. This orange sleeve-less blouse has a teardrop design in the front and the matching *morpankhi* motif of the sari is added at the borders to the design of the blouse.

BLOUSE (modern day)

The blouse is intricately embroidered with *resham*, **zari** and beads. Neckline and waist are embellished with a central floral motif. Combining net with brocade shows creativity of the designer.

Jama-zebi – The Sari Ensemble

Jama-zebi is an Awadhi expression to describe a costume as an ensemble, and the modern day sari is one such example. The modern day sari is illustrative of the contribution of the nawabs, in textiles and workmanship, and the British, in tailoring. While the sari had existed, it was only during this period that the sari ascended to the place it currently holds in women's Indian costumes. Its elegance upholds the nawabi nazakat, and its composition encapsulates age-old unstitched garments *antariya*/ dhoti (lower garment), *uttariya* (upper garment); the modern blouse as it evolved from the choli/*angiya*, the usage of the petticoat as an inner garment as a result of Western influence, and the rise of distinct female fashion over time.

'Creativity and inspiration are limitless. I find this limitless creativity in the way the Indian woman wears the sari. The way it is draped around the body is not only elegant and sensual, but totally different from the western perception of sensuality. This is what sets her apart, 'Roberto Cavalli (Tiwari, 2010).

Tracing its evolution, the word sari is derived from Sanskrit 'sati', which means 'strip of cloth' which was distorted to sari in Hindi. It was not worn with a blouse nor a petticoat. The upper corner was usually knotted firmly around the waist and the remaining folds of cloth would also be tucked into the waist. Over the time, the *antariya* and *uttariya* became one piece, with increased length sufficient to be worn as a sari. Gradually the unstitched clothes of ancient times were replaced by stitched garments. As seen earlier, the *stanapatta* led to the choli, which in turn evolved into the tailored blouse. The petticoat instead was introduced as an inner garment for the sari ensemble during the British Raj. A petticoat is a full-length skirt tied tightly at the waist. The petticoat, which was similar to the lehenga that was worn as an outer garment, became an undergarment for the sari. The petticoat became a central part of the sari ensemble, colours of the petticoats, initially only white, were increasingly matched with the colour of the sari in modern times. 'The origin of combining the petticoat with the sari can be traced to Calcutta in the 1870s, when Gyanodanandini, sister-in-law to Rabindranath Tagore, first introduced it (Kumar, 1999).' This combination was likely to have been inspired by the usage of underskirts by British women.

There are two main ways of draping the pallav of the sari. The *sidha* (correct) pallav style was considered the proper way of wearing the sari as it was inspired by the *odhni*/chunni and was prevalent in Awadh. The second style which has gained more popularity is the Nivi style, also known as the *ulta* (contrary or improper) pallav style, in which the pallav is draped over the left shoulder and left hanging —instead of coming from the back over the right shoulder and tucked at the back. The pallav is usually the most decorated part of the sari.

The sari continues to remain the most admired and popular garment in Uttar Pradesh and is today a statement of Indian feminine glamour.

Facing page, Left: This white and gold zari brocade sari from Varanasi is embellished with *sunehra* and *ruphala gota* work creating a Ganga-Jamuni effect, typical of Awadh.
Facing page, Right: Sari worn in *nivi* style in *ulta palla* style.

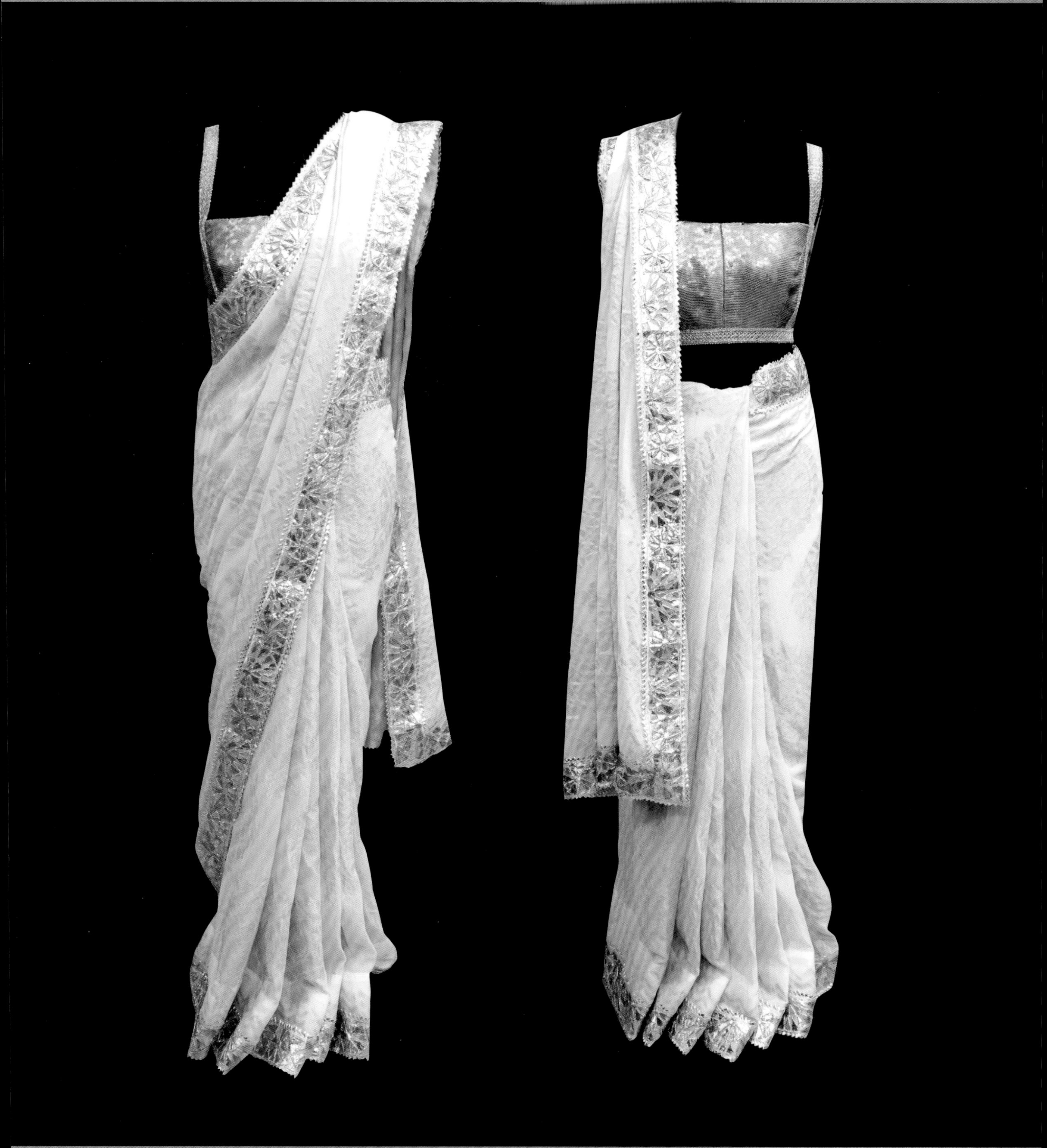

Lehenga/blouse/*odhni* ensemble

The lehenga/blouse/*odhni* ensemble has also undergone an increased amount of sophistication. In earlier times, although the three costumes (lehenga-choli-*odhni*) were worn together, they were simply assembled instead of being meticulously coordinated. As the garments started to be viewed as an ensemble, this further sparked innovations and creativity, new designs and new combinations. New variations are introduced in the style: A-line lehengas flow down in A-shape; circular lehenga is circular in shape and has a large circumference at the bottom; fish-tail lehenga sticks to the body from the waistline and flares down at the bottom; panelled lehenga gives the right amount of flare and a perfect fall. The cholis have also become shorter in length and are sometimes matched with crop tops and short coat-jackets.

With the evolution in fashion, there was increased focus on the harmony of materials, colours and motifs for each ensemble to create an alluring effect.

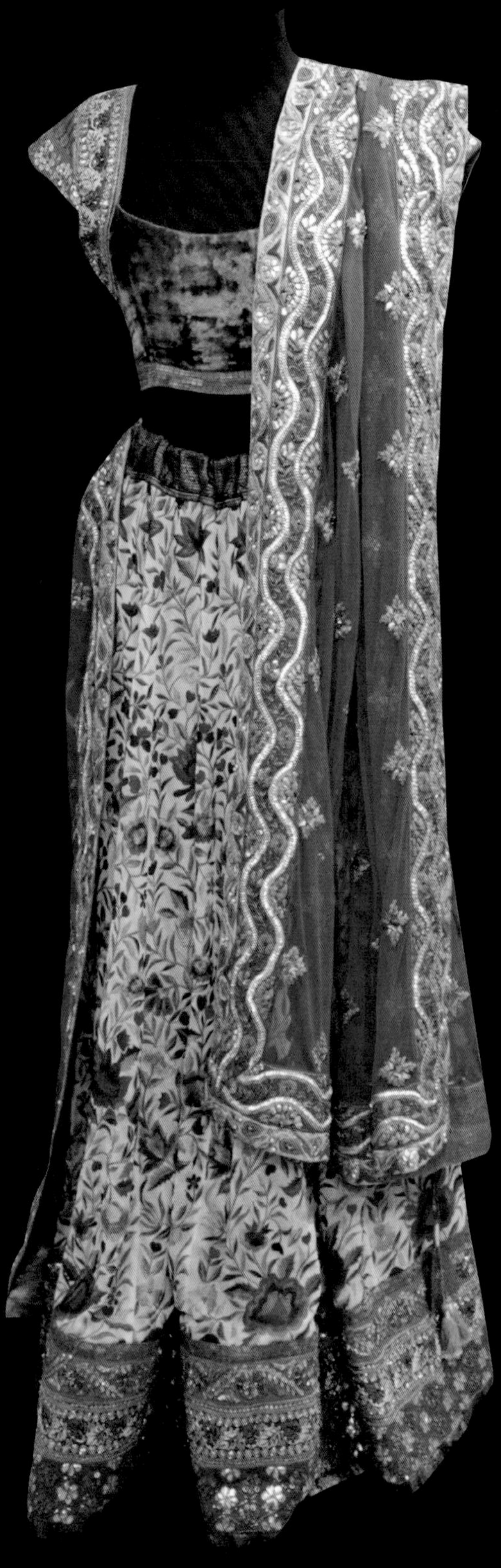

Fully embroidered *jaal* of this multi-coloured georgette lehenga has a richly embellished border in zardozi, *phool-patti ka kaam* and sequence work. *Laheriya* pattern of *gokru gota* encases floral *bel* motif of the matching orange tuille *odhni*. A green-tasselled ornamental *izarband* hangs from the contrasting violet brocade *nefa*. Choli style velvet blouse with leaf motif of the lehenga completes this contemporary lehenga-blouse-*odhni* ensemble, reflecting the traditional design and craftsmanship of Awadh.

FASHION TRENDS IN CONTEMPORARY LUCKNOW

Nawab Masood Abdullah and his wife Begum Almaas Abdullah, Lucknow fashion designers, very aptly described to me the contemporary trends in Awadh:

'These days, traditional garments are produced according to the latest designs, styles and cuts. The *angarkha*, which was mainly part of men's costume during the nawabi and British periods, is being re-introduced for women and is now presented with *bar ka paijama/bade paichon ka paijama* (Autumn-Winter 2008). We have innovated by combining various types of embroideries: for example, we integrated Parsi embroidery and chikan work with zardozi and ari-work. We took care to maintain the refinement of earlier times by using the very fine thread, size no. 100 instead of no. 60. This takes longer but when it is finished, it makes you feel happy.

'Fashion comes from the development in the field of yarn and availability of colours. Swarovski crystals, sequins and coloured stones have replaced the precious stones of the Nawabi Era. Bold colours and combinations like pink/ beige, beige/turquoise and dark maroon/henna green are being used once again. The bright shade of pink, earlier called *dehati* pink [pink used by villagers], is widely used by contemporary designers. Contemporary motifs are now architecturally inspired by the *jali* work and bel-*buti*s in the marble inlay work of Mughal monuments.

'Among the highlights of our work is the use of calligraphy in our creations. Religious iconography lends itself to be used in many interesting ways. We like to use Sufi themes in our garment creations and by using calligraphy on them, we seek to combine two different forms of art as well as give them a meaning beyond fashion. We also introduced *chikankari* embroidery on pashmina, which had not been done before. One particular stole was so richly embroidered that the surface was hardly visible.'

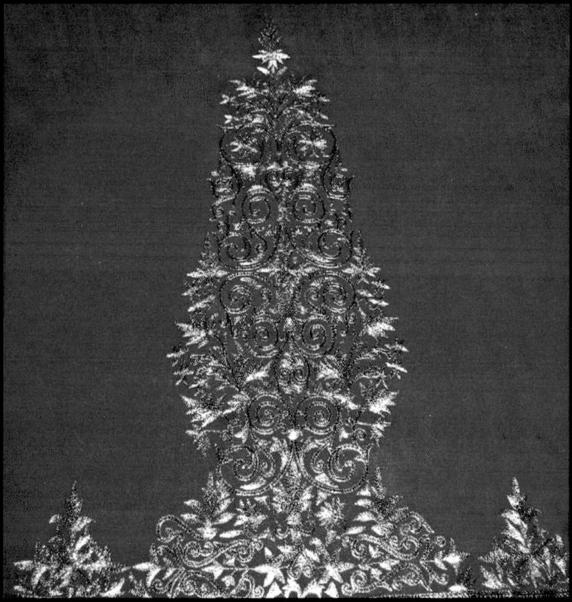

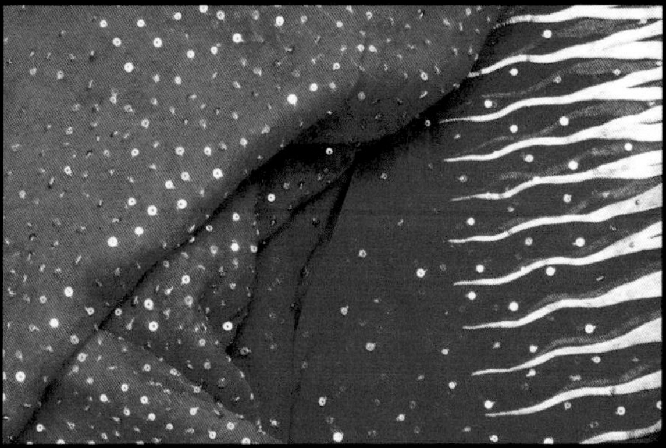

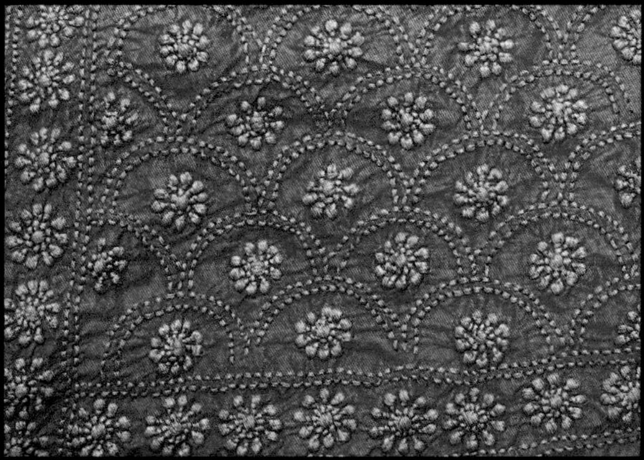

Topmost: A motif embroidered on bright orange sari with silver zari in *ari* work.
Centre: *Mukaish* work delicately decorates this pink shaded georgette sari.
Below: The *mahepusht* (fishscale) design in bright contrasting colours is revived in chikan embroidery.

EPILOGUE

On 15 August 1947, India gained independence from British rule and adopted a democratic form of government. In 1991, Prime Minister Narsimha Rao initiated reforms to liberalize the economic system. Today, India is much further integrated into the global economy and is the world's largest democracy.

As witnessed previously in the Nawabi Era and the British Raj, such dramatic changes in society are followed by equally remarkable changes in costumes, textiles, ornamentations, motifs and colours. The 'hippie' cult of the 1960s introduced new dresses such as bell-bottomed pants, flares, stretch pants and maxis.

With women entering the workforce, their costumes saw a wave of innovations in the last two decades, they adopted formal work-suits, knee-length dresses, cocktail dresses and evening gowns. There has been an increased fusion of traditional and Western costumes, more variety, new styles and modes of dressing. The introduction of Western costumes such as T-shirts, polo shirts, track-suits and especially jeans revived the unisex concept that existed in ancient times in Awadh, when both men and women used to wear similar clothes. Although the traditional costumes (*lehenga*, sari, *chunni*, churidar paijama, kurti) continue to exist from the olden times, these are now often combined with Western clothes and styles (such as a *kurti* with jeans).

With nostalgia, some extraordinary skills and beautiful materials that existed during the Nawabi Era are now lost. The fine muslins and Tanda *jamdanis* of Nawabi era have now disappeared. The Banaras brocades of real *zari* have become very expensive and *kinkhwab* brocades are difficult to find. *Mushru*, used for lehengas and kalidar paijamas, achkans and sherwanis are not at all produced. Nowadays, any intricate *jaal* covering the major surface of any fabric uses the term *jamavar*. The usage of the term is now identified with the design rather than with the intricate weaving craft of Kashmir made of Pashmina wool, used by nawabs for jamas and shawls.

The expertise of the artisans in ornamentations, developed over multiple generations and through the generous patronage of the nawabs of Awadh, has unfortunately been lost over the centuries such as *chatta-patti ka kaam* and *daraz ka kaam*. The crochet-work, lace and smocking introduced during the British Raj too have lost popularity in modern times.

The importance of headgear has now decreased significantly and the use of accessories like *rumals*, *khadau* and *patka* has also completely declined.

On a more positive note, many costumes have survived over the centuries and been enhanced in modern times. The traditional Khadi has maintained its popularity, but has no longer significant patriotic connotations. The silk-based textiles such as chiffon, georgette and net, introduced during the British Raj, are still very much in use. Although many organzas are woven presently with synthetic filament fibres, such as polyester or nylon, the most luxurious organzas are still woven in silk.

The screen printing industry replaced a large part of the block printing industry but block printing in Lucknow is regaining its popularity. However, it is no longer limited to *fard* (quilt covers) and *fatohi* (quilted garments).

There has been an effort at revival of the old textiles and forms of craftsmanship that were obscured since the end of the Nawabi Era. Many Indian designers have contributed to revive Awadhi workmanship and have recently taken *chikankari*, *zardozi and kamdani* to new heights. An innovation has been introduced into *chikankari* by using metallic gold and silver threads with sequins, traditionally performed white-on-white; it is now being done with coloured threads on white and also with white threads on coloured cloth. Another novelty is seen in the zardozi work, it is now being applied on cotton, net and georgette which were previously confined to velvet and silk only. However, the real gold and silver threads of the opulent nawabi period have been replaced with synthetic threads and *kamdani* is now done with silver-coated aluminium flat wires instead of pure silver flat wires.

Today, many contemporary designers, both Western and Indian, are finding inspiration from the Awadhi costumes, cuts and age-old traditional embroideries. Awadhi inspiration has found its way into Armani's *angarkha*, Ferrè's interpretation of the *lehenga* and Galliano's adaptation of the salwar-kurta/kameez.

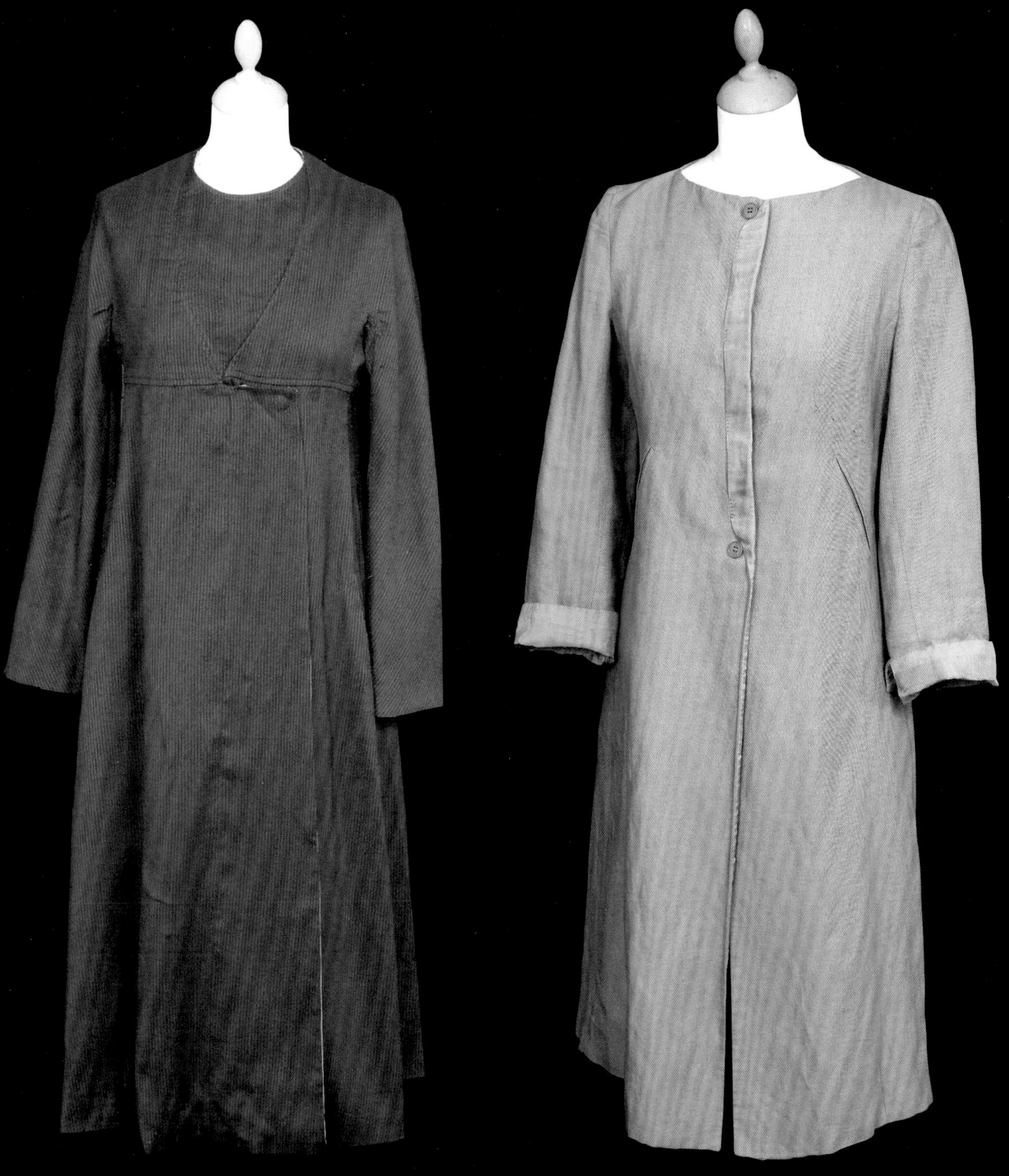

Left: This high-waist coat by Armani is inspired by angarkha with a central fastening with tie-cords. An inner flap or purdah can be seen with *ghundi* and *tukma* (cotton button and loop) type of fastening Bagalia is inserted to join the sleeves.
Right: An adoption of *achkan* by Giorgio Armani. The neck is in boat shape rather than collared round neck. It has two slanted pockets at waist level. Only first and last buttons are visible of the central fastening and the rest is concealed by a border.

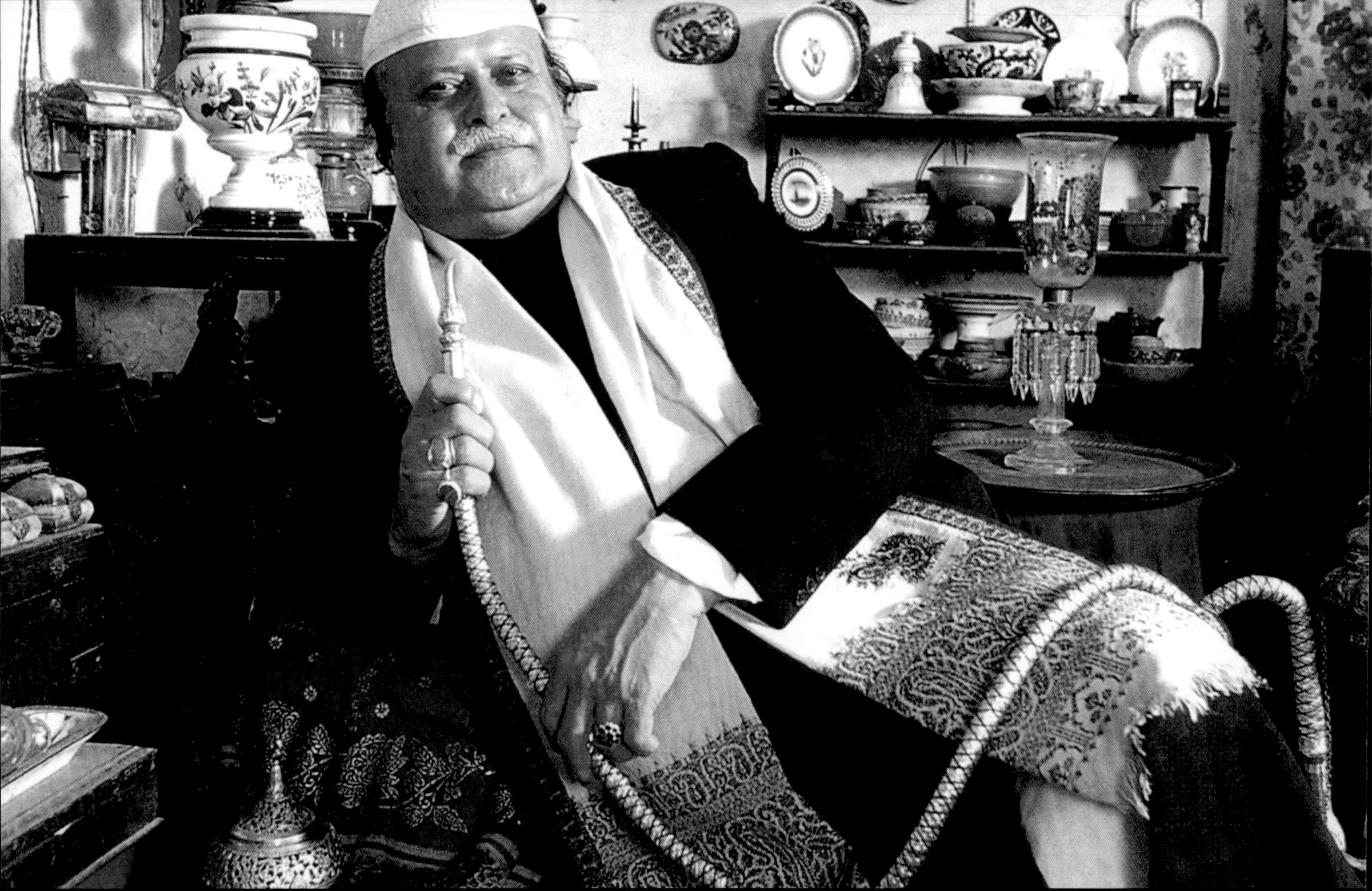

Nawab Mir Abdullah of Sheesh Mahal Lucknow, is wearing sherwani, *arz ka pyjama*, *dopalli* cap and a jamawar stole and enjoying his hukkah.

ACKNOWLEDGEMENTS

I would like to thank my father who taught me to dream before putting my ideas into words; Vinod, my husband, accompanied me to all impossible places; my son Chetan and daughter Tulika for standing by me like pillars during my whole endeavour to transform my idea into this book. Special thanks to Nawab Jafar Mir Abdullah, Nawab Masood Abdullah, Begum Almasood, Begum Hazira, Began Taj Ara, Dr Naqvi and Mr Vishnu Agrawal for their time. Dr S.N. Upadhaya, Dr I. P. Pandey, Dr Yogesh Pravin, Mrs Nusrat Naheed for their continuous assistance. I am grateful to Shri Indra Bhushan of Textile Block Printers Association for showing me the whole process involved in the art of block-printing and Mrs Rita Vishal, Director of the U.P. Institute of Design, Lucknow, for her help. Mrs Sadhana Swarup and Mrs Seema Kumar thank you for sharing with me the poetic feel of Awadh. I would also like to thank Mishika, my cousin's granddaughter, for her great help.

My special thanks go to Rajkumar Mohd Amir Naqi Khan of Basha state for sharing his experiences and extending his nawabi hospitality to me. He was also gracious enough to share not only valuable information but also photographs from his collection.

I am also grateful for the resources and valuable material I found at the Asiatic Library in Mumbai, the Lucknow State Museum, the National Museum in New Delhi, the National Handicrafts and Handloom Museum in New Delhi, the Asian Department at Victoria & Albert Museum and the British Library in London.

I would like to thank Parutosh, Maurizio Bianchi, Primo Ianmarino and Chetan for photographic shoots of my collection.

I am profoundly thankful to my publishing team for producing a wonderful book.

GLOSSARY

A

ab-i-rawan – running water
achkan – long-sleeved, knee-length coat with band collar, for men, fastened in the middle with buttons
ada – style
adda – wooden frame
alam pasand – kind of cap invented by Wajid Ali shah
ambi – unripe mango motif
amiya – raw mango
amrasi – a shade of saffron yellow resembling to the colour of ripe mango
angarkha – full-sleeved outer wear, open at the chest and tied in the front, covering the chest with an inner flap (purdah)
angiya – bodice like garment
anokhi – unique
antariya – unstitched garment used as lower garment
ari bel – diagonal stripes of creeper motif
arz ke paichon ka paijama – wide-legged paijama of straight cut, using arz
(the whole width of the fabric)
asafkhani – bodice with flare
asmani – a shade of sky blue
aughi – ladies shoes
aurebdar – bias-cut cloth

B

bachkani dhoti – child size dhoti
badami – almond (colour)
badhi – string of flowers worn in criss-cross manner across front and back
badla – flattened gold or silver wire wound on silk or cotton thread
badla-work – embroidery using badla
baft hawá – woven air
bagalia – triangular piece under the armholes
baingani – aubergine (colour)
baju-band – gold or silver arm band, studded with precious stones
balabar – an unfastened outer garment for men similar to the Persian cape
bandi – waistcoat
bandiyas – lady helpers
banke – dandy of Lucknow
bar ka paijama/ barey paichon ka paijama – wide legged paijama
basanti – lime yellow (colour)
batua – a pouch
batuiya – a smaller pouch
bel – a creeper pattern
bela – variety of jasmine flower
bel-patti – floral vine design
besandani – wash-basins
bichiya – toe-rings
bukka – mica flakes
buta – large flower motif
buti – small floral motif
butidar – flowers are scattered all over the surface

C

chaapakhana – printing workshop
chhader/ chadariya – an unstitched piece of cloth of varying materials and measurements used to drape the upper part of the body
chak – slit
chameli – jasmine flower
champa – magnolia flower
chanda – moon-shaped
chandan – sandalwood
chapka – ornament for the hair worn on the side
chapkan – knee-length coat for men. Upper half is similar to a Western style coat and lower part resembles an angarkha
chapta – flat thread
chariyon ki gote – straight vertical lines
chasak – decoration at the joints of paijamas and lahengas
chaugoshia – four-cornered cap
chiffon – plain weave in silk, with a twisted thread count of about 43 wrap/43 weft per centimeter.
chikankari – white-work embroidery from Lucknow
choga – a loose outer garment for men, of Turkish origin, worn over angarkha
choli – tight-fitting stitched bodice
chuna – lime
churi – glass bangles
churidar paijamas – paijama with bangle-like gathers at the ankles
chutki-wala gota – crinkled gota

D

dagla – full-sleeved quilted garment
danedar – grainy
dastar – turban of white cotton
dast-band – ornament for hand
Devnagri – Hindi script
dhani – yellowish green (colour)
dhanush – crumpled narrow gota
dhoop-chayyian – having warp and weft in two different colours (generally red and green) giving effect of light and shade
dhoti – unstitched cloth for covering the lower part of body draped in various ways
dil bahar – pleasing
doria -striped
dopalri – small-close-fitting cap, with two identical pieces of cloth stitched together with a curve at the top
dushalas – bigger shawls

E

ek vastra – single clothing

F

falsai – shade of purple (colour)
fardi buti – tiny dots
farji – sleeveless or short-sleeved coat-like garment, worn over a jama or angarkha
farshi paijama – wide-legged trailing paijama, worn with a kurti
farshi salaam – long bowed greetings
fatohi – sleeve-less jacket
ferozi – turquoise (colour)
fitas – cotton ribbons
furma – cardboard mould

G

gajji – satin-weave cloth
galis – narrow lanes
Ganga-Jamuni – used for the confluence of different colours of water of these two rivers
gharara – a variation of paijama
genda buti – marigold flower
ghatela – shoes with long toe, shaped

like an elephant's trunk, curving over the feet in a large spiral
gherdar – flared
ghundi – cloth-cased button
ghuttana – short paijama
gokhru – hoof-shaped
gopi chandni – pale yellow
gota – ribbon with flattened gilt wire in warp and weft in silk thread
gota-patti – small leaf shapes made of gota
gote – richly decorated lower part of a paijama or lahenga
gotdar – with broad border
gulab – rose
gulabi – rose (colour)
gulbandh – necklace
gul daudi – chrysanthemum flower
gulenar – red colour of pomegranate
ghungroos – tiny bells

H

hansli – a rigid circular necklace (from word hansa, meaning neck)
harsingar – flower
hathphool – ornament for hand
hina – myrtle

I

ingari – green
itr – perfume
izar – variation of paijama
izarband – ornated draw-string at the waist to hold paijamas or lahenga

J

jaal – an all-over pattern on a printed fabric or done by embroidery
jalpariya – fish
jama – full-sleeved outer garment for man with tight bodice and a flared skirt. Popular at Mughal court in Delhi and in the Court of Awadh during late eighteenth and early nineteenth century
jama-zebi – costume ensemble
jamdani – fine muslin with discontinuous supplementary-weft motifs
Jamevar – woven Kashmiri shawl in twill-tapestry weave
Jamun/jamuni – violet
Jaiphal – Nutmeg
Javitri – Mace
Jhalerdar – with frills
jhamak – mica flakes
jhilmil – band with a shimmering effect
jhulas – swings
jhumar – hair ornament worn on the side of the head
joda – set of clothes
juhi – variety of jasmine flower
juti – leather footwear, embroidered and with up-turned toes

K

kaccha – fugitive colour
khadau – wooden footwear
kafsh – shoes with heels
kairi buti – raw-mango motif
kajal – kohl
kakshya style – dhoti wrapped around each leg, like trousers
kalabattun – metallic thread made by wrapping gold or silver gilt thread around silk or cotton yarns
kalga buta – cypress-shaped motif
kalgi/sarpesh – head-ornament worn on turban, made of gold and precious stones
kali – gored panel, triangular pieces used to add volume to the garment
kalidar kurta – made up of gored pieces and kalis, thus becoming loose
kalidar paijama – paijama with several gored pieces or kalis, thus flared.
kalpvriksha – Ancient Indian tree symbolizing eternity, strength, fertility and creation
kamal – lotus flower
kamarband –- sash, tied over the jama at the waist, to hold a dagger or a sword
kamdani – embroidery using badla thread
kanni – double twill-tapestry weaving
karchob – wooden frame used for embroidery, also called adda
karchobi-work – embroidery done in kalabattun with muthias on karchob
kardhani – girdle
kare – thick bangles made of gold
kargha – loom
karnphool – earrings
kas – fastenings made of cloth
kasab – gold or silver wire
kattha – catechu
katori – cup-shaped sequins
kela silk – artificial silk
kewra – pandanus flower
kewra water – made of pandanus flower
kirmiz – scarlet
kharaun – footwear made of wood
khari work / verek work – adhesion of bukka (mica flakes) or gold dust to the printed fabric
khas – special fabrics made for royalty
khillat – a ceremonial robe of honour
kinari – decorated edging
kinkhwab / kimkhab / kamkhab – heavily brocaded silk fabric with gold and silver metal wires. Yellow silk is used under gold and white silk under silver. More than fifty percent of gold or silver work is visible
kiran – gold or silver fringe
kor – piping
kotha – chambers of courtesan
kullah / qaraquziburk/ qalpaq/ duwalghaburk – a skull-cap.
kundan – technique of setting gold
kurti – shorter than kurta

L

lachka – crumpled wide gota
lahriya – creating wave-like design on fabrics with tie and dye process of printing
laung – nose pin , clove
libaas – a dress
likhai – drawing of a design for brocades

M

mahepusht – fish scales
makhmal – velvet
malmul – muslin
malmul khas – of the finest quality
mandel/ mandi – headgear
maang-tika – head ornament
markeen – type of cotton
mashshata – ladies who helped begums in dressing
mashru or galta – twill fabric with silk warp and cotton weft
mathapatti – a head ornament
mehfil – soirees
minakari – enamelled work
misl – a set of garments
mirzai –- half-sleeved quilted upper-garment or over-garment
miyani – a triangular piece of cloth to join two leggings of paijamas
mohallas – a part of a city

mor-pankhi – a blend of blue and green (colour)
motia – jasmine flower
Muharaam – a Muslim festival
muga (antheraea assama) – the natural yellow gold silk of Bengal and Assam
mughalai paijama – of 'Mughal' cut
mughlania – artisans
mujra – music and dance performance by courtesans
mukaish-work – embroidered with badla
mukta silk – silk produced without the moth being killed inside the cacoon
mulmul – fine muslin of plain weave, woven in Bengal
mundaphool – flower
mushk – hibiscus abelmoschus
mushki – black
muthia – crochet type hook with a wooden round top

N

nada – drawstring
nafasat – sophistication
naib – provincial governor
naksh – a pattern
nakshband – a designer making patterns
narangi – orange (colour)
nayansukh – pleasing to the eye
Nawabs – Provincial Governor
nazakat- delicacy
nima/nimtana – a variation of kurta
nimcha – a short tunic
nishatkhana – courtesan's chambers
nukkadar – pointed

O

odhni – a veil approx. 2.7 m. long and 1 m. wide

P

paat – middle portion of paijama or lahenga
pagri – turban or headgear
paijeb – anklets
pallav – the ornated end-piece of the sari
pan-buti – of the shape of a betel leaf
panchgoshia – headgear having five corners
pari-khana – abode of fairies
pashm – wool
patka – a decorated waist band, the end parts remain hanging
pattha – plain gota
payal – ankle ornament
peshwaz – full-sleeved garment with bodice attached to a long skirt.
phool patti ka kaam – appliqué work
phalsa – Grewia asiatica
pistai – pistachio (colour)
pitambari – yellow-coloured
pote – small glass beads
pyazi – onion (colour)

R

rafoogar – master darner
rangrez – a person who dyes fabric
rani – magenta (colour)
rumal – large scarf used by men in Awadh

S

sadri – a sleeve-less jacket worn over a shirt or a kurta
salma – coiled, metallic wire used in zardozi type of embroidery
sarkar-i-ala – muslins made in Dacca for nawabs
saropa – full dresses
satlara – seven-stringed necklace
satrangi – of seven colours
sausani – plum (colour)
sawan – monsoon season
sehra – used for head decoration for men
shabnam – dew
shal – a shawl
shaluka – a tunic similar to kurta worn by women
sharara – a loose paijama worn by women
sheikhzadas – landlords
sheesham wood – delbergia sisso
silabchis – portable wash-basins
Shimla – headgear
sidha paijama – narrow paijama of straight –cut worn by Mughals
sidha pallav – end of the sari drooping over the right shoulder from the back
sitara-work – sequins work
stanapatta – a breast-band for women
suapankhi – parrot green
suba – province
subedar – head of a province
sufed – white
suhag – sign of being married
surahi – a type of terracotta vase generally used as water container
suthanne – a kind of paijama

T

tana – warp
Tanda jamdani – Jamdani fabric woven in the city of Tanda
tanzeb – that adorns the body
tara – star
taraanah – symphony
tarbuzi – crimson (watermelon colour)
tauk – a necklace
tawaif – a courtesan
tehzeeb – etiquette
tepchi – long running stitch
tercha – grouped in diagonal lines.
tika – an ornament for the forehead
tiki – flat metal discs used in zardozi embroidery
tilla – a type of thread
tojli – wooden spools
totai – parrot green (colour)
tukma – loop made of stringed cord to hold the ghundi
tukri ki gote – gote made of tukri (patchwork): aari chariyon ki gote – gote in diagonal shape; gilloriyon ki gote – triangular shaped gote; katari ki gote – semi circular shape; namak pare ki gote – diamond shaped gote; patake ki gote – square shaped gote; sitare ki gote – star shaped;
turanj – mango motif
turra – head ornament

U

uda – purple (colour)
ulta pallav – end part of sari drooping on the left shoulder from the front
uttariya – unstitched garment used as upper garment
uttu – thin strip of plain gota

V

Vedic – of the Vedas, the Hindu scriptures
verek-work – a technique of ornamentation where gold dust or mica flakes are applied on the fabric.

W

war – yard
wazir – minister

Z

zafrani – saffron (colour)
zard – yellow

BIBLIOGRAPHY

Amaresh Mishra, 'Lucknow Diary', *Diary Magazine*, 31 May 1999.

Aseh-ul-Matabai Tazkirah. *Mashahir-i-Kakori,* Lucknow, 1927.

Awadhwasi Lala Sitaram, *Ayodhya Ka Itihas*, Prayag, 1932.

Badana Tiwari, 'Eternal Romantic', *Vogue India*, January, 2010.

B. Meer Hassan Ali, *Observations on the Mussulmauns of India*, Edited with notes and an introduction by W. Crooke, second edition, 1917.

C. A. Silberrad, Monograph on Cotton Fabrics produced in the North Western Provinces and Oudh, 1898.

E. H. Hilton, *The Tourist's Guide to Lucknow,* E. H. C. Powell, London Printing Press, Lucknow 1911.

Geeta Mehta, *The Taj Magazine*, Vol. 34, No. 4, 2006.

John T. Platts, Dictionary of Urdu, Classical Hindi and English, Oxford University Press, 1974.

M. C. Pande, Bulletin of Museums and Archaeology, No.1, March 1968, p35.

Ritu Kumar. *Costumes and Textiles of Royal India,* Christie's Books, London, 1999.

Samuel Lucas , John Robert Taylor, *Dacoitee in Excelsis:* Or, *The Spoliation of Oude,* Faithfully Recounted (1923). Reprinted Kessinger Press, 2011.

Sharar, Abdul Halim, *Lucknow – The Last Phase of an Oriental Culture*, translated and edited by E. S. Harcourt and Fakkir Hussain, Oxford University Press, 2001.

S. N. Dar. *Costumes of India and Pakistan*, Munshiram Manohar Lal, Bombay 1969.

State Museum, Lucknow.

Stephen Yafa, *Cotton: The Biography of a Revolutionary Fiber,* Penguin Books, London, 2006.

Sudipta Dev, 'Lucknow: Then and Now', *Marg Publications,* 2003, p. 55.

Violette Graff (ed.). *Lucknow: Memories of a City,* Oxford University Press 1999.

W. H. Russell. *My Diary in the Years 1858-59.* 2 vols. London: Routledge, Warner and Routledge, 1860.

PHOTO CREDITS

Indra Swarup: pp. 137 (above left), 147 (extreme left)

Muzaffar Ali Collection: p. 21

Nawab Jafar Mir Abdullah: p. 85 (bottom)

Nawab Masood Abdullah: p. 151

National Handicrafts and Handloom Museum, New Delhi: pp. 42, 43, 45, 59, 64, 65, 66, 77, 113, 137 (above right and below),144, 145

National Museum of India, New Delhi: p. 44

Onita Boutique, London: pp. 7, 149,150,

Padma Rani: pp. 55, 112, 118

Paintings Galleries blogspot: 49 (Akbarnama: Paintings of Mughal Costumes, Ornaments and Cultural History of India)

Author's Personal Collection: pp. 3, 4,5, 7 (top, center, second from right, extreme right), 27, 29, 32, 33, 34, 35, 46, 47, 48, 52, 53, 54, 56, 60, 61, 62, 63, 64, 68, 69, 70, 71 (left), 72, 73, 74, 75, 76, 77 (topmost and centre), 79, 80, 81, 82, 83, 84, 86, 87, 88, 89, 90-95, 96, 98, 99, 100, 101, 102, 103, 104, 106, 107, 110, 111, 112, 113 (bottom), 114, 115, 116, 117, 119, 120, 121, 122, 123, 125, 126, 127, 128, 129, 130, 131, 132, 134, 135, 136, 137 (above centre), 138, 139, 140, 141, 144 (extreme left), 145, 146, 147 (centre and right), 153, 154

RajKumar Ali Naqi Khan: pp. 22, 23, 24

Rashmi Swarup: pp. 2, 7 (extreme left), 57, 108, 109, 113 (above left and right)

Roli Books Archive: p. 142

Sangeeta Bhatnagar and R. K. Saxena, *Dastarkhwan-e-Awadh*, Harper Collins Publishers, India, 1997: pp. 14, 85 (top)

State Museum Lucknow: pp. 1, 2, 3, 6 (top extreme right), 11, 12, 15, 16, 18, 19, 20, 26, 28, 29, 30, 31, 36, 37, 38, 39, 40, 41, 46, 50, 51, 58, 67, 71 (right), 77 (bottom) 78, 105, 144 (centre and right)

Textile Block Printers Association: p. 8

wikimedia.org: p. 124